Public Health Communication Challenges to Minority and Indigenous Communities

Kealeboga Aiseng
Rhodes University, South Africa

Israel A. Fadipe
Ajayi Crowther University, Nigeria

IGI Global
PUBLISHER of TIMELY KNOWLEDGE

A volume in the Advances in Linguistics and Communication Studies (ALCS) Book Series

Published in the United States of America by
IGI Global
Information Science Reference (an imprint of IGI Global)
701 E. Chocolate Avenue
Hershey PA, USA 17033
Tel: 717-533-8845
Fax: 717-533-8661
E-mail: cust@igi-global.com
Web site: http://www.igi-global.com

Library of Congress Cataloging-in-Publication Data

Names: Aiseng, Kealeboga, editor. | Fadipe, Israel A., editor.
Title: Public health communication challenges to minority and indigenous communities / edited by Kealeboga Aiseng, Israel Fadipe.
Description: Hershey, PA : Information Science Reference, [2024] | Includes bibliographical references and index. | Summary: "This book has a significant impact on the field of sociolinguistics, especially under contemporary circumstances involving the ongoing relationship between indigenous and colonial languages"-- Provided by publisher.
Identifiers: LCCN 2023048629 (print) | LCCN 2023048630 (ebook) | ISBN 9798369306246 (h/c) | ISBN 9798369306253 (s/c) | ISBN 9798369306260 (eISBN)
Subjects: LCSH: Communication in public health--Africa, Sub-Saharan. | Minorities--Medical care--Africa, Sub-Saharan | Indigenous peoples--Medical care--Africa, Sub-Saharan | COVID-19 Pandemic, 2020---Africa, Sub-Saharan.
Classification: LCC RA423.2 .P78 2024 (print) | LCC RA423.2 (ebook) | DDC 362.1089/97067--dc23/eng/20231229
LC record available at https://lccn.loc.gov/2023048629
LC ebook record available at https://lccn.loc.gov/2023048630

This book is published in the IGI Global book series Advances in Linguistics and Communication Studies (ALCS) (ISSN: 2372-109X; eISSN: 2372-1111)

British Cataloguing in Publication Data
A Cataloguing in Publication record for this book is available from the British Library.

For electronic access to this publication, please contact: eresources@igi-global.com.

Advances in Linguistics and Communication Studies (ALCS) Book Series

Abigail G. Scheg
Western Governors University, USA

ISSN:2372-109X
EISSN:2372-1111

Mission

The scope of language and communication is constantly changing as society evolves, new modes of communication are developed through technological advancement, and novel words enter our lexicon as the result of cultural change. Understanding how we communicate and use language is crucial in all industries and updated research is necessary in order to promote further knowledge in this field.

The **Advances in Linguistics and Communication Studies (ALCS)** book series presents the latest research in diverse topics relating to language and communication. Interdisciplinary in its coverage, ALCS presents comprehensive research on the use of language and communication in various industries including business, education, government, and healthcare.

Coverage

- Media and Public Communications
- Computational Linguistics
- Non-Verbal Communication
- Youth Language
- Dialectology
- Language in the Media
- Interpersonal Communication
- Forensic Linguistics
- Language and Identity
- Language Acquisition

IGI Global is currently accepting manuscripts for publication within this series. To submit a proposal for a volume in this series, please contact our Acquisition Editors at Acquisitions@igi-global.com or visit: http://www.igi-global.com/publish/.

The Advances in Linguistics and Communication Studies (ALCS) Book Series (ISSN 2372-109X) is published by IGI Global, 701 E. Chocolate Avenue, Hershey, PA 17033-1240, USA, www.igi-global.com. This series is composed of titles available for purchase individually; each title is edited to be contextually exclusive from any other title within the series. For pricing and ordering information please visit http://www.igi-global.com/book-series/advances-linguistics-communication-studies/78950. Postmaster: Send all address changes to above address.

Titles in this Series

For a list of additional titles in this series, please visit:
www.igi-global.com/book-series/advances-linguistics-communication-studies/78950

Quantitative Measures and Warranty Coverage of the Risk of Misinforming
Dimitar Grozdanov Christozov (American University in Bulgaria, Bulgaria)
Information Science Reference • copyright 2024 • 354pp • H/C (ISBN: 9781668488003) • US $220.00 (our price)

AI and Its Convergence With Communication Technologies
Badar Muneer (Mehran University of Engineering and Technology, Pakistan) Faisal Karim Shaikh (Mehran University of Engineering and Technology, Pakistan) Naeem Mahoto (Mehran University of Engineering and Technology, Pakistan) Shahnawaz Talpur (Mehran University of Engineering and Technology, Pakistan) and Jordi Garcia (Universitat Politècnica de Catalunya, Spain)
Information Science Reference • copyright 2023 • 308pp • H/C (ISBN: 9781668477021) • US $250.00 (our price)

Combining Modern Communication Methods With Heritage Education
Lia Bassa (Budapest Metropolitan University, Hungary & Foundation for Information Society, Hungary)
Information Science Reference • copyright 2023 • 317pp • H/C (ISBN: 9781668462171) • US $215.00 (our price)

Handbook of Research on Socio-Cultural and Linguistic Perspectives on Language and Literacy Development
Angela K. Salmon (Florida International University, USA) and Amparo Clavijo-Olarte (Universidad Distrital Francisco Jose de Caldas, Colombia)
Information Science Reference • copyright 2023 • 500pp • H/C (ISBN: 9781668450222) • US $270.00 (our price)

A Social-Scientific Examination of the Dynamics of Communication, Thought, and Selves
Seif Sekalala (Drexel University, USA)
Information Science Reference • copyright 2022 • 277pp • H/C (ISBN: 9781799875079) • US $205.00 (our price)

Narrative Theory and Therapy in the Post-Truth Era
Recep Yılmaz (Ondokuz Mayis University, Turkey) and Bozkurt Koç (Ondokuz Mayis University, Turkey)
Information Science Reference • copyright 2022 • 373pp • H/C (ISBN: 9781799892519) • US $240.00 (our price)

Handbook of Research on Communication Strategies for Taboo Topics
Geoffrey D. Luurs (Murray State University, USA)
Information Science Reference • copyright 2022 • 602pp • H/C (ISBN: 9781799891253) • US $295.00 (our price)

IGI Global
PUBLISHER of TIMELY KNOWLEDGE

701 East Chocolate Avenue, Hershey, PA 17033, USA
Tel: 717-533-8845 x100 • Fax: 717-533-8661
E-Mail: cust@igi-global.com • www.igi-global.com

Table of Contents

Detailed Table of Contents

This chapter examined the effectiveness of COVID-19 risk communication messages in indigenous languages vis-à-vis the promotion of safe practices in Ondo, Nigeria. The survey research design was used, and a questionnaire was randomly administered to 384 respondents in Akure, Ondo State. Findings showed that most of the respondents were exposed to COVID-19 risk communication messages and got their first information about it from social media. Furthermore, the study found that respondents were not receptive to COVID-19 messages passed across in indigenous languages. They prefer COVID-19 messages to pass across in the English language. The study recommended that there is a need to ensure that risk communication messages aired in indigenous languages are demystified in a way that the audience can easily understand and act upon. The use of indigenous languages should continue to be used and encouraged, especially for risk communication interventions such as COVID-19. This will go a long way in ensuring that the audience accepts it.

The first cases of Covid-19 in the world can be traced to 2019. However, in Kenya and a number of other East African countries, the first cases of the disease were documented in March 2020. As the day went on, the spread of the virus gained momentum causing panic in the country. Awareness messaging on Covid-19 led by the government and supported by health agencies became regular on the Kenyan media, especially on the radio, television, and mainstream newspapers. Messaging was mainly done in English, Kiswahili, and mother tongue with the earlier enjoying a skewed advantage. A portion of this messaging was done via video, composed locally and internationally. The objective of the study was to examine the strategies employed in this video communication to create awareness of Covid-19. The results demonstrate that in a substantial number of cases, the dissemination was hampered by wanting grammar, English to Kiswahili translational flaws, and unsuitable animatronics. The chapter contends that the Kiswahili video messaging mainly failed the test of communicative value.

The COVID-19 pandemic brought about unprecedented challenges to societies worldwide, compelling individuals and institutions to adapt rapidly to a new reality dominated by digital communication. Social media platforms emerged as essential channels for information dissemination, community building, and emotional expression during this global crisis. Language played a pivotal role in shaping these interactions, influencing the spread of information, the formation of online communities, and the impact of public health campaigns. This chapter explores the multifaceted role of language in social media during the COVID-19 pandemic. Firstly, it highlights the significance of language as a medium for facilitating

Public health communication is imperative to every livelihood including minorities. Language, however, remains one of the fundamentals of communication that can make the message reach the people. This chapter focuses on health awareness campaigns on Facebook community radio to analyse public health communication in Zimbabwe's minority languages. The authors used community radio platforms on the assumption that local languages such as minority languages can at least find space on community radio. However, a qualitative content analysis on radio content on Facebook reveals the dominance of Shona (major indigenous language) and English in public health communication by health authorities and representatives of the ruling party. There were a few exceptions of minority languages used in code-switch with English. Theorising effective communication to minorities, this chapter notes that governments should prioritise public health communication in minority languages through open collaborative networks by making use of language translation and community leadership in health awareness campaigns.

Chapter 9
Public Health Communication and Language Policy at Rhodes University During the COVID-19 Pandemic 130
Zikhona Mamase, Rhodes University, South Africa
Kealeboga Aiseng, Rhodes University, South Africa

The COVID-19 pandemic offered unprecedented obstacles to public health communication worldwide. Pandemic revealed disparities and significant gaps in access to public health information for those not proficient in English, potentially leading to the exclusion of indigenous language speakers and minority communities from issues of national interest, including vital COVID-19 updates. This chapter examines the case study of Rhodes University in the Eastern Cape, South Africa and explores the institution's language policies and practices during the pandemic. The institution grapples with linguistic diversity, where English is the primary language of teaching and administration. The study explores language, public health communication, and inclusion at Rhodes University. It seeks to find linguistic and cultural contestations during this time by evaluating the university's response to the pandemic through language. The study uses document analysis to understand how Rhodes University's language practices impacted public health communication during the pandemic.

Chapter 10
Amplifying the Health Concerns of Minoritized Groups in Nigeria Using Documentary 143
Abigail Ogwezzy, University of Lagos, Nigeria
Akpan Samuel Unwana, University of Lagos, Nigeria
Ogechi Okanya Cookey, Edwin Clark University, Nigeria
Iniobong Courage Nda, University of Uyo, Nigeria

Several studies have shown that most highly placed government officials in the Ministry of Health in Africa do not bother to get to the hinterlands, slums, or inner cities where there are poor people, and socially excluded people, because according to them, these are hard-to-reach areas; and additionally due to the spate of insecurity in the continent. In the case of Nigeria, it has also been revealed that these top government health officials prefer a situation where they are briefed by their media aids who must have gone to have a one-on-one encounter with these minority groups, by capturing their plights on camera, especially in this era of rising insecurity in the country. This chapter explores the role of documentaries in amplifying the health concerns of these minority groups in Nigeria. The study uses social shaping theory in explaining concepts, themes, and constructs. Findings are shared.

Societies structure their communication relationships in a variety of ways. The Akan in Ghana have a peculiar way of communicating issues relating to their sexuality. They find it difficult mentioning the real names of the human sex organs; they prefer employing various metaphors to signify these. It is not clear what the reasons are and how feasible this becomes when they (Akan) are confronted with reporting reproductive health since it is usually considered important for patients to indicate specific parts of the body that ail for appropriate diagnosis and healthcare. The study investigated how the Akan communicate sexuality generally, and how this affects their reporting of reproductive health issues. It was grounded on the rhetorical sensitivity theory. A multiple case study was employed for the study. In all, eight respondents were sampled and were categorised into two as cultural respondents and medical respondents. Cultural respondents comprised the Fante ethnic group of the larger Akan group. One respondent each was selected from three Fante traditional communities.

The COVID-19 disease presents an imminent danger that requires immediate action as it could be deadly. Vaccines against COVID-19 are considered to be of great importance to prevent and also to control, but there are challenges, one of which is uncertainty about public acceptance of the vaccine. The study looked at audience perception of COVID-19 vaccination and its effect on the behavioural responses of respondents in Oyo West Local Government. The study was anchored on the perception theory and the behaviour theory. The multistage probability sampling technique was adopted. The study found out that the COVID-19 vaccination awareness was not enough, thereby making the social media to have the upper hand by passing false rumours about the vaccine in order to get the people discouraged thereby leading to their non-challan behaviour and superstitious beliefs. The study concluded that the masses should be educated on the need to get vaccinated and therefore recommended that there should be more awareness on the COVID-19 vaccination to prevent future infections and deaths.

This chapter examines the views and perspectives of journalists on the role played by Radio Zimbabwe in informing refugee residents at Tongogara Refugees Camp in Zimbabwe about COVID-19. Also, the chapter examines their views and perspectives on the potential of Radio Zimbabwe and its COVID-19 message in creating a sense of belonging for the refugees. Its theoretical toolkit is drawn from the social responsibility theory and public sphere theory. Empirical data were drawn from in-depth interviews with 12 purposively selected radio journalists from Zimbabwe. The chapter established that Radio

Zimbabwe's jingles, news, and announcements on COVID-19 were not directed at refugees; thus, it was argued that the radio station did not adequately inform refugees residing at Tongogara Refugee Camp. Also, the chapter fleshes out Radio Zimbabwe's mediation of COVID-19 failed to fan a sense of belonging in refugees. Instead, the way Radio Zimbabwe handled COVID-19 strengthened the minority and marginalised identity in Zimbabwe.

Using framing as a springboard and critical discourse analysis as the methodology, this chapter aims to conduct a thoroughgoing exegesis of two speeches that were made by Oppah Muchinguri between the 14th of March 2020 and the 16th of January 2021. This chapter seeks to critically explain the influence of social, political, religious, and cultural factors on opinion leaders' attitude to COVID-19 and show the extent to which they represent perceptions of Zimbabweans regarding the virus and what should be prioritized between privacy of journalists' sources and the public interest. The chapter also adds to the huge corpus of studies on society's conceptualization of COVID-19 and urges stakeholders to avoid unsubstantiated claims and to use their influence to rally behind experts' advice in dealing with the pandemic.

This chapter examines the communication and language experiences of African migrants in Cape Town public health facilities in South Africa, exploring strategies they employ to navigate language and communication challenges they may encounter in the healthcare system. About 2.9 million migrants, predominantly Africans, live in South Africa, and their movement to South Africa has brought linguistic diversity and linguistic and cultural complexity, creating unique communication dynamics in healthcare settings. This mainly qualitative research draws on the responses of African migrants from various African countries purposively selected and surveyed to explore their lived experiences and perspectives. The study explores how African migrants experienced language use and communication, considering differences between migrant experiences in South African health institutions and their home countries and offering recommendations to improve communication in health facilities and, consequently, enhance the experiences of African migrants in South African health institutions.

Fact-checking and media literacy promoting organisations are now more committed than ever to combatting misinformation in Africa. The challenge, however, is that they have been publishing the bulk of their contents in colonial legacy languages of the African countries, thereby losing the opportunity to enlighten

Preface

AN OVERVIEW OF THE SUBJECT MATTER

In an increasingly interconnected world, public health communication plays a pivotal role in shaping the well-being and future of societies. It serves as the bridge between health practitioners, policymakers, and the general public, facilitating the dissemination of vital information, promoting awareness, and encouraging behavioral changes that can lead to healthier lives. However, while the significance of public health communication is undeniable, it is not without its complexities, especially when addressing the diverse needs of minority and indigenous communities.

WHERE THE TOPICS FITS IN THE WORLD TODAY

This book, *Public Health Communities Challenges to Minority and Indigenous Communities*, delves into the intricate dynamics of public health communication, focusing on the hurdles these marginalized and often underserved groups face. It recognizes the imperative of considering the unique cultural, linguistic, and social contexts that influence health perceptions, access to care, and the efficacy of communication strategies.

The challenges confronting minority and indigenous communities in public health communication are numerous and multifaced. Language barriers, historical mistrust of healthcare systems, disparities in access to care, and socioeconomic inequities are just a few obstacles these communities grapple with. Moreover, the impact of globalization and urbanization on traditional ways of life for indigenous groups adds a layer of complexity to the issues.

This book attempts to shed light on these challenges while celebrating the resilience and resourcefulness of minority and indigenous communities in the face of adversity. It brings together a collection of insightful chapters authored by experts, scholars, and practitioners in public health, communication, media, sociology, and anthropology. Each chapter offers a unique perspective on the intricacies of public health communication and its profound impact on minority and indigenous communities in Africa.

A DESCRIPTION OF THE TARGET AUDIENCE

The book's core objective is to serve as a resource for academics, practitioners, policymakers, and anyone interested in improving the relationship between the health and well-being of minority and indigenous communities and communication. It provides an opportunity for dialogue and learning, offering valuable insights into the unique challenges and successes that have emerged in public health communication.

A DESCRIPTION OF THE IMPORTANCE OF EACH OF THE CHAPTER SUBMISSIONS

In the chapter "Digital Public Sphere's Role in COVID-19 Mitigation in Zimbabwe," the authors investigate the dynamics of government and citizen interaction in Zimbabwe concerning the COVID-19 pandemic, with a particular emphasis on the digital public sphere. As technology emerges as vital in information dissemination, understanding the balance between official government sources and informal channels is pivotal. Using qualitative interviews, the authors examined the influence of these channels on public perceptions. The study underscores the significance of tailored communication strategies, considering socio-economic, linguistic, and digital divides. The findings have broad implications for future pandemic response strategies, emphasizing the importance of trust, clarity, and accessibility of information.

The authors of the chapter "Psychological Well-Being and Language Learning During the COVID-19 Pandemic" propose evidence-based interventions and strategies to enhance the psychological well-being of language learners and educators in similar crises in the future. It also looks at the psychological well-being of language learners and educators, specifically examining the challenges and opportunities that emerged during this unprecedented time. Additionally, it puts forth a set of evidence-based interventions and strategies to fortify the mental and emotional health of both language learners and educators. These proposed measures serve as a proactive blueprint to navigate similar crises that may arise, ensuring a more resilient and adaptive educational ecosystem.

The chapter "Effectiveness of COVID-19 Risk Communication Messages in Indigenous Languages and the Promotion of Safe Practices in Ondo State, Nigeria" examined the effectiveness of COVID-19 risk communication messages in indigenous languages vis-à-vis the promotion of safe practices in Ondo, Nigeria. The survey research design was used, and a questionnaire was randomly administered to 384 respondents in Akure, Ondo State. Findings showed that most respondents were exposed to COVID-19 risk communication messages and got their first information from social media. Furthermore, the study found that respondents were not receptive to COVID-19 messages passed across in indigenous languages. They prefer COVID-19 messages to pass across in the English language. The study recommended that there is a need to ensure that risk communication messages aired in indigenous languages are demystified in a way that the audience can easily understand and act upon.

The chapter "Kiswahili Video Messaging on COVID-19 Awareness in Kenya" examined the strategies employed in video communication to create awareness of COVID-19. The results demonstrate that in a substantial number of cases, the dissemination was hampered by wanting grammar, English to Kiswahili translational flaws, and unsuitable animatronics. The chapter contends that the Kiswahili video messaging mainly failed the test of communicative value.

The authors of the chapter "The Role of Language in Social Media During the COVID-19 Pandemic" explore the multifaceted role of language in social media during the COVID-19 pandemic. The chapter highlights the significance of language as a medium for facilitating real-time updates and news dissemination. The chapter asserts that governments, health organizations, and news outlets utilized language to convey critical information, ranging from infection rates and safety measures to vaccination updates, reaching a diverse and vast audience worldwide. This chapter also examined how language was a crucial tool in combating misinformation.

In "Cultural Perspectives on Health Communication: The Case of Katkari Tribals in Western Maharashtra, India," the authors contend that Public Health Communication becomes crucial for tribal, as it can empower them with vital information and resources to address the high prevalence of diseases, lower life expectancies, thus reducing health disparities. Effective delivery of health information can promote better access to healthcare services and improve overall health outcomes within these communities.

The chapter "President's Speech and Terminology Used During the COVID-19 Pandemic: The Interpretation of Linguistic Meaning in Context and Situational Context" investigates the interpretation of the South African President's terminologies during family meetings in a linguistic and situational context. The authors argue that most South African people do not know how to write and speak English. However, the COVID-19 information was delivered in English. Therefore, it excludes those who do not know English, with special reference to Setswana speakers.

The authors in "Public Health Communication and the Exclusion of Minority Languages in Zimbabwe: Analysis of Community Radio Awareness Campaigns in Facebook Posts" used community radio platforms as case studies on the assumption that local languages, such as minority languages, can at least find space, on community radio. However, a qualitative content analysis on radio content on Facebook reveals the dominance of Shona (a major indigenous language in Zimbabwe) and English in public health communication by health authorities and representatives of the ruling party.

The chapter "Public Health Communication and Language Policy at Rhodes University During the COVID-19 Pandemic" asserts that the COVID-19 pandemic offered unprecedented obstacles to public health communication worldwide. The pandemic revealed disparities and significant gaps in access to public health information for those not proficient in English, potentially leading to the exclusion of indigenous language speakers and minority communities from issues of national interest, including vital COVID-19 updates. This chapter examines the case study of Rhodes University in the Eastern Cape, South Africa, and explores the institution's language policies and practices during the pandemic.

In the chapter "Amplifying Health Concerns of Minoritized Groups in Nigeria Using Documentary," the authors state that several studies have shown that most highly placed government officials in the Ministry of Health in Africa do not bother to get to the hinterlands, slums, or inner cities where there are poor people, and socially excluded people because according to them, these are hard-to-reach areas; and additionally due to the spate of insecurity in the continent. The chapter explores the role of documentaries in amplifying the health concerns of minority groups in Nigeria.

The authors of "Communicating Sexuality and Reporting Reproductive Health Issues Among the Akan" investigated how the Akan communicate sexuality generally and how this affects their reporting of reproductive health issues. It was grounded in the rhetorical sensitivity theory. A multiple case study was employed for the study. In all, eight (8) respondents were sampled and were categorized into two groups: cultural respondents and medical respondents. Cultural respondents comprised the Fante ethnic group of the larger Akan group. One respondent each was selected from three Fante traditional communities.

The chapter on "Audience Perception of COVID-19 Vaccination and its Effect on the Behavioural Responses of Respondents in Oyo West Local Government" found out that COVID-19 vaccination awareness was not enough, thereby making the social media have the upper hand by passing false rumours about the vaccine in order to get the people discouraged thereby leading to their non-challan behaviour and superstitious beliefs. The study concluded that the masses should be educated on the need to get vaccinated and therefore recommended that there should be more awareness of the COVID-19 vaccination to prevent future infections and deaths.

In the chapter "COVID-19 Messages and High-Risk Areas," the authors examine the views and perspectives of journalists on the role played by Radio Zimbabwe in informing refugee residents at Tongogara Refugees Camp in Zimbabwe about COVID-19. Also, the chapter examines their views and perspectives on the potential of Radio Zimbabwe and its COVID-19 message in creating a sense of belonging for the refugees. Its theoretical toolkit is drawn from social responsibility and public sphere theories.

The author of the chapter "Framing of Opinion Leaders' COVID-19 Stance(s) on Society" uses framing as a springboard and critical discourse analysis as the methodology to conduct a thoroughgoing exegesis of two speeches that Oppah Muchinguri made between the 14th of March 2020 and the 16th of January 2021. This chapter seeks to critically explain the influence of social, political, religious, and cultural factors on opinion leaders' attitudes to COVID-19, show the extent to which they represent perceptions of Zimbabweans regarding the virus, and what should be prioritized between the privacy of journalists' sources and the public interest.

In the chapter "Navigating Borders," the author examines the communication and language experiences of African migrants in Cape Town public health facilities in South Africa, exploring strategies they employ to navigate language and communication challenges they may encounter in the healthcare system. The chapter explores how African migrants experienced language use, communication, and differences between migrant experiences in South African health institutions and their home countries. It also offers recommendations to improve communication in health facilities and, consequently, enhance the experiences of African migrants in South African health institutions.

The authors of the chapter "The Justification for Publishing Media Literacy and Fact Checks in African Indigenous Languages" review the efforts of three purposively selected Nigerian fact-checking organizations in reaching media publics who are not likely to be English-literate or on the internet. Key findings are that the indigenous-speaking public prefers audio-visual content to texts, and funds significantly impact the efforts of media literacy organizations in reaching the indigenous public.

The chapter "Participatory Intervention in Eliminating Harmful Traditional Practices: A Review of Female Genital Mutilation Practices in Nigeria and South Africa" intends to broaden the theoretical discourse (democratic participant theory), seeking to highlight participatory interventions to put an end to harmful traditional practices in selected African countries (Nigeria and South Africa). Primarily, it intends to explore the concept of participation and dialogue by incorporating the concerted effort of all, particularly that of this practice's cultural adherents/perpetrators. Thus, in order to achieve a colossal decline in female genital mutilation in Africa, active participation/involvement of cultural adherents is pertinent.

In the chapter "Impact of Town Criers Using Indigenous Yoruba Language in COVID-19 Awareness on Radio for Behavioral Change Among Rural Dwellers in Lagos," the authors carried out a study to show the roles of the new fusion between the indigenous and traditional media (Traditional town criers and radio) using indigenous Yoruba language in creating the awareness of COVID-19 among select rural dwellers in Lagos state. This study revealed a novel scene where traditional town criers were brought into language radio stations to create awareness for COVID-19 using the Yoruba language. Therefore, this chapter investigates the impact the fusion between the traditional town criers as an indigenous media and radio as a traditional media had on select minoritized rural dwellers in Lagos state during the pandemic.

HOW THE BOOK IMPACTS THE FIELD AND CONTRIBUTES TO THE SUBJECT MATTER

While the communication challenges facing minority and indigenous communities are undeniable, this book seeks to emphasize the potential for positive change. It highlights successful initiatives, innovative approaches, and stories of resilience, demonstrating how effective public communication can empower these communities and improve health outcomes.

This book is not merely an academic endeavor but a testament to the ongoing commitment to improving the lives of those who have long been marginalized. It is a call to action for researchers, practitioners, and policymakers to work collaboratively toward solutions that prioritize the health, well-being, and communication of all members of society, regardless of their cultural, ethnic, or linguistic backgrounds.

We hope the insights and perspectives presented in this book will inspire new conversations, initiatives, and policies that honour the diversity and resilience of minority and indigenous communities while striving for healthier and more equitable societies. As we journey through the following chapters, we encourage our readers to approach this material with an open heart and inquisitiveness. The stories and strategies within these pages hold the potential to transform public health communication for the better and, in doing so, to enhance the lives of countless individuals and communities.

Kealeboga Aiseng
Rhodes University, South Africa

Israel A. Fadipe
Ajayi Crowther University, Nigeria

Chapter 1
Digital Public Sphere's Role in COVID-19 Mitigation in Zimbabwe:
Government-Citizen Engagement

Kedmon Nyasha Hungwe
Michigan Technological University, USA

Ashley R. Rakatsinzwa
Flexi Academy, South Africa

Felix Mukono
Midlands State University, Zimbabwe

ABSTRACT

This research investigates the dynamics of government and citizen interaction in Zimbabwe concerning the COVID-19 pandemic, with a particular emphasis on the digital public sphere. As technology emerges as a vital player in information dissemination, understanding the balance between official government sources and informal channels is pivotal. Using qualitative interviews, the authors examined the influence of these channels on public perceptions. The results highlighted a lack of trust in the government, reliance on informal networks for counternarratives, and widespread misconceptions about the virus. The study further underscores the significance of tailored communication strategies, considering socio-economic, linguistic, and digital divides. The findings have broad implications for future pandemic response strategies, emphasizing the importance of trust, clarity, and accessibility of information.

INTRODUCTION

In this study, we explore the crucial dynamics of government and citizen engagement and participation in responding to the spread of COVID-19 in Zimbabwe. A focal point of our investigation is the

DOI: 10.4018/979-8-3693-0624-6.ch001

significant role played by the digital public sphere in these efforts. We investigate the intricate interplay between official government information sources and informal channels of information dissemination. By analyzing the influence of these sources on public perceptions and behaviors, the research aims to provide valuable insights into the challenges of managing information flow during a crisis and the consequent implications for public health outcomes. Moreover, understanding the dynamics of information dissemination can aid policymakers in developing more effective communication strategies that address misinformation, build trust, and foster more inclusive and culturally sensitive approaches to crisis response and containment efforts.

There is a growing consensus that the global community "failed its test of preparedness and response to the COVID-19 pandemic" (Frieden, Buissonnière, & McClelland, 2021). Moreover, experts predict that global pandemics are likely to recur in the future, and a substantial proportion of people are expected to experience an extreme pandemic like COVID-19 within their lifetime (Marani, Katul, Pan, & Parolari, 2021; Osterholm, 2020).

The epidemic unfolded in a distinctive era characterized by the emergence of the "digital public sphere" (Schäfer, 2015). This concept denotes the online realm that facilitates public discourse, discussions, and debates on matters of interest and concern. It encompasses various digital spaces, including social media platforms, online forums, blogs, news websites, and more, where citizens can engage in the roles of information consumers, distributors, and creators. In Zimbabwe, cellphone technology has played a particularly significant role in shaping the digital public sphere, with applications like WhatsApp becoming indispensable tools for communication. As technology continues to rapidly evolve, it is evident that the digital public sphere will assume an increasingly crucial role in shaping societies' responses to future pandemics.

BACKGROUND

Context plays a critical role in influencing how individuals seek information and determine whether to use it or not. As noted by Rauchfleisch, Vogler, & Eisenegger (2021), during times of crisis, like a pandemic, the public sphere undergoes a shift into "crisis mode." In the realm of related research, Chatman made significant contributions to our comprehension of how personal factors and social norms intertwine to shape the reception and interpretation of information. This understanding was gained through insightful ethnographic studies focusing on marginalized and disadvantaged populations.

The first COVID-19 case in Zimbabwe was officially announced by the Ministry of Health on March 21, 2020. This case involved an individual who had recently traveled from the United Kingdom. By August 12, 2020, the number of reported cases had reached 4,893, with 122 fatalities. Consequently, the Zimbabwean government declared COVID-19 a "formidable epidemic disease" through the implementation of Public Health Regulations. According to the constitution, the state was obligated to take all available preventive measures, including education and public awareness programs, to curb the spread of the disease. Furthermore, the declaration also necessitated the equitable allocation of resources to prioritize healthcare services.

During the pandemic, a crucial aspect of the context revolved around the citizenry's profound emotional involvement in the situation. This emotional investment manifested in various anxieties related to illness and the fear of potential illness. Additionally, the challenges of loneliness due to isolation and social distancing, along with increased stress from adapting to new routines and grappling with financial and employment insecurities, further compounded the situation. Moreover, feelings of depression arose as a consequence of reduced physical activity, disrupted daily routines, and a sense of loss.

The pandemic's impact was significantly intensified by socio-economic disparities. Livelihoods were disrupted, leading to a rise in the number of citizens facing extreme poverty (Larsson et al., 2023; World Bank, 2023). These factors profoundly influenced the discourse within the digital public sphere. The effectiveness, viability, and usefulness of this digital sphere relied on the development of authentic and rational discussions. It's crucial to acknowledge the dual role of the state: not only as a contributor to the digital information sphere but also as a regulator shaping the context in which the digital sphere emerged (Mazzoleni, Gianpietro et al., 2015).

The research findings revolve around three key thematic issues. First, we explore a lack of public confidence and trust in the government. We examine how this influenced public response and the role of the digital public sphere in this dynamic. We analyzed the role of informal networks as citizens consumed, generated, and distributed counternarrative content in the digital sphere amidst an ever-changing and uncertain environment. Finally, we demonstrate how the public's understanding of the nature of Covid-19 and its associated preventative measures was fraught with misconceptions. This was despite the fact that core segments of the public believed they had a clear grasp of the information communicated.

The research conducted by Afrobarometer is among several sources shedding light on a problem of distrust in government information about the pandemic (Kugarakuripi & Ndoma, 2022). The study revealed that fewer than half of adults trusted the government's statistics on COVID-19 infections and deaths, as well as its ability to ensure the safety of COVID-19 vaccines. Notably, vaccine hesitancy was particularly prevalent among individuals who relied on social media as their primary news source. In contrast, other research conducted during the same period indicated that social media messaging from "trusted sources," which were often non-governmental entities, significantly influenced individuals' knowledge and related behaviors (Bowles, Larreguy, & Liu, 2020).

The lack of trust in vaccines emerged as a significant issue. Several reports highlighted slow uptake, even among healthcare practitioners. The likelihood of individuals accepting vaccinations was notably linked to their confidence in vaccine safety. Notably, there was a prevailing distrust of vaccines, particularly those of Chinese origin (McAbee, Tapera, & Kanyangarara, 2021; Mhute, Mangeya & Jakaza, 2021). Social media played a role in amplifying these concerns, as we examine media communication to gain deeper insights into these issues.

RESEARCH QUESTION

How did the integration of information from multiple sources, including government channels and informal social media platforms influence the public's comprehension, attitudes, and adherence to virus containment measures, with a particular focus on the role of indigenous communities in this process?

METHODOLOGY

The objective of the methodology was to critically assess the communication of COVID-related information and its subsequent interpretation and comprehension within a specific underprivileged urban community. Considering the linguistic diversity of the study area, a decision was made regarding the languages in which the survey would be available. English and Shona, being the predominant languages of the region, were chosen to cater to the linguistic preferences of the residents. This dual-language approach ensured that respondents could articulate their views in the language they were most comfortable with, enhancing the authenticity and depth of their responses.

For data collection, we gathered information shared by government sources and informal social media channels. Our focus was on the period between 2020 and 2021. In the process of gathering data, a total of 45 interviews were conducted. The majority, 39 in total, were in-person interviews, allowing for a direct, face-to-face interaction with the respondents. The remaining 6 interviews were conducted via WhatsApp, leveraging the available technology and expanding the size of the sample. The characteristics of responses from both the in-person and WhatsApp-based interviews were largely similar. Given this overarching similarity, it was deemed appropriate to combine the responses into a single consolidated group.

The state broadcaster's online video content emerged as a principal source of information. In this digital age, other online sources from non-governmental organizations were inevitably encountered. However, they are not part of this study, which focuses on understanding perceptions about government-sponsored messaging.

The analysis of the survey data focused on items that illuminated the respondent's understanding of COVID-19, its transmission, the sources from which the respondents learned their information, and most importantly, their perceptions regarding the clarity and effectiveness of government-sponsored messages. For the social media analysis we examined self-reported uses, and views, comments, and content communicated. This set of data was used to corroborate the interpretations from the survey, which was the source of data.

Central to this research was understanding how language practices intertwined with imbalances in power dynamics. Pragmatics, as described by Yule (1996), delves into the conveyance and comprehension of meaning between a sender and a receiver. We recognized that Zimbabwe showcases a phenomenon called linguistic diglossia. "Diglossia" refers to a scenario in which one language community employs two distinct dialects or languages for different purposes. Under this setup, one dialect or language, termed as the "high" variety (H variety), is utilized in official, literary, and formal contexts. The "low" variety (L variety) is used in everyday, informal conversations in that same context. Within the linguistic landscape of Zimbabwe, English is an H-variety language, while local languages including Shona, isiNdebele, Tonga, Kalanga, among others hold a subordinate position (Chimhundu 2006, Veit-Wild 2006, Mashiri 2002).

PROFILE OF RESPONDENTS

Demographic data included employment status, gender, education level, and age. Employment status offered insights into economic trends and the population's well-being. Gender data helped in examining social, cultural, and economic patterns. Education level acted as an indicator of an individual's knowledge, literacy, and socio-economic positioning. Age data provided a perspective on the life stages of individuals. Collectively, these indicators were intended to help in forming an understanding of the population's characteristics.

With respect to employment status, most respondents were in the informal sector of the economy. Out of all respondents, 32 or 78% found their livelihoods within this sector. A total of 5, which translates to

12.2%, were without jobs, while only two individuals were part of the conventional formal workforce. However, ambiguity remained for three participants whose employment status was not determined.

Turning to the educational background, the data indicate a literate population, with 29 (69%) of the respondents having completed four years of secondary schooling and acquiring the Zimbabwe Ordinary Level Certificate. Additionally, 11 participants, or 11.9%, had earned the Advanced Level Certificate, which represents a commitment to six years of secondary education. An additional six had a college-level certification. On the other end of the spectrum, two had some secondary education that didn't extend beyond four years.

Age-wise, the profile of our respondents was predominantly young, mirroring the general demographic trend observable in Zimbabwe. The largest age group was those between 20 and 30 years, with 24 participants or 54.5%. The next substantial group fell into the 31-40 years bracket, with 12 or 27.3%. Five were aged above 40, while the youngest category, those under 20, included three individuals.

Examining gender distribution, a near balance was achieved. Of the respondents, 23 were females, and there were 20 males. This balance was also evident in the linguistic preferences for survey response. English was the preferred choice for 25 respondents, whereas 20 favored Shona. A trained field worker, fluent in both English and Shona, translated all Shona responses into English.

In summary, the critical features of the demographic were the relatively young age of mostly under-employed young generation, striving to make a living in an economy that was already challenging before the onset of the pandemic.

RESULTS

The results discussion centers on the sources of information utilized, participants' self-evaluation of their comprehension of pandemic-related information, and the insights they acquired about the pandemic.

Sources of Information Used by the Participants

Participants in the survey were posed the question: "Which information sources did you depend on to get updates on COVID-19?" The results are presented in Table 1.

The data highlights the predominant influence of broadcast media among the surveyed group. The Zimbabwe Broadcasting Corporation, a state-controlled organization, has been the primary broadcaster for both TV and radio. Information about COVID-19 was disseminated via news segments and regular updates. The study also points out a notable reliance on supplementary media, especially posters and billboards placed in public areas, with hospitals and clinics as key locations for these displays. The diminished role of newspapers is also evident. Given Zimbabwe's economic challenges and the people's daily struggles for livelihoods, there was a clear preference for broadcast media over print media, which would involve additional costs.

When asked, "Did you use social media to obtain information about Covid?", 44 out of 45 respondents affirmed their use of social media. The lone individual who refrained from using social media remarked, "I tried as much as possible to avoid the fallacies of these platforms." This same individual also avoided local sources, stating a preference for information from the World Health Organization, CNN, and Al Jazeera. This respondent stands out from the majority, possessing a college degree and seemingly having

Table 1. Which information sources did you depend on to get updates on COVID-19?

Source	Frequency
Television	31*
Radio	23
Posters/Billboards	16
Clinics/Hospitals	15
Workplaces	6
Neighbors/Friends/Social Groups	5
Workplace	6
Police Announcements	4
Road Shows	4
Newspapers	3
Schools	3
Others+	6

*Essentially local television. Includes single mentions of foreign media sources: British Broadcasting Corporation (BBC), Al Jazeera, South African Broadcasting Corporation (SABC), and Cable News Network (CNN).

+ Includes banks, supermarkets, articles, & government, internet search.

access to the internet and other informational sources. Table 2 summarizes the respondents' engagement with social media.

WhatsApp emerged as the dominant social media app. The app is designed to handle erratic internet connections, ensuring messages are sent once there's a signal. It's also compatible with affordable feature phones. The app also supports a range of content, from photos, and videos, to documents, and audio messaging. It also allows for free international messaging, which is vital in regions where families are spread across borders. Given these features, it's understandable that WhatsApp has dominated as the preferred messaging app, not only in Zimbabwe, but in other African countries. In Zimbabwe, consistent usage of YouTube poses a financial burden due to the nation's widespread poverty and elevated unemployment levels. Additionally, it demands higher data expenses and necessitates stronger network connections. The data confirms the infrequent use of YouTube. However, the state broadcasting services did create a YouTube channel where Covid-19 updates were posted weekly from October 1, 2020, to August 2021.

Table 2. Uses of with social media for COVID-19 information

Source	Frequency
WhatsApp	42
Facebook	34
Instagram	6
Twitter	4
YouTube	2
TikTok	1
Google Search	1

Dr. Agnes Mahomva, the Chief Coordinator of the National Response to Covid-19 in the Office of the President and Cabinet, produced and presented the complete series of videos (ZBC News, 2021). Before being uploaded to the YouTube channel, these videos were broadcasted live on television. Dr. Mahomva is a medical practitioner of international repute.

The average number of views for the 24-video playlist was 741, which is low considering the national population of 15.99 million (as of 2021). There are two standout videos in the YouTube playlist. First, President Mnangagwa appeared in a video in mid-March 2021 to promote vaccination. A separate news program had previously shown him getting vaccinated at Victoria Falls on March 24, 2021. The YouTube video was titled "Get Vaccinated Now, Together We Will Conquer". The President stated: "We have lost many of our loved ones. I am here to tell you that you and I have a role to play." This video garnered 2,600 views, which, though low, was the highest for the national broadcaster's YouTube channel.

The second most-watched video was a presentation by Dr. Agnes Mahomva, dated January 14, 2021 (ZBC News, 2021). The number of views was 1,500. Although the number was low, it nevertheless indicated higher than average interest, and a trend that could be consolidated. Dr. Mahomva highlighted that Zimbabwe was experiencing a second wave of the epidemic. She voiced concerns about non-compliance with guidelines, like wearing facemasks and social distancing. Super spreader events, especially during the Christmas period, were a threat to public health. The standout feature of this presentation was a short documentary that captured non-compliance in the "high density suburb" of Mabvuku, a suburb of Harare, the nation's capital city. In Zimbabwe, a "high-density suburb" describes residential areas where homes are smaller and situated closer together compared to the expansive layouts of low-density suburbs. These neighborhoods predominantly house the working class and, in recent times, have seen an influx of economically disadvantaged individuals, leading to overcrowded conditions and pressure on the amenities. The documentary depicted daily routines and behaviors. Dr. Mahomva's presentations were typically limited do the presentation of data regarding infection numbers, recoveries, and fatalities. International patterns and collaborations, especially with entities like the WHO, were a recurring theme. Governmental strategies addressing the COVID pandemic were prominently discussed, complemented by preventive measures. The use of visuals and occasional graphs enriched the content, ensuring it was clear, well-presented, and scientifically rooted. Nonetheless, the material might not have been relatable for the everyday Zimbabwean, partly due to its lack of contextual nuances and variety. Motivating people on actions such as social distancing, isolation, and quarantine would be particularly challenging in areas with dense populations where the quest for space and adequate housing was a daily hurdle.

Nevertheless, the limited data on audience response suggests strategies that could potentially boost audience engagement: The first is the active engagement from leadership at the highest level as was shown by the spike in interest in the President's video episode. The second approach emphasizes crafting media messages that include the daily lives and routines of everyday people, as showcased in the documentary. Overall, the data indicates a relatively weak uptake of data-intensive platforms like YouTube. In an epidemic-type situation, these platforms may have limited value, and a thorough cost-benefit analysis is essential. It might be more effective to channel investments into local media production, adopting a documentary-style method, and streamline the scientific/technical details to focus on the most crucial aspects. The goal would be to not only inform, but to engage and motivate.

Our research is limited to what was broadcast on television and presented in English. We couldn't locate archival sources of Dr. Mahomva's program in local languages. Sign language translation was available, and there were periodic reports on the epidemic in local languages during local news broadcasts. Additionally, interview data indicated that participants had access to information in local languages. Still,

Table 3. Reasons why the information presented through government sources was not clear

• "People were not clear about the issue of vaccines. People were not convinced that they were safe and believed that the government needed funding from the World Health Organization."
• "Information that came from the government was biased especially on the number of cases and deaths. The members of public felt that figures were exaggerated."
• "Sometimes it was not easy to understand when they used force to control people."
• "Not really as there were a lot of difficult words used which were not easy to understand at times."
• "Information from the government was not clear. For instance, information on number and deaths was not clear."
• "Information about vaccination was not easy to understand especially the issue of type of vaccine, significance of number of doses and, it's safety."
• "Only information about vaccines was difficult to understand and it caused a lot of people to resist vaccination believing that it was a mark of the beast."

the predominant view was that English language sources dominated, as evidenced by the President's presentation being in English.

Clarity of Information

The respondents were asked the question, "Did you find the information that came from the government to explain Covid easy to understand?" A majority of 25 persons reported finding the information clear and easy to understand. Nineteen (19) did not find it easy to understand. One person did not give a clear answer. We examined the data to find out why the information presented was not clear. Table 3 indicates the pattern of responses. Several of these were raised multiple times, by different people.

There were persistent questions about vaccine safety, and Dr. Mahomva was aware of them. One recurring query was about the primary sourcing of vaccines from China and, to a lesser extent, from Russia. According to her, many were asking, "Why only the Chinese vaccine?" (ZBC News, 18 February 2021). The main question was, "Is the Sinovac vaccine safe?" Many believed it was developed too hastily. Her response was both candid and technical. She emphasized that the standard approval process was adhered to, stating, "It may not be possible to have all the data that would normally be available before approving a drug." The vaccine was released as part of a "public health emergency." In the March 4, 2021, update, Dr. Mahomva addressed the ongoing vaccine hesitancy. She delved into details about how vaccines function, including the development of antibodies, and discussed potential side effects like rashes, fevers, and chills. She emphasized that severe effects were rare and manageable, adding, "All medicines can have side effects." A comment on the video highlighted the continuous concerns about vaccines. The viewer's comment was:

"Still not convinced. I mean accepting vaccines from another country like Russia and China is no, no. Are you telling me the Covid-19 variant in Zimbabwe is the same as the variant in Russia? I don't think so. Why isn't Africa coming up with its own? Donation of vaccine means Zimbabwe is a test lab. Period." (March 4, 2021)

It should be noted that the typical Zimbabwean audience, most of whom are poor with limited health-care provision, are generally unaccustomed to receiving detailed medical information like that provided about Covid vaccines. This lack of familiarity made it challenging for them to trust the official scientific information. Dr. Mahomva was on stronger ground when she pointed out that the Vice President, who

Table 4. What do you know about how COVID-19 is spread?

- "Covid-19 is spread through contact with the infected person. It is also spread through the air when coughing and sneezing."
- "Covid-19 is spread through hand shaking and through breathing contaminated air."
- "Covid-19 is spread through handshakes. It is also spread through breathing contaminated air."
- "Covid-19 is spread through touching people infected by Covid-19 with bare hands."
- "Covid-19 is usually spread through shaking hands with different people in public spaces. It is also caused by sneezing and coughing without covering one's mouth."
- "Covid-19 Spread through attending funerals and other over-crowded gatherings."
- "It is spread through air when infected person coughs. Also, through hand shaking."
- "It is spread through saliva when sharing the same beer or drink with the infected person. It is also spread through shaking hands."
- "It is spread through sharing beer with the infected person. It is also spread through hand shaking."
- "It spreads through saliva and public gatherings, in buses and through contact."
- "Through sneezing or coughing in public spaces without covering your mouth."
- "Covid-19 is spread through public gatherings, attending funerals of people deceased with "Covid-19. It also spread through shaking hands."
- "It is spread through handshakes or any other form of contact with the infected person."

also served as the Minister of Health, had been vaccinated. The broadcast vaccination of the President, and his appearance to urge vaccination did create a spike in interest, as already noted.

Language Issues

It was clear that the survey respondents had encountered information on Covid-19 in their language, as well as in English. However, there was a perception that the presentations were predominantly in English, and a greater use of local languages would have been preferred. Based on our analysis of the messages, the issue was not just about the use of English, but the uses of technical language, and jargon, and scientific terms. For instance, Dr. Mahomva employed terms like "genomic sequencing" (ZBC News, June 10, 2021), which would be beyond the comprehension of the general population, many of whom only have a secondary education. In the same presentation, detailed data were flashed on screen under the title "Our World Data" to display global vaccination statistics. The information was dense, and it appeared briefly. The local relevance remained ambiguous. It wasn't clear who the intended audience for this data was. Moreover, mentions of Covid-19 variants lacked sufficient context and pertinence. Additionally, much time was dedicated to policy and governmental activities, and did not resonate with the everyday individual. Technical terms like "post-cabinet briefing" (June 10, 2021) would not be meaningful to the average person trying to understand and navigate the challenges of the pandemic. In summary, while the efforts were commendable, the data points out areas that needed review and refinement.

Additional insights came from an analysis of the responses from the 25 persons who believed that the information on Covid from the government was 'easy to understand.' We focus on the answers to the question, "What do you know about how Covid-19 is spread"" The data indicate that respondents tended to overestimate their understanding of the messages. Respondents clearly provided answers that indicated misconceptions, or limited understanding. The listing in Table 4 highlights the range of these responses.

The answers, although not irrelevant, provided a grossly incomplete picture of the epidemiology of COVID-19, as well as the critical role of social distancing and face masks. Upon further exploration, this discrepancy seemed to stem from a shallow understanding of the nature of COVID-19 transmission. A majority of respondents likened it to the flu. This perspective is evident in the responses to the question, "What do you know about COVID-19?" The following set of responses represent this point of view.

• "Covid -19 is a virus that causes illness such that a person can get a flu or fever." • "Covid-19 is just a flu. In fact, is just another version of flu that came more stronger, and it is caused by a virus." • "Covid-19 is pandemic that is caused by a virus which is just like flu." • "Covid-19 is an illness caused by a virus that cause flu-like symptoms." • "Covid -19 is virus that lives in human body and when it is not controlled, it caused harm even to death." • "Covid is a disease similar to flu. The only difference is that Covid-19 kills people and Is more dangerous than flu." • "Covid is a disease that is caused by a virus like flu." • "Covid-19 is a disease which causes flu symptoms, and it is dangerous such that it kills especially the old age." • "Covid-19 is a flu- like disease it is a global pandemic that caused millions of death all over the world." • "Covid-19 is a global pandemic that killed millions of people." It is a strong flu." • "Covid-19 is just a flu. In fact, is just another version of flu that came more stronger, and it is caused by a virus." • "Covid-19 is pandemic that is caused by a virus which is just like flu." • "Covid-19 is a disease that is caused by viruses such as a flu virus."

Table 5. What do you know about COVID-19?

The answers reflected the prevailing view that COVID-19 was a type of flu. However, equating COVID-19 with the flu is problematic. While both are respiratory illnesses with some overlapping symptoms, COVID-19 has demonstrated a higher potential for severe outcomes and long-term complications, even among younger age groups. The World Health Organization (WHO) has consistently emphasized that, while many people worldwide have built immunity to seasonal flu strains, COVID-19 is a novel virus to which no one had prior immunity, leading to more widespread outbreaks.

The transmission dynamics of COVID-19 also differ, making its containment more challenging. Moreover, likening COVID-19 to the flu can result in public complacency. Such comparisons could lead people to dismiss it as "just another flu," thereby underestimating its severity and the critical nature of mitigation measures like vaccination, masking, and social distancing.

Dr. Mahomva's presentations consistently stressed the importance of mask-wearing. Although there was significant adherence to wearing masks, many wore them incorrectly. Typically, masks only covered the mouth, aligning with responses about coughing, saliva, and other transmission methods. A video from the television documentary aired on Dr. Mahomva's program highlighted the incorrect usage of masks, even by the police. Additionally, social distancing was often neglected. Part of this neglect might stem from the belief that physical contact was the primary transmission method and that airborne spread was only a concern when individuals displayed symptoms like coughing. One crucial element missing from the public's understanding was the concept of asymptomatic transmission of COVID-19. This refers to the spread of the virus from individuals who are infected but do not show any symptoms of the disease. Our review of the messaging on COVID indicated a lack of focus on this aspect.

BEYOND MAINSTREAM MEASURES: COUNTERNARRATIVES OF COVID-19 PREVENTION

It is evident from the data that the population surveyed was most immediately more concerned with daily livelihood issues than with the Covid-19 pandemic itself. The mandates for face masking and the recommended use of sanitizers became a burden on their already strained finances and resources. Lockdowns pushed many out of employment. Most of these individuals, with only a few exceptions, were engaged in the informal sector. Their understanding or concern for guidelines on the isolation of infected individuals, or the quarantine was limited. Furthermore, their places of work in the informal

Table 6. What are some of the challenges you faced in following the COVID-19 preventative measures?

• "There was no housing and transport that was suitable for social distance. Lack of money to buy Covid-19 materials such as masks and hand sanitizers."
• "During Covid-19 there were a lot of problems such as lack of money to buy preventive materials like masks and hand sanitizers."
• "Jobs were hard to find during the Covid - 19 pandemic. Also, we had no money to purchase Covid-19 preventive materials such as hand sanitizers and face masks."
• "During Covid-19 pandemic there was scarce resources in terms of money to purchase basic Commodities. Even preventive facilities such as masks were expensive."
• "Challenges include restricted movement to and from work, hunger and starvation, lack of facilities."
• "Challenges include restricted movement to and from work, hunger and starvation, lack of facilities."
• "Money was difficult to find during Covid-19. Hand sanitizers and face masks were also difficult to find during Covid-19 lockdowns."
• "Sanitizer was expensive to purchase because of economic harsh conditions. It was also difficult to move from one place to another which caused shortage of food and other basics in many household."
• "Shortage of masks and hand, sanitizers, hunger & starvation during lock downs."
• "Shortage of masks and hand, sanitizers, hunger & starvation during lock downs."

sector were bustling and crowded, lacking well-designed operational spaces. We refer again to the video documentary aired on Dr. Mahomva's program in January 2021 to illustrate this point. Table 6 presents the range of responses obtained for the question, "What are some of the challenges you faced in following the Covid-19 preventative measures?"

Overall, the practicalities of complying with health guidelines posed severe challenges for these populations. In response, they crafted their own narratives and strategies to manage and cope. These counter-narratives primarily focused on informal remedies, diverging significantly from recommended preventative measures such as social distancing, face masking, and isolation. These alternatives were highlighted in responses to the question, "Which alternative cures or remedies did you come to know about? Were they effective?" Table 7 is a represents the answers. Some responses repeat the same point with some extension.

Table 7. Which alternative cures or remedies did you come to know about? Were they effective?

• "Drinking lemons and eucalyptus leaves to maintain alkalinity in the body. It was helpful in reducing the chances of infection."
• "Exercises like jogging, drinking herbs, vaccination and using flu tablets. These were helpful to some extent."
• "Herbs such as *zumbani*+ helped people to people to reduce the risk of Covid-19."
• "Measures on social media were true and effective e.g., surrounding the bed with chopped king onion to avoid blocking nasal passages, and steaming/*kufukira.* * The measures worked."
• "Remedies such as using pealed King Onions and drinking lemon and ginger syrup were helpful in reducing the impact of Covid-19."
• "Steaming of herbs such as *zumbani.*+ Exercising everyday."
• "Steaming of herbs was helpful in reducing the risk of Covid-19."
• "The remedies that were trending on social media about preventing the spread of the virus include using eucalyptus leaves, lemons, and others."
• "There were remedies that circulated on social media platforms. Such as steaming lemons in hot water. It was helpful to some extent."
• "We usually got information about sleeping while facing downwards to avoid blocking of nostrils or nasal passage. Also steaming with an open mouth to allow the steam to penetrate the lungs."
• "Yes, they are helpful. For instance, the use of lemons and exercises. Steaming as well as exercises."
• "*Zumbani,*+ eucalyptus leaves, mint leaves, guavas, inhaling onions, ginger and lemons, steaming."

*"Steaming lungs" is not a recognized medical treatment or procedure. It involves inhaling steam from hot water and is believed to ease symptoms of colds, flu, and sinus infections.

+*Zumbani*, scientifically known as Lippia javanica, is a plant native to Zimbabwe. During the pandemic, it became widely known due to its lemon-like aroma. The leaves of the plant were used as a herbal tea. The information was widely spread though the social media.

SUMMARY

The Zimbabwe Broadcasting Corporation (television and radio) were the most cited as sources of update information on the Covid-19. Supplementary media, such as posters and billboards, played a secondary role, while newspapers were notably absent from the responses. When asked about the sources, it is notable that social media were not mentioned (Table 1). However, when asked directly if they used social media to obtain information on COVID-19, all but one of the respondents indicated that they did (Table 2). Our understanding is that they depended on the official sources (primarily television and radio) for authoritative information on the status of the pandemic, regulations, and preventative measures, including information on such things as vaccines. However, regarding their coping mechanisms, in their personal spaces, they turned to social media, which they seemed to regard as a quasi-authoritative source. A "quasi-authoritative source" in this case, would mean a source that appears, feels, or is perceived as authoritative but isn't fully or officially recognized or endorsed. The information on social media focused more on alternative remedies that were deemed the best fit. In that sense, they were able to say that they depended on official sources, but only to a degree. The tendency to think of the Covid-19 as a type of flu, reinforced the motivation to engage in counternarratives and practices.

One way to mitigate the challenge of counternarratives would be to enhance the quality of the official sources, making the information more relatable. A significant barrier identified was the heavy reliance on English in state broadcasts coupled with the regular use of technical terminology and bureaucratic jargon. Although most of the target audience felt they grasped the conveyed messages, their responses to queries about the nature and spread of COVID indicated a different reality. A critical misconception was equating Covid-19 to the flu. Another critical, and related gap was a lack of appreciation of the role of asymptomatic transmission.

For this segment of the population, COVID-19 prevention measures felt more burdensome than the disease itself. Practical issues like the cost of masks and sanitizers, impact of lockdowns, and the dynamics of the informal sector made compliance very difficult. As a result, alternative preventative narratives emerged, focusing on informal remedies like "steaming lungs" and the use of the plant *zumbani*, which many came to believe in.

LIMITATIONS OF THE RESEARCH

This research provides insights into communication strategies concerning COVID, but it's essential to recognize some contextual and methodological limitations.

A primary limitation relates to the geographical scope. The research was concentrated in a specific region of Zimbabwe and targeted one linguistic group. This specificity raises concerns, especially given Zimbabwe's rich linguistic diversity.

Non-governmental actors were involved in the digital realm, as showcased by Zimbabwean youth partnering with the non-profit organization Voluntary Service Overseas (VSO). Using platforms like Twitter, WhatsApp, Facebook, and radio, they worked to identify and correct COVID-19 misinformation (Murewanhema, Burukai, Chireka, & Kunonga, 2021). The discourses arising from these channels highlight the potential of building a complementary digital public space to counter public health threats. Yet, our research still uncovered consistent misconceptions. Thus, the effectiveness and scope of these efforts seems to have been constrained. The data suggest that people primarily engaged with information within their informal circles, whether due to preference, access, or both. This topic certainly merits further exploration. Moreover, the study touches upon the intersection of cultural and economic influences, especially among socioeconomically disadvantaged groups. Their gravitation towards alternative preventative narratives calls attention to the interplay of cultural beliefs, economic constraints, and health behaviors. There's a clear need for more comprehensive research to investigate this dynamic further.

CONCLUSION

This study contributes to the body of literature that focuses on public health factors associated with the COVID-19 pandemic in both an African and Zimbabwean context. The studies include Dzinamarira, Nachipo, Phiri, & Musuka (2021) focusing on the COVID-19 vaccine roll-out in South Africa and Zimbabwe. The study emphasized the need to address community readiness, apprehensions, and vaccine hesitancy. Iyamu et al. (2022) investigated the influence of social media on preventive measures, specifically highlighting the use of face masks. Mutanga, Ureke & Chani (2021) concentrated on the nexus between social media and the COVID-19 pandemic, evaluating the public's reactions. Mackworth-Young et al. (2021) focused on community perspectives concerning Zimbabwe's response to COVID-19. Bowles, Larreguy & Liu (2020) examined strategies for countering misinformation related to COVID-19 disseminated via WhatsApp.

We conclude by advocating for studies centered on user needs, communication strategies, and barriers to understanding. The COVID-19 pandemic has underscored the importance of timely, accurate, and comprehensible information dissemination. While many studies have focused on misinformation, addressing and countering this (Bowles, Larreguy & Liu, 2020), misinformation is only part of a broader, more intricate issue. There is a clear need for research that investigates user needs, communication strategies, and barriers to understanding critical information. Several studies on public health have adopted this user-centered approach (Adekunle & Mohammed, 2022; Ngondo & Klyueva, 2022; Mason et al., 2022).

In this regard, recognizing the diversity of audiences and their unique informational needs is essential. Audiences typically span various demographics, each with its own set of informational requirements. Factors such as age, cultural background, educational level, and regional distinctions influence how information is interpreted and acted upon. Addressing these specific needs ensures inclusivity, enhancing the reach and impact of information. While generic, one-size-fits-all approaches might be convenient and more easily produced, they often fall short. Tailored communication strategies are more effective at engaging audiences, ensuring that information is not only shared but also understood, leading to desired actions. Misinformation, though pervasive, isn't always the primary concern. Our study suggests that even accurate information can be challenging for the average person to grasp, especially when presented with scientific data or guidelines. Additionally, our study identified the issue of false confidence when individuals mistakenly believe they have grasped essential information. Overcoming these barriers to communication is essential, ensuring that reliable information is not only readily available but also easily understood.

In designing communication strategies, the significance of socioeconomic and linguistic factors cannot be understated. Furthermore, establishing effective communication pathways is fundamental to building trust. Strategies developed from a user-needs perspective foster trust between information distributors, like health organizations or governments, and the broader public. This trust is particularly valuable during health crises, where adherence to guidelines can have life-altering implications. Another crucial consideration is the digital divide. Our research emphasizes a noticeable trend: a reduced reliance on data-intensive platforms like YouTube. Not every demographic has equal digital access, especially concerning social media. Acknowledging and addressing the challenges posed by the digital divide, particularly the costs associated with data, are vital to ensuring that communication strategies are as effective as possible.

REFERENCES

Adekunle, T. B., & Mohammed, W. F. (2022). Communication in context: How culture, structure, and agency shape health and risk communication about COVID?19 in Ghana. World Medical & Health Policy, 14(2), 437-444.

Bates, M. J. (2010). Information behavior. Encyclopedia of library and information sciences, 3, 2381-2391.

Bowles, J., Larreguy, H., & Liu, S. (2020). Countering misinformation via WhatsApp: Preliminary evidence from the COVID-19 pandemic in Zimbabwe. *PLoS One*, *15*(10), e0240005. doi:10.1371/journal.pone.0240005 PMID:33052967

Chimhundu, H. (2006). Languages and Cultures of Marginalized Groups: Challenges of Inclusion in Higher Education. Paper presented at the International Conference on the Transformation of Masvingo State University to Great Zimbabwe National University, Great Zimbabwe Hotel.

Dzinamarira, T., Nachipo, B., Phiri, B., & Musuka, G. (2021). COVID-19 vaccine roll-out in South Africa and Zimbabwe: urgent need to address community preparedness, fears and hesitancy. Vaccines, 9(3), 250.

Fishman, J. (1972). *The sociology of language: An interdisciplinary social science approach to language in society*. Newbury House.

Frieden, T. R., Buissonnière, M., & McClelland, A. (2021). The world must prepare now for the next pandemic. *BMJ Global Health*, *6*(3), e005184. doi:10.1136/bmjgh-2021-005184 PMID:33727280

Iyamu, I., Apantaku, G., Yesufu, Z., Oladele, E. A., Eboreime, E., Afirima, B., ... Mpofu, M. (2022). Is social media, as a main source of information on COVID-19, associated with perceived effectiveness of face mask use? Findings from six sub-Saharan African countries. Global Health Promotion, 29(3), 86-96.

Kugarakuripi, J., & Ndoma, S. (2022). Lack of trust in government, reliance on social media may drive vaccine hesitancy in Zimbabwe. Findings from the most recent Afrobarometer survey in Zimbabwe

Larsson, L., Chikwari, C. D., Simms, V., Tembo, M., Mahomva, A., Mugurungi, O., ... Kranzer, K. (2023). Addressing sociodemographic disparities in COVID-19 vaccine uptake among youth in Zimbabwe. *BMJ Global Health*, *8*(7), e012268. doi:10.1136/bmjgh-2023-012268 PMID:37407229

Mackworth-Young, C. R., Chingono, R., Mavodza, C., McHugh, G., Tembo, M., Chikwari, C. D., ... Ferrand, R. A. (2021). Community perspectives on the COVID-19 response, Zimbabwe. Bulletin of the World Health Organization, 99(2), 85.

Marani, M., Katul, G. G., Pan, W. K., & Parolari, A. J. (2021). Intensity and frequency of extreme novel epidemics. *Proceedings of the National Academy of Sciences of the United States of America*, *118*(35), e2105482118. doi:10.1073/pnas.2105482118 PMID:34426498

Mashiri, P. (2002). Shona–English Code-Mixing in the Speech of Students at the University of Zimbabwe. *Southern African Linguistics and Applied Language Studies*, *20*(4), 245–262. doi:10.2989/16073610209486314

Mason, C., Lazenby, S., Stuhldreher, R., Kimball, M., & Bartlein, R. (2022). Lessons learned from implementing digital health tools to address COVID-19 in LMICs. Frontiers in Public Health, 10, 859941.

Mazzoleni, G. (2015). The International Encyclopedia of Political Communication. London: Wiley Blackwell.

McAbee, L., Tapera, O., & Kanyangarara, M. (2021). Factors associated with COVID-19 vaccine intentions in eastern Zimbabwe: A cross-sectional study. *Vaccines*, *9*(10), 1109. doi:10.3390/vaccines9101109 PMID:34696215

Mhute, I., Mangeya, H., & Jakaza, E. (2021). Endangering the endangered: Impact of fake covid-19 social media communications in Zimbabwe. *Pharos Journal of Theology*, *102*(2), 1–11. doi:10.46222/pharosjot.102.211

Murewanhema, G., Burukai, T. V., Chireka, B., & Kunonga, E. (2021). Implementing national COVID-19 vaccination programmes in sub-Saharan Africa-early lessons from Zimbabwe: A descriptive cross-sectional study. *The Pan African Medical Journal*, *40*(1). Advance online publication. doi:10.11604/pamj.2021.40.180.30824 PMID:35018213

Mutanga, M. B., Ureke, O., & Chani, T. (2021). Social media and the COVID-19: South African and Zimbabwean netizens? response to a pandemic. Indonesian Journal of Information Systems, 4(1), 1-14.

News, Z. B. C. (2021). Covid-19 Weekly Update [Video playlist]. YouTube. https://www.youtube.com/playlist?list=PL-R_K60Fu927gvzDlcNRtVoLKoKbG_J6N

Ngondo, P. S., & Klyueva, A. (2022). Toward an ubuntu-centered approach to health communication theory and practice. Review of Communication, 22(1), 25-41.

Osterholm, M. T. (2020). Preparing for the next pandemic. In *The Covid-19 Reader* (pp. 11–20). Routledge. doi:10.4324/9781003141402-2

Patton, M. Q. (2002). *Qualitative Research and Evaluation Methods*. Sage.

Rauchfleisch, A., Vogler, D., & Eisenegger, M. (2021). Public Sphere in crisis mode: How the COVID-19 pandemic influenced public discourse and user behaviour in the Swiss twitter-sphere. *Javnost (Ljubljana)*, *28*(2), 129–148. doi:10.1080/13183222.2021.1923622 PMID:34393592

Schäfer, M. S. (2015). Digital public sphere. The international encyclopedia of political communication, 15, 1-7.

Yule, G. (1996). *Pragmatics*. Oxford University Press.

Chapter 2
Psychological Well-Being and Language Learning During the COVID-19 Pandemic

Josephine Atieno Otiende
https://orcid.org/0009-0006-9478-0184
Daystar University, Kenya

ABSTRACT

The COVID-19 pandemic has reshaped the landscape of education worldwide, leading to a significant shift towards remote learning and virtual classrooms. Language learning, an essential component of education, has also undergone a drastic transformation during this period. This chapter proposes evidence-based interventions and strategies to enhance the psychological well-being of language learners and educators in similar crises in the future. It also looks at the psychological well-being of language learners and educators, with a specific focus on examining the challenges and opportunities that emerged during this unprecedented time. Additionally, it puts forth a set of evidence-based interventions and strategies aimed at fortifying the mental and emotional health of both language learners and educators. These proposed measures serve as a proactive blueprint to navigate similar crises that may arise in the future, ensuring a more resilient and adaptive educational ecosystem.

1. INTRODUCTION AND BACKGROUND

Exploring the impact of the COVID-19 pandemic on language and education can be an intriguing area for research, as it has brought unprecedented challenges and opportunities in these domains. The COVID-19 pandemic has disrupted traditional education systems globally, compelling a rapid shift to remote learning environments. The spread of this epidemic has had a significant impact on the education sector.

In a precautionary measure to safeguard public safety and health, the government mandated the closure of all schools and higher education institutions. Consequently, the traditional in-person teaching and learning activities were halted during the period of movement restrictions. To ensure the uninterrupted

DOI: 10.4018/979-8-3693-0624-6.ch002

continuity of education, educators swiftly transitioned to conducting classes through online platforms (Rosli & Bakar, 2021).

According to the World Health Organization (2023) the global impact of the COVID-19 pandemic on education has been profound, affecting over 150 countries and impacting the learning of 1.6 billion students worldwide. In response to this unprecedented challenge, numerous nations swiftly adopted various forms of remote learning as an emergency measure. While the aim was to ensure access for all students, the outcomes were not universally successful. With the progression of the pandemic, education strategies have adapted accordingly. Presently, in numerous regions, schools have partially or fully resumed in-person instruction.

The COVID-19 pandemic according to Rosli & Bakar(2021) necessitated the adoption of online learning platforms, posing novel challenges to language learners and educators. The abrupt transition from traditional face-to-face instruction to virtual classrooms has triggered various psychological issues for both students and teachers. Throughout the period of home-based teaching and learning, school educators and teachers, in particular, grappled with a multitude of pressures. These included adapting to online work, navigating diverse student frustrations, contending with the unpredictability of internet access, and managing their own personal life responsibilities.

Amid the COVID-19 pandemic, the adoption of online learning platforms, as highlighted by Rosli and Bakar (2021), brought forth a new set of challenges for language learners and educators alike. The sudden shift from conventional face-to-face instruction to virtual classrooms gave rise to various psychological concerns for both students and teachers. Throughout the period of home-based teaching and learning, educators, in particular, faced a multitude of pressures. These encompassed adapting to online work, addressing diverse student frustrations, contending with the unpredictability of internet access, and balancing these demands with their own personal life responsibilities. In addition to these challenges, educators had to grapple with the need for innovative and engaging teaching strategies that could effectively translate to the online environment. They had to rapidly acquire technical proficiency in using various digital tools and platforms, while also finding ways to maintain a sense of connection and community among their students. Furthermore, teachers had to navigate the emotional well-being of their students, recognizing the potential impact of the pandemic on their mental health and providing the necessary support and resources.

2. STATEMENT OF THE PROBLEM

Following the unprecedented upheaval of the COVID-19 pandemic, schools around the globe have largely resumed regular operations. However, the realm of education remains in a phase of recuperation, diligently evaluating the impact incurred and extracting invaluable insights from the experience. The pandemic's toll according to UNESCO (2020) was felt by over 1.5 billion students and young individuals, with those in the most precarious circumstances bearing the brunt of the crisis. Regrettably, strides previously taken towards achieving the objectives outlined in the 2030 Education Agenda have been regrettably reversed.

In the wake of the COVID-19 pandemic, the world witnessed a profound impact on mental health, with a spectrum of symptoms ranging from insomnia and anxiety to depression and frustration (Shigemura et al., 2020). This toll extended to the dedicated professionals at the frontlines, grappling with uncertainty about their safety and shouldering an unprecedented caseload. These challenges not only underscore the critical importance of psychological well-being but also shed light on its pivotal role in learning, motivation, and language acquisition. Recognizing the profound psychological implications of this global crisis in the realm of language education is paramount in devising effective strategies to support both learners and educators alike.

Behavioral, psychological, psychosocial, and mental health symptoms such as insomnia, anxiety, insomnia, depression, frustration, and hysteria were some of the effects of COVID-19 (Shigemura et al., 2020). Professionals also experience psychological suffering due to various factors. These included uncertainty about having a safe workplace, leading to heightened stress levels. This manifested in symptoms like irritability, insomnia, sadness, and demoralization. Additionally, the lack of adequate time for rest, coupled with exhaustion from dealing with a rising number of cases, further contributed to psychological distress (Guangming and Grupo Diretor Central, 2020; Theorell, 2012; Ryall, 2020). This therefore is an indication that psychological well-being significantly influences the learning process, motivation, and language acquisition. (Nesen & Bakar, 2021; Fancourt et al., 2020 Therefore, understanding the psychological implications of the pandemic in the context of language education is crucial for designing effective strategies to support learners and educators.

In the aftermath of the COVID-19 pandemic, the world witnessed a profound impact on mental health, with a wide spectrum of symptoms ranging from insomnia and anxiety to depression and frustration (Shigemura et al., 2020). This toll extended to the dedicated professionals at the frontlines, who grappled with uncertainty about their safety while bearing an unprecedented caseload. These challenges not only underscore the critical importance of psychological well-being but also shed light on its pivotal role in learning, motivation, and language acquisition. Recognizing the profound psychological implications of this global crisis in the realm of language education is paramount in devising effective strategies to support both learners and educators alike.

Furthermore, understanding the nuanced interplay between mental health and effective language education is crucial. Research has shown that psychological well-being not only impacts an individual's ability to learn and acquire language but also influences their motivation and engagement in the learning process (Nesen & Bakar, 2021; Fancourt et al., 2020). Therefore, prioritizing mental health support for learners and educators within the context of language education is not only a compassionate response to the challenges posed by the pandemic but also a strategic investment in the overall success and well-being of the education community.

3. PURPOSE OF THE CHAPTER

The purpose of the proposed chapter is to examine the intricate relationship between psychological well-being and language learning amidst the challenges posed by the COVID-19 pandemic. The chapter aims to investigate how the sudden shift to remote learning and virtual classrooms during the pandemic has affected the mental health and well-being of both language learners and educators. The chapter will review a variety of sources of secondary data including content analysis. This will involve the analysis of online content related to psychological well-being and language learning during the COVID-19 Pandemic. The chapter seeks to shed light on the psychological struggles faced by individuals in the language learning process and explore potential solutions to mitigate the negative impacts.

4. CHAPTER OBJECTIVES

The primary objectives of this chapter were as follows:

- To explore the psychological challenges faced by language learners during the COVID-19 pandemic.
- To investigate the coping mechanisms adopted by language learners to overcome the psychological impact of remote learning.
- To examine the experiences and psychological well-being of language educators while adapting to virtual teaching environments.

5. LITERATURE REVIEW

Psychological Challenges of Remote Learning

One of the primary concerns of the chapter is to identify the psychological challenges that language learners and educators encounter during the transition to remote learning. The sudden change in the learning environment, reduced social interaction, and the isolation caused by online education might have had adverse effects on mental health, affecting motivation, engagement, and overall well-being. (Segre et al., 2021).

Psychological well-being is a multidimensional construct, delineated from various perspectives (Hupert & So, 2013; Diener et al., 2010). Scholars generally concur that individuals experiencing psychological well-being are characterized by a positive emotional state. As posited by Sinha and Verma (1992), it encompasses the amalgamation of distinct facets, including confidence, self-control, a sense of significance, freedom from feelings of failure, anxiety, and loneliness.

Psychological well-being encompasses a life that is characterized by both a sense of contentment and effective functioning (Huppert, 2009). In essence, sustainable well-being doesn't necessitate a perpetual state of feeling good; experiencing challenging emotions like disappointment, failure, and grief is a natural part of the human experience. What truly matters for long-term well-being is the ability to navigate and manage these negative or painful emotions.

Remote learning refers to an educational setting where the storyteller or information source is not physically present in a conventional classroom. Instead, information is delivered through technology, allowing for two modes of engagement (Infoscipedia, 2023). Synchronous learning facilitates real-time peer-to-peer interaction and collaboration, while asynchronous learning involves self-paced activities conducted independently of the instructor. This versatile approach to education enables students to access and process information from various locations and at their own pace, adapting to individual learning styles and circumstances.

According to the COVID-19 pandemic presented numerous challenges for families worldwide. (Magson et al., 2020). In Hong Kong, according to Ye et al., (2023), the pandemic prolonged school closures required young students to adapt to remote learning for over a year, potentially impacting their mental well-being. A total of 700 primary school students in Hong Kong (with a mean age of 8.2) participated in an online survey where they reported on their emotional experiences, feelings of loneliness, and their perception of their academic self-concept (Ye et al., 2023). Additionally, 537 parents provided information on their own levels of depression and anxiety, their perception of their child's depression and anxiety, and their level of social support. Responses from both students and parents were analyzed within the context of the family unit.

The findings from the students' responses according to (Ye et al., 2023) revealed that positive emotional experiences were inversely associated with feelings of loneliness and positively linked to COVID-19. Furthermore, the results from the paired samples indicated that, during the year-long societal lockdown and remote learning period, socioemotional factors were correlated with the mental health conditions of both primary school students and their parents.

Coping Mechanisms and Resilience

The section is concerned with understanding the coping mechanisms adopted by language learners and educators to navigate the challenges of remote language learning. By examining these coping strategies, this chapter aims to identify factors that contribute to resilience and positive mental health during times of crisis.

In accordance with the findings of Gore, Bloem, Patton, Ferguson, and Joseph (2014), it is emphasized that amidst pandemics, certain students effectively navigate the demands of online education by assuming their responsibilities and actively seeking both social and academic assistance. Liang and Chen's (2012) parallel research reveals that a portion of students in their study resorted to detrimental coping mechanisms, including self-isolation, alcohol consumption, and drug use, as a means of dealing with the stress induced by the rigors of online teaching and learning. This underscores that students may resort to adverse coping strategies to grapple with the anxiety stemming from pandemics and the shift to online education.

During the COVID-19 pandemic, Dohaney et al. (2020) provide a systematic delineation of coping mechanisms and resilience exhibited by both individuals and institutions. Resilient individuals demonstrate characteristics such as flexibility, adaptability, collaborative skills, digital literacy, quick decision-making, and pedagogical proficiency. On the institutional level, factors contributing to resilience encompass effective communication strategies, strong leadership, well-defined emergency response plans, provision of support for faculty, fostering a sense of community, and motivation. These elements collectively contribute to the ability of individuals and institutions to effectively cope with and bounce back from the challenges posed by the pandemic.

A study by Raghunathan et al., (2022) involved a survey assessing the resilience levels of 102 teachers hailing from three distinct countries: India, Malaysia, and Fiji. It sought to examine how the Covid-19 pandemic influenced their capacity to persist in the teaching and learning process as well as measure their resilience levels. Coping mechanisms for stress in this model encompassed variables like institutional support, peer support, and student support. Teachers exerted substantial effort to enhance their proficiency in techniques for engaging learners in online education. This included mastering live session technologies, adept use of mobile devices, navigating Learning Management Systems (LMS), and becoming proficient in lecture recording. They also dedicated time to acquire video editing skills and underwent a shift in mindset to ensure the optimal support of their students. These findings hold significant relevance to internal resilience, as they represent the fundamental competencies that profoundly influenced teaching and learning in a remote online educational setting and were affirmed by Kimhi et al. (2020), Connor and Davidson (2003).

Experiences of Language Educators

Another concern of the chapter is to explore the experiences of language educators during the pandemic. As they adapted their teaching methods to online platforms, they might have faced unique challenges and opportunities related to student engagement, communication, and support, all of which could have implications for their own well-being.

The findings from both interviews and questionnaires in a study by Muliyah et al. (2022) underscored the formidable task faced by teachers in leveraging digital technology to extend education beyond the confines of school premises and into the homes and devices of Indonesian students. This necessitated a fundamental reevaluation of teaching approaches, prompting educators to devise fresh and innovative avenues for students to engage with curriculum mandates.

Engaging in online learning offered numerous advantages, including heightened flexibility and fostering a sense of connection and interaction between teachers and students, irrespective of their respective time zones and physical locations. (Hwang et al., 2021). In essence, online learning provides students with the opportunity to tailor their learning environment to suit their individual preferences and needs, promoting a personalized educational experience. In addition, it facilitates access to a diverse range of digital resources and materials, enriching the learning process with multimedia content and interactive tools.

Impact on Language Acquisition

Negative emotions like worry, fear, tension, and anger, especially, have the potential to impede a learner's optimal learning capacity and significantly hinder their language acquisition abilities (Ran et al., 2022). Conversely, positive emotions like self-esteem, empathy, motivation, and enjoyment can position learners in an optimal state for language learning, significantly smoothing the learning process. Second language learners endowed with higher emotional intelligence exhibit greater proficiency in impulse control, stress management, and maintaining a positive outlook in the face of challenges and frustrations. This therefore means that an altered learning environment influences language proficiency levels and that pandemic-induced stress and anxiety affects language acquisition and is supported by (ZOU et al., 2022).

Designing Interventions for Well-Being

Evidence-based interventions and strategies to promote psychological well-being in the context of language learning during crises is crucial. By identifying effective approaches, this chapter aims to provide guidance to educational institutions and policymakers to better support learners and educators in similar situations. When considering psychosocial interventions, García-Álvarez et al., (2021) assert that the strategies to be formulated may align more effectively with an approach that prioritizes health promotion and addresses risk factors for prevention, particularly in the primary prevention of psychopathology. This statement suggests that when designing psychosocial interventions, it is recommended to focus on strategies that promote overall mental and emotional well-being. This approach should also target factors that can lead to the prevention of mental health issues, especially in their early stages, before they develop into more serious psychopathological conditions. In essence, the emphasis is on proactively fostering mental health and addressing potential risk factors to prevent the onset of psychological disorders.

Teacher well-being is a multi-faceted concept encompassing physical, psychological, and spiritual health, along with factors related to occupational attachment, stability, commitment, and overall satisfaction (Granziera et al., 2021). The well-being of teachers, therefore, means considering various aspects of their health and job-related factors. It goes beyond just physical health and includes their mental and emotional well-being, as well as their sense of purpose and satisfaction in their work. Additionally, it takes into account their level of attachment to their profession, the stability they experience in their role, and their overall commitment to their job. All of these elements together contribute to the overall well-being of a teacher. This comprehensive understanding is crucial for addressing and promoting the health and satisfaction of learners and educators during pandemics.

Long-Term Implications and Future Preparedness

The long-term implications of the pandemic on language education and psychological well-being are important for several reasons: 1) Understanding the long-term effects allows educational institutions to adapt and implement strategies that ensure continued quality education. This includes developing effective online learning platforms and resources, which may continue to be relevant even after the pandemic. 2) Recognizing the lasting impact on psychological well-being highlights the need for sustained mental health resources and support for both students and educators. This can help mitigate the potential long-term effects of the pandemic-related stressors.3) Governments and educational authorities can develop policies and plans that take into account the enduring effects of the pandemic on education and mental health. This may involve budget allocations, infrastructure improvements, and curriculum adjustments.

The lessons learned from this experience can inform future preparedness for potential disruptions in education and what measures can be taken to ensure the well-being of students and educators in similar situations. This can hence contribute valuable insights to the fields of language education, providing a comprehensive understanding of the interplay between psychological well-being and language learning during the COVID-19 pandemic.

Lessons learned from this experience that can inform future preparedness for potential disruptions in education are affirmed by García-Álvarez et al.,(2021) whose intervention encompasses eight modules that guide participants through a formative exploration of positive psychology, facets of well-being, character strengths, positive education techniques, mental styles, resilience and optimism, as well as the integration of mindfulness with self-regulation. Additionally, it covers emotional management, empathy, and compassion which is part of Psychological Well-being that will enhance the psychological well-being of language learners and educators in similar crises in the future.

6. THEORETICAL FRAMEWORK

Social Cognitive Theory

This theory, proposed by Albert Bandura, emphasizes the importance of social interactions, observational learning, and self-regulation in the process of learning. In the context of language learning during the COVID-19 pandemic, social cognitive theory suggests that learners can observe and model language behaviors even in remote or online settings. Additionally, Bandura (2008) affirms that self-regulation skills, including setting goals, monitoring progress, and providing self-feedback are crucial for autonomous language learning.

In the context of language learning during the COVID-19 pandemic, the application of Social Cognitive Theory, proposed by Albert Bandura, is evident in several ways: 1) Observational Learning: Social Cognitive Theory emphasizes the role of observational learning, where individuals learn by observing the behaviors of others. In online learning environments, learners can still observe their teachers and peers through video lectures, discussions, and recorded sessions. They can model proper language usage, pronunciation, and communication strategies, even in virtual settings. 2) Modeling and Imitation: Even in remote learning settings, instructors can employ modeling techniques by providing clear and effective demonstrations of language usage. They can use videos, audio recordings, and interactive platforms to showcase proper pronunciation, sentence structure, and communication strategies, allowing learners to imitate and internalize these skills. 3) Social Interaction and Collaboration: Social Cognitive Theory underscores the importance of social interactions for learning. Through online forums, discussion boards, and virtual classrooms, learners can engage in collaborative activities, practice conversational skills, and receive feedback from peers and instructors. This facilitates a sense of social connectedness and provides opportunities for social learning.

7. METHOD

The research paper employed a secondary research methodology, also known as desk research, which involved reviewing a diverse range of existing data sources. This approach relied on well-established and previously vetted data. The collected data was meticulously tailored to align with the specific requirements of the researcher. As noted by Yin (2014), the choice of secondary research was motivated by the availability of reliable sources. This method utilized pre-existing data from reputable sources, enhancing the credibility and trustworthiness of the information gathered.

This chapter looked into the adjustments made by teachers and parents in response to virtual learning demands during the initial COVID-19 school closures in spring 2020 (Cohen et al., 2022). The investigation focused on scrutinizing families' day-to-day routines, encompassing parents' emotional states and their assessments of the significance of these routines at two distinct time intervals. A total of thirty-two parent-child pairs participated in this research (mean child age = 78 months, 50% male; 47% Latinx/Hispanic; 28% Spanish-speaking). These participants were drawn from a school district in Southern California, known for serving a diverse demographic. The research employed a daily diary texting protocol employing an experience sampling method (ESM), which involved participants providing responses five times per day over a span of five days (Cohen et al., 2022).

Throughout this period, families predominantly engaged in mealtime activities, involving both meal preparation and consumption, while spending time together. Notably, families hailing from lower socioeconomic backgrounds expressed higher appraisals for academic activities, social skills, and life skills when compared to their counterparts from higher socioeconomic backgrounds. Additionally, parents reported experiencing a greater frequency of positive emotions as opposed to negative emotions. These findings bear significant implications for educators, suggesting avenues to address potential learning setbacks by leveraging children's learning experiences and the adaptations made by families to their everyday routines during the COVID-19 pandemic.

In another study Rasmussen et al. (2022) of 2907 students invited, 637 (22%) responded with 288 of the respondents (45%) providing a response to at least one of the three open-ended questions. Three major themes associated with the impact of the pandemic on psychosocial well-being and learning were identified: psychosocial impact of the pandemic, adjustment to new modes of teaching and learning, and concerns about course progression and career. These themes were underpinned by lack of motivation to study, feeling isolated, and experiencing stress and anxiety that impacted on students' well-being and their ability to learn and study. Domains such as health, psychological well-being and effect of COVID 19 on learners were assessed. The study revealed four pivotal themes pertaining to the psychosocial repercussions of the pandemic: diminished motivation, the profound influence of isolation and the worldwide health crisis on students' mental well-being, the weight of concurrent responsibilities on students' capacity to concentrate and participate in educational endeavors, and an elevated level of resilience demonstrated by the students (inclusive of pertinent quotes supporting each theme) (Rasmussen et al.,2022).

In another study by (Villani et al., 2021) A cross-sectional survey was conducted in the immediate aftermath of the initial lockdown period. The survey was administered through 90 questionnaires on the personal websites of undergraduate students at the Università Cattolica del Sacro Cuore. To assess engagement, anxiety symptoms, and depression symptoms, the Patient-Health-Engagement-Scale, Self-Rating-Anxiety-Scale, and Self-Rating-Depression-Scale was utilised. The study comprised a sample of 501 individuals, among whom 35.33% exhibited symptoms of anxiety, while 72.93% displayed symptoms indicative of depression. Impressively, over 90% of respondents demonstrated a robust grasp of preventive measures, even though more than 70% grappled with the challenge of being unable to physically meet with friends and partners.

In another study by Watts & Pattnaik (2022) they documented the adverse effects of COVID-19 on the comprehensive development of children. This qualitative study delved into the viewpoints of teachers and parents concerning the repercussions of physical and social distancing measures, as well as school closures, on the socioemotional growth of children. The investigation took place during the autumn of 2020 and involved a diverse sample, including four U.S. preschool teachers (instructing 4-year-olds), four international preschool teachers (engaging with 4 and 5-year-olds), three U.S. kindergarten teachers (overseeing 5-year-olds), and four U.S. parents of 4 and 5-year-olds. Interviews were conducted via Zoom. Participants revealed that the social limitations experienced by children, including a dearth of friendships, the absence of peer-driven learning and communication, diminished playtime, and restricted social interactions, had a profound impact on their offspring's socialization skills, higher-order cognitive development, mental well-being, and overall activity levels. The study captured the experiences of learners and educators during the COVID-19 period. Other learners experienced social deprivation, loneliness and anxiety. Other changes in learner behavior, such as increased restlessness and a reduction in opportunities for social interaction and physical activity were witnessed. Still, a few others were cranky with emotions like fear, apprehension, sadness, feeling lost, and experiencing stress, being cautious, and struggling with emotional regulation. A handful had attention-seeking mannerisms. The teachers also mentioned that some learners were frightened, uneasy, despondent, disoriented, anxious, troubled, vigilant and struggling with emotional regulation. Some children became overly dependent on their parents during the pandemic. This excessive reliance on parents resulted in behaviors like neglecting proper hygiene, struggling with independence, sulking, requiring assistance with daily tasks, and displaying a lack of motivation. There were also delayed motor skills, feelings of anxiousness, along with a deficiency in the cultivation of vital abilities like resolving conflicts, problem-solving, and fostering creative thinking amongst learners.

Search terms and key themes included Psychological Well-being, Language, Learning, COVID, COVID-19, remote learning and virtual classrooms, language learners and educators.

Significance of This Chapter

This chapter aims to provide valuable insights into the psychological impact of the COVID-19 pandemic on language learners and educators. By understanding the challenges faced by these individuals during remote learning, the study will help educational institutions and policymakers design targeted interventions and support systems to promote psychological well-being in future crises. Additionally, the research findings contributed to the development of evidence-based guidelines for educators to enhance student engagement, motivation, and language acquisition in virtual classrooms.

Key Outcomes and Results

The study done by Rasmussen et al.,(2022) was based on the impact of covid-19 on psychosocial well-being and learning for Australian undergraduate students. The prevailing psychosocial consequence of COVID-19 most frequently reported by respondents was a notable decline in motivation towards their academic pursuits. Participants recollected experiencing a noticeable lack of drive, subsequently influencing their ability to focus and actively participate in teaching and learning endeavors. From this study, it was concluded that;

1) The prevailing psychosocial consequence of COVID-19 most frequently reported by respondents was a notable decline in motivation towards their academic pursuits. Participants recollected experiencing a noticeable lack of drive, subsequently influencing their ability to focus and actively participate in teaching and learning endeavors.
2) Participants conveyed grappling with a range of emotional challenges, including anxiety, depression, and stress, stemming from various sources. These sources encompassed feelings of isolation and apprehension about their academic progress, financial stability, the psychosocial strain on their families during clinical placements, and additional worries like travel restrictions linked to the global pandemic. Moreover, a prevalent sentiment of helplessness emerged, notably in terms of feeling cut off from familial and support networks throughout the lockdown phase.
3) Students grappled with a multitude of competing factors that significantly impacted their capacity to concentrate and actively participate in the learning process. These encompassed apprehensions about work, potential unemployment, and family matters, as well as financial constraints. Additionally, the responsibilities associated with remote schooling, including home-based learning, posed a substantial challenge. Furthermore, concerns regarding the risk of contracting COVID-19 further compounded these difficulties.
4) A notable positive outcome emerged from the study: participants attested that enrolling in undergraduate studies amidst the pandemic resulted in a marked boost in their resilience. They discovered an inherent fortitude while navigating their individual circumstances, university protocols, and government directives within a dynamic and swiftly evolving environment.

The study done by Watts & Pattnaik (2022) was on the perspective of educators on the influence of the COVID-19 pandemic on learners' socio-emotional health. All participants acknowledged socio-emotional difficulties in their children following the pandemic. The participants' responses highlighted psychological challenges including feelings of "loneliness due to a lack of friendships," "absence of peer learning and communication," "reduced playtime," and "limited opportunities for socialization with peers especially when language development failed to occur through interaction with other fellow learners.

8. FINDINGS

From the Rasmussen et al.,(2022) study, participants acknowledged a transitional phase characterized by the adoption of novel modes of teaching and learning, a response to the imperative of physical distancing measures and social constraints. This adjustment period yielded four discernible themes: the implementation of adaptable teaching methods and fresh strategies; enhanced study methodologies; a reduction in in-person classes; and an evaluation of the effectiveness of teaching approaches and techniques that aid psychological well-being.

From the Rasmussen et al.,(2022) study, The prevailing psychosocial impact of COVID-19, most frequently cited by respondents, was a notable decrease in motivation towards their academic pursuits. Participants recounted experiencing a distinct lack of drive, consequently influencing their ability to concentrate and actively engage in teaching and learning activities. Secondly, Participants disclosed grappling with a spectrum of emotional challenges, encompassing anxiety, depression, and stress arising from feelings of isolation and concerns about their studies, financial stability, and the psychosocial strain on their families during clinical placements. Additionally, other apprehensions, including those related to travel restrictions in the global pandemic context, were prevalent. A prevailing sentiment of helplessness emerged, particularly in terms of feeling estranged from familial and support networks during the lockdown period. Thirdly isolation because of geographical distance brought about by the effects of the pandemic brought about mental and psychological instability to the learners.

From the Watts & Pattnaik (2022) study, there was absence of social connections, limited peer-based learning and communication, diminished play opportunities and restricted socialization with peers, leading to social deprivation among learners. There was also lack of creative thinking skills and problem solving skills amongst students and learners.

The above findings from the three studies are supported by Mahmud et al., (2021)who affirm that schools play a critical role in restoring children's socio-emotional health. Although learners have experienced severe academic learning loss during the pandemic, the post-pandemic curriculum must keep a strong socio-emotional and practical life skills focus. Teachers and educators need to implement child-focused play and instructional activities even while maintaining proper hygiene and social distancing practices. Educators also need to maximize outdoor activities as well as art, movement, and music activities by skillfully integrating these activities into their curriculum. The findings of the present study and studies by other researchers suggest a need for training teachers and parents to restore children's psychological well-being of language learners and educators in similar crises in the future.

9. CONCLUSION

This chapter aims to shed light on the psychological challenges and opportunities faced by language learners and educators during the COVID-19 pandemic. By examining the impact of the pandemic on their well-being and learning experiences, this chapter contributed to the development of effective strategies to support language education in times of crisis. Ultimately, it is hoped that this research will aid in creating resilient and adaptable language learning environments that can thrive amidst future uncertainties.

This study enriched existing feedback literature by unveiling three adaptive strategies for enhanced teachers and learners to optimize their psychological well-being and language learning post the COVID-19 Pandemic and this was affirmed by Rasmussen et al.,(2022).

In essence in all studies enlisted, participants recognized a phase of adaptation to novel modes of teaching and learning, implemented in response to mandates for physical distancing and social limitations. This adjustment period yielded four distinct themes: the adoption of adaptable teaching methods and innovative strategies; enhancements in study methodologies; a reduction in in-person classes; and an evaluation of the effectiveness of teaching strategies.

Firstly, by engaging in internal dialogues with learning materials, generating inquiries, and actively seeking answers from various sources (e.g., online courses, websites), participants can serve as their own instruments to garner valuable feedback on their learning. Secondly, the deliberate establishment of a virtual space through online platforms or communication tools (e.g., email) enabled participants to promptly receive feedback from diverse sources and revisit it at their own convenience. Lastly, maintaining a resilient mindset and exploring alternative avenues for obtaining feedback that align with their needs and expectations proved vital, particularly in cases of dissatisfaction with existing online feedback practices. These strategies exemplified their adeptness in critical thinking and autonomy in seeking feedback, illustrating their commitment to overseeing their professional development as self-regulated learners as affirmed by (Zimmerman, 2005).

Based on the findings of this research, the following recommendations are proposed to enhance the psychological well-being of language learners and educators in similar crises in the future:

- Enhance psychosocial support and incorporate inventive teaching approaches, including adaptable delivery modes and interactive online methods.
- Implement supplementary measures to bolster student motivation and participation in their educational endeavors, such as specialized counseling services and opportunities for social networking.
- Ensure transparent and timely communication of risk management protocols during clinical placements to alleviate stress and anxiety among students.

Schools play a critical role in restoring children's socio-emotional health. Although children have experienced severe academic learning loss during the pandemic, the post-pandemic curriculum and virtual lessons must keep a strong socio-emotional and practical life skills focus. (Davis et al., 2022). Preschool teachers need to implement child-focused play and instructional activities even while maintaining proper hygiene and social distancing practices. Teachers need to maximize outdoor activities as well as art, movement, and music activities by skillfully integrating these activities into their curriculum. The findings of the present study and studies by other researchers suggest a need for training educators, teachers, and instructors to restore learners' and students psychological well-being.

REFERENCES

Bandura, A. (2008). *Social Cognitive Theory of Mass Communication*. Routledge.

Cohen, S., Guerra, A. W., & Miguel, J. (2022). Erratum to "social class and emotional well-being: Lessons from a daily diary study of families engaged in virtual elementary school during COVID-19.". *AERA Open*, *8*. doi:10.1177/23328584221095854

Connor, K. M., & Davidson, J. R. T. (2003). Development of a new resilience scale: The connor-davidson resilience scale (CD-RISC). *Depression and Anxiety*, *18*(2), 76–82. doi:10.1002/da.10113 PMID:12964174

Davis, C. R., Baker, C. N., Osborn, J., & Overstreet, S. (2022). Understanding teacher self-efficacy to address students' social-emotional needs in the COVID-19 pandemic. *Urban Education, 004208592210998*. Advance online publication. doi:10.1177/00420859221099834

Dohaney, J., de Róiste, M., Salmon, R. A., & Sutherland, K. (2020). Benefits, barriers, and incentives for improved resilience to disruption in university teaching. *International Journal of Disaster Risk Reduction*, *50*, 101691. doi:10.1016/j.ijdrr.2020.101691 PMID:32509512

García-Álvarez, D., Soler, M. J., & Achard-Braga, L. (2021). Psychological well-being in teachers during and post-covid-19: Positive Psychology Interventions. *Frontiers in Psychology*, *12*, 769363. Advance online publication. doi:10.3389/fpsyg.2021.769363 PMID:34975659

Gore, F., Bloem, P. J. N., Patton, G. C., Ferguson, J., & Joseph, V. (2014). *Global burden of disease in young people aged 10–24 years: a systematic analysis*. Routledge.

Granziera, H., Collie, R., & Martin, A. (2020). Understanding teacher wellbeing through job demands-resources theory. *Cultivating Teacher Resilience*, 229–244. doi:10.1007/978-981-15-5963-1_14

Guangming, P. (2020). Mais de 3.000 Equipes Médicas em Hubei Foram Infectadas no Estágio Inicial da Epidemia, Atualmente não há Relatos de Infecção Entre as Equipes de Assistência Médica. https://politics.gmw.cn/2020-03/06/content_33626862.htm

Huppert, F. A. (2009). Psychological well-being: Evidence regarding its causes and consequences. *Applied Psychology. Health and Well-Being*, *1*(2), 137–164. doi:10.1111/j.1758-0854.2009.01008.x

Hwang, G.-J., Wang, S.-Y., & Lai, C.-L. (2021). Effects of a Social Regulation-based online learning framework on students' learning achievements and behaviors in mathematics. *Computers &amp. Computers & Education*, *160*, 104031. doi:10.1016/j.compedu.2020.104031

Infoscipedia. (2023). *What is remote learning*. IGI Global. https://www.igi-global.com/dictionary/character-development/97112

Kimhi, S., Marciano, H., Eshel, Y., & Adini, B. (2020). Recovery from the COVID-19 pandemic: Distress and resilience. *International Journal of Disaster Risk Reduction*, *50*, 101843. doi:10.1016/j.ijdrr.2020.101843 PMID:32953439

Liang, R.Y.H., Chen, D.T. (2012). Online learning: Trends, potential and challenges. Academic Press.

Magson, N. R., Freeman, J. Y., Rapee, R. M., Richardson, C. E., Oar, E. L., & Fardouly, J. (2020). Risk and protective factors for prospective changes in adolescent mental health during the COVID-19 pandemic. *Journal of Youth and Adolescence*, *50*(1), 44–57. doi:10.1007/s10964-020-01332-9 PMID:33108542

Mahmud, S., Mohsin, Md., & Dewan, Md. N., & Muyeed, A. (2021). *The Global Prevalence of Depression, Anxiety, Stress and Insomnia among General Population during COVID-19 Pandemic: A Systematic Review and Meta-Analysis*. doi:10.21203/rs.3.rs-1136589/v1

Muliyah, P., Aminatun, D., & Septiyana, L. (2022). Teaching in pandemic: Teachers' experiences during coronavirus outbreak. *Journal of Research on Language Education*, *3*(1), 1. doi:10.33365/jorle.v3i1.1894

Nesen, J. N., & Bakar, A. Y. A. (2021). Coping strategies for parents with special need children during COVID-19 lockdown in Malaysia. *Journal of Management Information and Decision Science*, *24*(SI1), 1–9.

Raghunathan, S., Darshan Singh, A., & Sharma, B. (2022). Study of resilience in learning environments during the COVID-19 pandemic. *Frontiers in Education*, *6*, 677625. Advance online publication. doi:10.3389/feduc.2021.677625

Rasmussen, B., Hutchinson, A., Lowe, G., Wynter, K., Redley, B., Holton, S., Manias, E., Phillips, N., McDonall, J., McTier, L., & Kerr, D. (2022). The impact of covid-19 on psychosocial well-being and learning for australian nursing and midwifery undergraduate students: A cross-sectional survey. *Nurse Education in Practice*, *58*, 103275. doi:10.1016/j.nepr.2021.103275 PMID:34922092

Rosli, A. M., & Bakar, A. Y. (2021). The Mental Health State and psychological well-being of school teachers during COVID-19 pandemic in Malaysia. *Bisma The Journal of Counseling*, *5*(3), 182–195. doi:10.23887/bisma.v5i3.42015

Segre, G., Campi, R., Scarpellini, F., Clavenna, A., Zanetti, M., Cartabia, M., & Bonati, M. (2021). Interviewing children: The impact of the covid-19 quarantine on children's perceived psychological distress and changes in routine. *BMC Pediatrics*, *21*(1), 231. Advance online publication. doi:10.1186/s12887-021-02704-1 PMID:33985448

Shigemura, J., Ursano, R. J., Morganstein, J. C., Kurosawa, M., & Benedek, D. M. (2020). Public responses to the novel 2019 coronavirus (2019-ncov) in Japan: Mental health consequences and target populations. *Psychiatry and Clinical Neurosciences*, *74*(4), 281–282. doi:10.1111/pcn.12988 PMID:32034840

Unicef, OECD, & UNESCO. (2020, January 1). *Education: From school closure to Recovery*. UNESCO.org. https://www.unesco.org/en/covid-19/education-response

Villani, L., Pastorino, R., Molinari, E., Anelli, F., Ricciardi, W., Graffigna, G., & Boccia, S. (2021). Impact of the COVID-19 pandemic on psychological well-being of students in an Italian university: A web-based cross-sectional survey. *Globalization and Health*, *17*(1), 1–14. doi:10.1186/s12992-021-00680-w PMID:33823897

Watts, R., & Pattnaik, J. (2022). Perspectives of parents and teachers on the impact of the COVID-19 pandemic on children's socio-emotional well-being. *Early Childhood Education Journal*. Advance online publication. doi:10.1007/s10643-022-01405-3 PMID:36285153

World Bank Group. (2023, March 30). *Remote learning during COVID-19: Lessons from Today, principles for Tomorrow*. World Bank. https://www.worldbank.org/en/topic/edutech/brief/how-countries-are-using-edtech-to-support-remote-learning-during-the-covid-19-pandemic

Ye, F. T.-F., Gao, X., Sin, K.-F., & Yang, L. (2023). Remote learning and mental health during the societal lockdown: A study of primary school students and parents in times of covid-19. *BMC Public Health, 23*(1), 1106. Advance online publication. doi:10.1186/s12889-023-16040-9 PMID:37286984

Yin, R. K. (2014). *Case study research: Design and methods*. Sage Publication.

Zimmerman, B. J. (2005). Attaining self-regulation: A sociocognitive perspective. In M. Boekaerts, P. R. Pintrich, & M. Zeidner (Eds.), *Handbook of self-regulation* (pp. 13–39). Elsevier Inc.

Zou, R., Zeb, S., Nisar, F., Yasmin, F., Poulova, P., & Haider, S. A.ZOU. (2022). The impact of emotional intelligence on career decision-making difficulties and generalized self-efficacy among university students in China. *Psychology Research and Behavior Management, 15*, 865–874. doi:10.2147/PRBM.S358742 PMID:35422664

KEY TERMS AND DEFINITIONS

Coping Mechanisms: Refer to the various psychological, behavioral, and emotional strategies that individuals employ to manage and adapt to stress, adversity, or challenging situations.

COVID-19: Short for "Coronavirus Disease 2019," is an infectious respiratory illness caused by the novel coronavirus SARS-CoV-2. It was first identified in December 2019 in the city of Wuhan, Hubei province, China, and it quickly spread globally, leading to a pandemic.

Educator: Is a person who is professionally trained and skilled in providing instruction, guidance, and support to learners in various educational settings. Educators can work in formal institutions such as schools, colleges, and universities, or in informal settings like community centers, museums, or online platforms. Their primary goal is to facilitate learning and development in individuals, helping them acquire knowledge, skills, and values that contribute to their personal and intellectual growth. Educators may include teachers, professors, trainers, tutors, mentors, and other professionals dedicated to fostering education and nurturing the potential of their students.

Language Learning: Refers to the process of acquiring the ability to communicate in a new or foreign language. This can involve developing skills in speaking, listening, reading, and writing, as well as understanding the cultural context in which the language is used. Language learning can occur through various methods, including formal instruction in classrooms, self-study with books or language learning apps, immersion in a native-speaking environment, or a combination of these approaches. It is a complex cognitive and social endeavor that requires practice, exposure, and often, a certain degree of cultural adaptation.

Learner: A learner is an individual who is engaged in the process of acquiring knowledge, skills, or competencies through study, experience, or instruction. Learners can be of any age and come from various educational backgrounds. The term encompasses students in formal educational settings like schools and universities, as well as individuals engaging in self-directed or informal learning.

Psychological Well-Being: Refers to a person's overall mental and emotional state characterized by a sense of contentment, fulfillment, and a positive outlook on life. It encompasses a person's ability to effectively cope with the challenges and stresses of daily life, build and maintain positive relationships, and experience a sense of purpose and meaning. Psychological well-being is not merely the absence of mental health disorders, but rather a state of positive mental health.

Remote Learning: Refers to a form of education where students and instructors are geographically separated and interact primarily through digital platforms and technologies. It allows for the continuation of educational activities even when physical attendance at a traditional classroom setting is not possible or practical, such as during situations like the COVID-19 pandemic. Remote learning encompasses a wide range of methods including online classes, video conferencing, virtual lectures, digital assignments, and collaborative online platforms.

Resilience: Refers to the ability of an individual or a system to bounce back, adapt, and recover effectively from challenges, setbacks, or adversities. It involves the capacity to withstand and navigate through difficult circumstances, maintain mental and emotional well-being, and continue functioning or even thrive despite facing adversity. Resilience encompasses qualities like mental fortitude, emotional strength, adaptability, and a proactive approach to problem-solving.

Well-Being: Refers to a state of overall health, happiness, and prosperity in various aspects of an individual's life. It encompasses physical, mental, emotional, and social dimensions.

Chapter 3
Effectiveness of COVID-19 Risk Communication Messages in Indigenous Languages and the Promotion of Safe Practices in Ondo State, Nigeria

Babatunde Adeyeye
https://orcid.org/0000-0002-9485-2444
North-West University, South Africa

Abiodun Salawu
https://orcid.org/0000-0002-1687-4621
North-West University, South Africa

ABSTRACT

This chapter examined the effectiveness of COVID-19 risk communication messages in indigenous languages vis-à-vis the promotion of safe practices in Ondo, Nigeria. The survey research design was used, and a questionnaire was randomly administered to 384 respondents in Akure, Ondo State. Findings showed that most of the respondents were exposed to COVID-19 risk communication messages and got their first information about it from social media. Furthermore, the study found that respondents were not receptive to COVID-19 messages passed across in indigenous languages. They prefer COVID-19 messages to pass across in the English language. The study recommended that there is a need to ensure that risk communication messages aired in indigenous languages are demystified in a way that the audience can easily understand and act upon. The use of indigenous languages should continue to be used and encouraged, especially for risk communication interventions such as COVID-19. This will go a long way in ensuring that the audience accepts it.

DOI: 10.4018/979-8-3693-0624-6.ch003

INTRODUCTION

Since Corona Virus Disease (COVID-19) was discovered in December 2019, substantial attention has been devoted to countering the wave of conspiracy theories, myths, and misinformation that are peddled about the disease (Depoux et al., 2020; Naffi, Davidson & Jawhar, 2020; Lucas, Targema, Jibril, Sambo, & Istifanus, 2020). Misinformation or lack of credible information during pandemics may affect the decision of the populace on what to do regarding daily socio-economic activities, as can be seen during the recent COVID-19 pandemic. Credible and adequate information during a pandemic is a situation where messages are shared with stakeholders including the citizens in a transparent and accountable manner, that is, everyone must understand what is going on. The reason for this is to cover the communication gap between the sender of the information and the receiver of the information so it does not generate mistrust among them. This will reduce the risk that may be attracted by the pandemic (Heras, Jambrino, Rando, & Iglesias, 2022). However, there is a need for everyone to be alert and aware of the information and disinformation they are subject to. For instance, amid the COVID-19 pandemic, there was a lot of disinformation and misinformation that brought fear and emotional disturbance to society (Heras, Rando, Jambrino & Paniagua, 2020).

Outbreaks of diseases generally impact the socio-economic life of people across the globe as evident with the COVID-19 pandemic. Credible and reliable information in this period is vital in reducing the pandemic by encouraging individuals to keep safe. To educate the public as much as possible about the pandemic, transmission routes, risk factors, preventive measures, and treatment options, risk communication interventions are a key part of the emergency response to Covid 19 in Nigeria. These interventions are carried out through a variety of communication channels, including electronic media, interpersonal communication channels, and print media. Therefore, the risk communication messages in indigenous languages emphasize the promotion of personal and community hygiene, keeping a safe distance of one meter from others, carrying sanitiser, frequently washing hands with water and soap, and avoiding close contact with anyone who is ill or exhibiting symptoms. These warnings also stress the importance of taking the following precautions: if you feel sick, stay at home and quarantine yourself; if you have any concerning symptoms, please seek medical attention; avoid using public transportation while you're sick; and if you're at a higher risk of contracting a serious illness, it's best to stay inside.

The traditional Yoruba town of Akure has existed in Nigeria for a very long time, well before the arrival of British colonial power there. Up until the 19th century, when it became a part of the Benin Kingdom, Akure was a sovereign state. In 1894, the territory was brought under the rule of Great Britain. Ondo State, in the South-Western region of Nigeria, is where the city is situated. The current, moderately sized urban centre was established as the provincial capital of Ondo province in 1939 and as the state capital and seat of local government in 1976. The city is roughly located 50°15' east of the Greenwich Meridian and 70°15' north of the equator. The distance between Lagos, Nigeria's commercial centre, and Akure is around 350 kilometres while the distance to the Federal Capital Territory is around 700 kilometres.

The effectiveness of risk communication interventions for COVID-19 19 especially in Ondo State is worth investigating. Ideally, it is expected that all receivers of the risk communication messages in indigenous languages must be able and capable of understanding and decoding the meaning of the messages sent to them and the message should be able to persuade the receivers to change their attitudes or their behaviours regarding specific cause/s or threats associated with an event. However, since risk communication interventions are targeted at the public in distress situations, particularly outbreak scenarios, there has been a growing interest in the effect of tension on public understanding and interpretation of risk communication messages in indigenous languages to make informed decisions (Ilesanmi, et al., 2023; Adebisi, Rabe & Lucero-Prisno, 2021; Winograd et al.,2021, Tambo, et al.,2021). The study is guided by the following objectives: to find out the level of exposure the audience has towards COVID-19 messages in indigenous languages; ascertain the level of audience receptiveness towards COVID-19 messages in indigenous languages; and identify the outcome of COVID-19 risk communication messages which were passed across indigenous languages in Ondo State.

THE PLACE OF THE MEDIA IN RISK COMMUNICATION

Since health issues are varied and take many different forms depending on a person's physiological makeup and lifestyle, public health is one of those fields where people lack adequate understanding. In the area of risk communication for health, the media is crucial to risk communication interventions. According to WHO (2017), news outlets are frequently the first and even the only places to learn about dangers. The public can obtain fundamental facts and information through the media, which can also be used to explain rumours and false information and, when necessary, guarantee that the public is aware of infection prevention techniques and what to do if they or someone they know becomes ill (WHO, 2017). Because of their ability to quickly reach a large and diverse audience, the mass media have remained a reliable method of distributing information about health risks. Additionally, they have the power to change how people perceive risk and behave to lessen societal harm.

Health risk communication is essentially the broadcast of information that educates the public on the underlying causes of illnesses, purported hazards, the level of attention it warrants, and the necessary precautions to be taken (Gesser-Edelsburg & Shir-Raz, 2016). Aiming to enhance knowledge and awareness of health risks as well as to encourage attitudinal change to alter behaviour, health risk communicators generally seek to deliver the appropriate information. The media is used in public health to encourage the dissemination of fundamental information about various diseases, the modification of health-related beliefs and values, and the adoption of new healthy behaviours (Catalán-Matamoros, 2011). As a result, Ugande (2008) writes that the mass media are very potent tools in the hands of awareness creators as they play an influencing role in contributing to public opinion formation.

To warn readers about potential health dangers and persuade them to take preventative actions that lower the risk, disease outbreak messages are often written (Manno, Lively, Manno, Cheng & Lau, 2018). Through daily newscasts, PSAs, talk programmes, editorials, features, comments, and other media that distribute health risk information, the health risk messages seek to alter public perception and behaviour (Manno, *et al.,* 2018). The impression of a health danger and subsequent behaviour have both been found to be affected, either directly or indirectly, by the mass media (Kott & Limaye, 2016). At the individual level, messages may have an impact on how decisions are made (Wakefield, Loken, & Hornik, 2010). When messages are exposed to individuals and the media sets the conversational topic for health issues, behaviour change is induced. Additionally, even if a person is not directly exposed to the message, behaviour modifications that become social standards may have an impact on their decisions (Wakefield, *et al.,* 2010).

Therefore, the media actively collaborates with health officials to simultaneously acquaint broad masses with the necessary information. Given that face-to-face health communication tactics take longer, involve a lot of human resources, and can only reach a small number of people, the mass media thus help to increase the audience reach. By giving specific problems a certain amount of publicity, the mass media sets the agenda for public conversation and influences how the public feels about certain issues. It should come as no surprise that Uwom and Oloyede (2014) claim that the media is one of the most important sources of health-related information and can influence how we think about and debate health. Given that educated conversation and contribution are byproducts of accurate information, the media gives the audience enough knowledge to think about as their thoughts spark their discourse on health issues.

The fact that persuading the public to adopt behaviours and communicating this to them is essential to disease containment makes infectious disease outbreaks inherently newsworthy (Fung & Caircross, 2006). During a disease outbreak, the mass media act as the main channels via which public health organizations communicate information to the general population (Kott & Limaye, 2016). Additionally, academics believe that the media is the main source of information.

AN OVERVIEW OF LANGUAGE USE IN ONDO STATE

Although numerous dialects are spoken by the state's hinter communities, Yoruba is the most widely spoken native language among Ondo state's population. These dialects are also related to standard Yoruba since they share genetic roots with Yoruba. according to the Ondo state's linguistic status as determined by its speakers' cumulative usage. Although it is now considered a standard language, it is still mostly a regional and local language in most places (Ben-Enukora, 2020; Ayeomoni, 2011).

In Nigeria, the Yoruba language is one of the three official main languages. In addition to two other West African nations, the Republic of Benin and Togo, it is spoken in the southwest of Nigeria. In Nigeria alone, there are about 15 million native speakers of the language, and an additional 5 million speak it in addition to their mother tongue. Speaks in Oyo, Lagos, Ondo, Osun, Ekiti, Ogun, certain portions of Kwara state, and a tiny piece of Edo state, the language is spoken in southwest and south-central Nigeria. It is a tonal language, just like other native languages, with three surface tones: high, mid, and low (Ayeomoni, 2011)

Nigeria's sociolinguistic diversity has made language planning and policy exceedingly complicated (Brann 1995). Nigeria only has a few clear language regulations that are targeted at the educational sector, in contrast to some multilingual countries that have formal policies for the language used throughout different public institutions. Thus, in addition to English, which is the state's official language, Yoruba, which is spoken in Ondo state, is the second language. Brann (1995) goes on to highlight the lack of language policy papers in Nigerian institutions, while in certain trilingual and bilingual countries, indigenous languages are used for a variety of public services, including security, health care, and transportation (Obukadeta, 2019).

One noteworthy aspect is that although most Nigerian language plans seek to recognise the country's linguistic variety as evidenced in the multiplicity of dialects spoken in Ondo state, none is as extensive and complete as the educational policy. Furthermore, the majority of the language sections found in the various policy documents seem ambiguous and frequently ignore Nigeria's intricate sociolinguistic environment.

EMPIRICAL REVIEW

Obiorah (2021) started a conversation about the function of Nigerian indigenous languages in COVID-19. He used digital media for data collection and used Salawu's approach to developing communication in native languages. His research's findings demonstrated that medical research, health education, and media briefings on national television all employ indigenous languages from Nigeria to propagate COVID-19 prevention strategies. Ude-Akpeh and Onyima (2020) studied how the usage of native language and authority figures affected the way COVID-19 messages were transmitted to rural residents in South-East Nigeria. The study affirms that rural residents in the Southeast zone can better understand and follow COVID-19 pandemic communications and preventative actions if authority figures and native languages are used.

Fadipe and Salawu (2021) explored the use of African Indigenous language media to improve people's use of coronavirus health messages. COVID-19 digital sources, health message kinds, and other related topics. They discovered that respondents were receiving preventive COVID-19 health messages on social exclusion and personal hygiene from a majority of interactive digital sources, with little or no African Indigenous language media incorporated into the health message. Nevertheless, it is important to combat the dissemination of false information through digital platforms.

Abubakari, Assem and Amankwah (2021) analyzed how the Kusaal-speaking populations in Ghana's Upper East Region are educated on the COVID-19 safety measures using indigenous language and song. Findings demonstrate that the music conveys promise and hope in the ability of ancestor deities to travel back in time at times of tragedy to ease their followers' pain.

Fadipe and Salawu (2022) examined how Yoruba native music artists promoted health issues related to the COVID-19 outbreak in Nigeria and the implications on the welfare of their fans. The musicians pushed for strict adherence to personal hygiene and compliance with government health regulations during the COVID-19 pandemic. They argued that Yoruba music creators must use cultural allusions that can capture the social realities of their audience to make more compelling arguments about the origins, impacts, and remedies to health issues like the COVID-19 pandemic.

Amenaghawon and Salawu (2022) focused on the promotion of local Afro-hip-hop music in Nigeria to a wider audience in the fight against COVID-19 infodemics. To inform, mobilize, and create an agenda for society in the reduction of COVID-19, they call for the use of indigenous music, particularly Afro-hip-hop, in the dissemination of true and verified information.

All the efforts of the researchers of the studies are highly commendable. A cursory look at the studies reveals that issues relating to the application of indigenous languages to risk communication messages related to COVID-19 were de-emphasized especially as it relates to safe practices. Furthermore, no study has been done to assess the effectiveness of COVID-19 risk communication messages in indigenous languages and the promotion of safe practices in Ondo State, Nigeria. This research gap is the bottom line of a study of this nature to improve on the above shortcomings.

THEORETICAL FRAMEWORK

Model of Indigenous Language for Development Communication

The Salawu model of indigenous language for development communication has been chosen as the model for this study. Salawu introduced this concept in 2015, and it states that information should be obtained and given in indigenous languages. Salawu (2015) asserts that the data should be obtained in L1 and provided to the speaker in L1. Below is a presentation of the language's developmental communication structure.

The Source is a change agent in the concept, and it might be a development agency, a nongovernmental organization, a government agency, or a media organization. The Message is primarily focused on development and is written in the indigenous language of the community for which the development program is intended. The language is owned by the receiver(s). They can express themselves better in this language and understand the development messages better, allowing for more robust interaction between them and the Source.

The illustration above depicts the assumption that the media will gather information in indigenous languages and communicate the message to the audience (language owners) in the same indigenous language. Television, radio, the internet, or social media could all be used as a channel.

Questions and answers, as well as instructions and orientations for indigenous peoples, must all be given in the indigenous language, according to this paradigm. In other words, information should not be obtained in Yoruba and then be conveyed in a language such as English or Chinese. This paradigm has the advantage of establishing a link between media and language users.

The motive for using this theory is to emphasize the need for communicators to include indigenous languages at the very beginning of the communication process. This would make sure that the original meaning of the message is not lost in interpretation

Figure 1. Model of indigenous language for development communication (Salawu, 2001 cited in Salawu 2015)

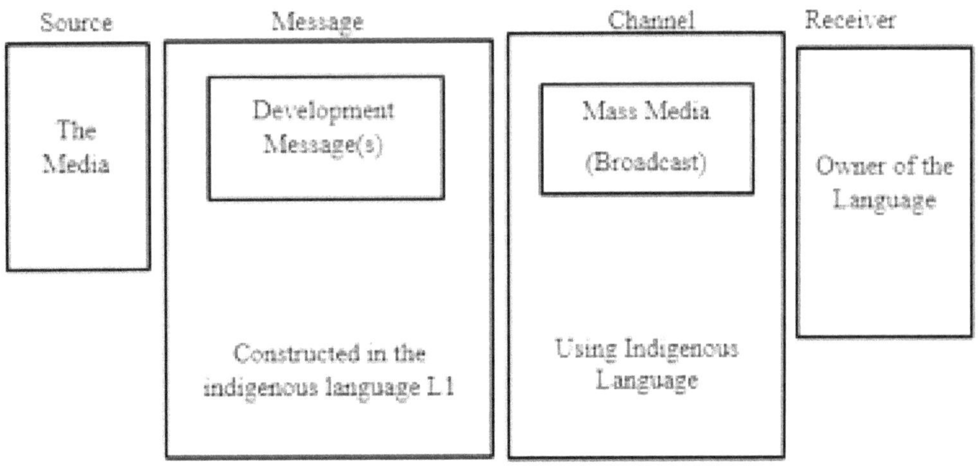

THEORY OF PLANNED BEHAVIOUR

The likelihood that a person will engage in a health behaviour (in this example, COVID-19 preventative measures) is correlated with the degree of that person's intention to engage in the behaviour, according to the Theory of Planned Behaviour (TPB). A behavioural intention demonstrates a person's resolve to act and is the outcome of the interaction of many different factors. According to the TPB, a person's attitudes about the behaviour, sense of subjective group norms on the behaviour, and degree of self-perceived control over the behaviour are all elements that directly affect intentions to engage in health behaviour (Fishbein, 2002).

As a behavioural model, the TPB is frequently employed. It helps us understand how people's behaviour might alter. The paradigm predicts intentional behaviour since it suggests that activity is preplanned (Ajzen, 1991). The Theory of Reasoned Action is a similar model that gave rise to the TPB (Ajzen & Fishbein, 1975). The realization that behaviour is not always voluntary and under our control led to the TPB's renaming. As a result, the theory was renamed to reflect the addition of perceived behavioural control to the model.

Any choice a person makes is influenced by three different types of factors, according to the Theory of Planned Behavior: behavioural beliefs (beliefs about the likely outcomes of the practised behaviour), normative beliefs (beliefs about other people's normative expectations), and control beliefs (beliefs about one's normative expectations) (beliefs about the presence of factors that may enable or obstruct the performance of the behaviour). Behavioural beliefs, control beliefs, and normative beliefs, which are impacted by perceived social pressure or subjective norms, can have a positive or negative impact on attitudes toward a certain behaviour. The subjective norm, perceived control, and good behaviour increase with a person's drive to complete the task at hand.

The theory of planned behaviour becomes a relevant frame because it adheres to instructions during the COVID-19 context, on a variety of health behaviours such as physical distance, mask-wearing, hand washing, travel intentions, and intentions to get a COVID-19 vaccination. Because limiting social connections is classified as an avoidant and unnatural activity that is more difficult to conduct, it is predicted that intentions, attitudes, social norms, and perceived control for hand washing will be higher.

METHODOLOGY

The quantitative method of research was applied in gathering data from the sample. A survey was used to obtain information from the sample. The survey is a quantitative research method used to collect data from a pre-determined group of respondents to gain data and substance about a subject matter. According to the UN World Urbanisation Prospects (2023), the city has 475,286 residents.

This sample size was ascertained from a total population of 475, 286 using the Krejcie and Morgan (1970) sample size determination table, which was calculated using this formula:

Where:
n= Sample Size
X2 =- Chi-Square for the specified confidence level at 1 degree of freedom
N = Population Size
P = Population proportion (.50 in this table)

ME = desired Margin of Error (expressed as a proportion)

Additionally, Krejcie and Morgan (1970) recommended the use of the next highest value if the researcher's exact population size is not listed in the table. The value in the next column is the sample size that is required to generate a margin of error of ± 5% for any population proportion. Consequently, the study employed for this study 5% margin of error within the 95% confidence level.

Simple random sampling and systematic sampling were employed during the selection process from the cluster areas. The survey respondents were randomly selected from district areas comprising fifteen clusters within Akure the state capital namely: Aponmu, Gbogi, Isikan, Ijomu, Obanla, Lisa, Oda, Odopetu, Aro, Uro, Oke-Aro, Oshodi, Owode, Isolo, Imuagun

These zones were further stratified into urban, semi-urban and rural categories based on the outlook of the environment. Because the number of households cannot be ascertained within the districts, every 8th building in each row of a street was randomly selected for the study. Therefore, 2 buildings each were randomly selected in a street. Only one eligible respondent (adult female or male, aged 18 and above) in a building will be eligible to participate in the study. In the absence of an eligible individual on the day of the visit, a repeat visit is made to the same building. This was done till all the questionnaire was exhausted.

Data obtained from this study will be analysed by Statistical Package for Social Sciences (SPSS). Also, a simple percentage would be used for the calculation and interpretation of data. This will facilitate easy understanding when reading the interpreted results. The content validity of the questionnaire was ensured in this study by dividing the variables into specific themes that respondents could easily relate to.

The reliability of the research route was established by using the pre-test reliability method and Cronbach alpha. The Cronbach's alpha was used for the overall value of all items, and it resulted in .838

RESULTS

It analyzed the data in order of the research questions of the study. The demographic data was first analyzed before proceeding to analyse the research questions while the findings were discussed with previous studies from other authors. However, out of the 400 questionnaires distributed, 378 were properly filled, retrieved, coded and subjected to analysis.

Demographic Data

A majority (52.4%) were male while 47.6% were female. Age distribution showed that 13.7% were between the ages of 16-20 years, and 41.7% were between the ages of 21-30 years. 29.6% were between 31-40 years while 15% were above 41 years. This means that most of the participants were between the ages of 21-20 years.

Source of Knowledge of COVID-19 Messages

Details of the data where respondents first got information concerning COVID-19 and their first source of information. It was discovered that the majority (40.7%) of the respondents first got information about COVID-19 from social media, this was followed by 31.7% of participants who first got information concerning COVID-19 on television. However, 19.3% of respondents first got their information concerning COVID-19 from Word of Mouth. Few respondents 8.4% of the participants first got information concerning COVID-19 on the radio. Hence, it can be said that most of the participants got their first information about COVID-19 from social media.

Audience Exposure to COVID-19 Messages Passed Across Indigenous Languages

Findings show that the majority of the respondents (51.8%) disagree that they have heard about risk communication messages in their indigenous languages and fully understand the messages. In contrast, 48.2% affirm that they understand these messages as compared to the English language. This is an indication that even though the respondents may have been exposed to risk communication messages in their indigenous languages, they did not understand the messages as against those aired in the English language. The implication of these results may be due to the familiarity of the respondents with the English language. Also, it may be due to poor understanding of their indigenous language, compared to their understanding of the English language.

Audience Receptiveness Towards COVID-19 Messages Passed Across Indigenous Languages

Based on audience receptiveness towards COVID-19 messages passed across indigenous languages, it was revealed that most of the participants (53.7%) were not willing to share information about COVID-19 in their native dialect. On the other hand, 24% were willing to share the information while 22.3% were undecided. Also, 55.5% of participants which represent the majority did not believe that COVID-19 should be passed across indigenous languages, 25.1% think otherwise while 19.4% were indifferent. These results imply that audiences are not receptive to COVID-19 messages passed across in indigenous languages. They prefer COVID-19 messages to pass across in the English language.

The Outcome of COVID-19 Messages That Were Passed in Indigenous Languages

Based on the outcome of COVID-19 messages passed in the indigenous language, it was revealed that the majority (49.8%) of the participants did not obey the COVID-19 messages in the indigenous language about social distancing. Also, few (17.2%) agree that they will obey the COVID-19 messages in indigenous languages related to the washing of hands frequently. Likewise, 18% which represents a few of the participants believe that they will obey COVID-19 messages in indigenous languages related to vaccination. The results also showed that 45% did not obey COVID-19 messages in indigenous languages related to sneezing into their inner elbow. Also, 46.8% of the participants did not obey the COVID-19 messages in indigenous languages related to wearing a face mask. 43.1% disagree with compliance with COVID-19 messages in indigenous related to using hand sanitiser. Finally, 40.2% of the respondents disagreed on their compliance with COVID-19 messages in indigenous languages related to travel restrictions. This result implies that the participants were not willing to obey indigenous messages related to COVID-19. The result is not surprising because the majority of the participants already indicated that they preferred messages in English to the indigenous language, this may be their reason for non-compliance.

To be sure of the outcome of the study, the mean value was used to gauge the response of the participants. The average response should be 3.00 but the grand mean (2.52) is well below 3.00 which indicates that participants did not obey COVID-19 messages in indigenous languages.

DISCUSSIONS

The focus of this study was to assess the audience's knowledge of COVID-19 risk communication messages in indigenous languages in Ondo State with the objectives of finding out the level of exposure the audience has towards COVID-19 messages in indigenous languages, ascertaining the level of receptiveness the audience has towards COVID-19 messages in indigenous languages and identifying the outcome of COVID-19 risk communication messages which were passed across in indigenous languages in Ondo State. Findings from the study revealed that most of the respondents got their first information about COVID-19 from social media which is still their current source of information.

Audience Exposure to COVID-19 Messages Passed Across Indigenous Languages

The findings showed that most of the participants had not heard of COVID-19 messages in their dialect while 97 participants disagreed and stated that they fully understood COVID-19 messages in their language better than those in the English language. This finding entails that they are not exposed to COVID-19 messages passed across indigenous languages and the few that are exposed may not have a full understanding of the messages being passed across to them. The implication of these results may be due to the familiarity of the respondents with the English language and possibly because the majority of the respondents were first-degree holders who must have understood the English language to a great extent because English is the major language that is used in delivering lecturers in higher institutions. The findings of Ajepe and Ademowo (2016) correlate with this study by affirming the fact that the English language has dominated the national space and it has become difficult for most of the Nigerian population to participate in national development. This may be the reason why most of the participants were not interested in the COVID-19 message passed in the indigenous language.

Therefore Ene (2007) submitted that education through the indigenous languages in Nigeria will stimulate learners for productivity more than the foreign language and make learning more functional. Also, it may be due to poor understanding of their indigenous language, compared to their understanding of the English language. This gives reference to Salawu's 2001 model of indigenous language for development communication which proposed that information should be gathered and delivered in indigenous language which would ensure the originality of the message. It also depicts the assumption that the media will gather information in indigenous languages and communicate the message to the audience (language owners) in the same indigenous language. Television, radio, the internet, or social media could all be used as a channel. Questions and answers, as well as instructions and orientations for indigenous peoples, must all be given in the indigenous language, according to this paradigm. In other words, information should not be obtained in Yoruba and then be conveyed in a language such as English or Chinese. This paradigm has the advantage of establishing a link between media and language users.

Audience Receptiveness Towards COVID-19 Messages Passed Across Indigenous Languages

It was shown that most of the participant (137) were not willing to share information about COVID-19 in their native dialect. The majority (119) did not believe that COVID-19 should be passed across indigenous languages. These results imply that audiences were not receptive to COVID-19 messages passed across in indigenous languages. They preferred COVID-19 messages to be passed across in the English language. The result is not surprising because English is Nigeria's official language and probably the participants were not well conversant with their indigenous language.

The findings are in sync with Olaoye (2013) who discovered that there are significant difficulties in making the best use of indigenous languages, and the reason for this is because of the variety of minority languages and linguistic desertification. The results of the current study have proved that there is a need for the government to start using indigenous languages to communicate with the citizens and do everything within its power to make them interested in speaking and hearing indigenous languages. Eze (2006) thinks that this action would reduce illiteracy and make them contribute to the betterment of society which includes adhering to COVID-19 messages. Hostility toward COVID-19 in indigenous languages can also be due to attitude problems. Obinyan (2010) attributed attitude problems to when individuals consider speaking and studying English, the language of elites to be more respectable and acceptable than their indigenous language.

This finding can be related to the theory of planned behaviour which examines adherence to instruction during the COVID-19 context. It justifies the fact that the audience already knows what type of message they would adhere to and those they would ignore, in this case, the audience's mind is programmed to be receptive to messages in English.

The Outcome of COVID-19 Messages That Were Passed in Indigenous Languages

Most of the participants were not willing to obey messages passed across to them in the indigenous language. They were not willing to obey social distancing, frequent hand washing, vaccination, sneezing into the inner elbow, wearing of face mask, use of hand sanitiser and travel restrictions if the information is passed to them in their indigenous language. Overall, their mean score was 2.52 which is below 3.00. Hence it was concluded that the respondents were not willing to obey COVID-19 messages passed across in indigenous languages. The results contradict the findings of Obiorah (2021) who concluded that Nigerian indigenous languages could be very significant in passing across COVID-19 information. The theory of planned behaviour backs up the fact that validates the fact that the audience already knows which messages they will pay attention to and which they will disregard; in this situation, the audience's mind is pre-programmed to respond to communications in English and disregard those in indigenous languages.

CONCLUSION AND RECOMMENDATIONS

In this course of study, and from analysis of the data gathered from the research, it can be concluded that the audience is more receptive and compliant to COVID-19 messages passed across in English compared to those passed across in indigenous languages. The study concludes that a good number of respondents do not have exposure to COVID-19 risk communication messages in indigenous languages via conventional media but social media and the few that are exposed do not have a full understanding of the messages being passed across to them.

Based on the findings of the study and the conclusions reached, the following recommendations are made:

i. There is a need to ensure that risk communication messages aired in indigenous languages are demystified in a way that the audience can easily understand and act upon.
ii. The use of indigenous languages should continue to be used and encouraged, especially for risk communication interventions such as COVID-19. This will go a long way in ensuring that the audience accepts it. Furthermore, it should be extended beyond mainstream media to social media.
iii. The audience is also encouraged to accept the use of indigenous languages in the airing of risk communication messages to promote and preserve the cultural heritage of the people.

REFERENCES

Abubakari, H., Assem, I. S., & Amankwah, A. S. (2021). Framing of COVID-19 safety protocols in Kusaal musical health communication: Language and literary analysis. *Language & Communication*, *81*, 64–80. doi:10.1016/j.langcom.2021.09.002 PMID:36540773

Adebisi, Y. A., Rabe, A., & Lucero-Prisno, D. E. III. (2021). Risk communication and community engagement strategies for COVID-19 in 13 African countries. *Health Promotion Perspectives*, *11*(2), 137–147. doi:10.34172/hpp.2021.18 PMID:34195037

Adzer, V. C. (2012). Factors militating against the development of indigenous languages: The TIV language in perspective. *Journal Of Igbo Language & Linguistics*, *5*, 76–79.

Ajepe, I., & Ademowo, A. J. (2016). English language dominance and the fate of indigenous languages in Nigeria. *International Journal of History and Cultural Studies*, *2*(4), 10–17.

Ajzen, I. (1991). The theory of planned behaviour. *Organizational Behavior and Human Decision Processes*, *50*(2), 179–211. doi:10.1016/0749-5978(91)90020-T

Ajzen, I. (2002). Perceived behavioural control, self-efficacy, locus of control and the Theory of Planned Behaviours. *Journal of Applied Social Psychology*, *32*(4), 665–683. doi:10.1111/j.1559-1816.2002.tb00236.x

Amenaghawon, F., & Salawu, A. (2022). Mainstreaming Afro-hip-hop Music in Redressing the Spread of Infodemics on COVID-19. In Indigenous African Popular Music, Volume 2: Social Crusades and the Future (pp. 239-255). Cham: Springer International Publishing. doi:10.1007/978-3-030-98705-3_14

Ayeomoni, O. M. (2012). A Lexico-syntactic Comparative Analysis of Ondo and Ikale Dialects of the Yoruba Language. *Theory and Practice in Language Studies*, *2*(9). Advance online publication. doi:10.4304/tpls.2.9.1802-1810

Ben-Enukora, C., Oyero, O., Okorie, N., Oyesomi, K., & Adeyeye, B. (2020). Effectiveness of Yoruba language radio jingles in promoting knowledge, attitude and practices regarding Lassa fever among women in Ondo state, Nigeria. *Journal of Public Health in Africa, 11*(2). Advance online publication. doi:10.4081/jphia.2020.1323 PMID:33680412

Catalán-Matamoros, D. (2011). The role of mass media communication in public health. *Health management-Different approaches and solutions*, 399-414.

de Las Heras-Pedrosa, C., Jambrino-Maldonado, C., Rando-Cueto, D., & Iglesias-Sánchez, P. P. (2022). COVID-19 study on scientific articles in health communication: A science mapping analysis in web of science. *International Journal of Environmental Research and Public Health, 19*(3), 1705. doi:10.3390/ijerph19031705 PMID:35162726

de Las Heras-Pedrosa, C., Rando-Cueto, D., Jambrino-Maldonado, C., & Paniagua-Rojano, F. J. (2020). Exploring the social media on the communication professionals in public health. Spanish official medical colleges case study. *International Journal of Environmental Research and Public Health, 17*(13), 4859. doi:10.3390/ijerph17134859 PMID:32640598

Depoux, A., Martin, S., Karafillakis, E., Preet, R., Wilder-Smith, A., & Larson, H. (2020). The pandemic of social media panic travels faster than the COVID-19 outbreak. *Journal of Travel Medicine, 27*(3), taaa031. doi:10.1093/jtm/taaa031 PMID:32125413

Emeka-Nwobia, N. U. (2015). The place of indigenous Nigerian languages in National development. *Research on Humanities and Social Sciences, 5*(12), 112–116.

Eze, O. J., Ajah, B. O., Nwonovo, O. S., & Atama, C. S. (2022). Health sector corruption and COVID-19 outbreak: Evidence from Anambra and Enugu States, Nigeria. *Journal of Contemporary African Studies, 40*(1), 34–46. doi:10.1080/02589001.2021.1921129

Fadipe, I. A., & Salawu, A. (2021). Influence of African Indigenous language media in COVID-19 digital health messaging. *Catalan Journal of Communication & Cultural Studies, 13*(2), 267–284. doi:10.1386/cjcs_00053_1

Fadipe, I. A., & Salawu, A. (2022). 'Coronavirus, you are a Stranger,'Examining Yoruba Indigenous Music in the Quest to Tackle COVID-19 Pandemic. *Journal of African Films and Diaspora Studies, 5*(1), 75–99. doi:10.31920/2516-2713/2022/5n1a4

Fishbein, M., & Ajzen, I. (1975). *Belief, attitude, intention, and behaviour: An introduction to theory and research.* Addison-Wesley.

Fung, I. C. H., & Cairncross, S. (2006). Effectiveness of handwashing in preventing SARS: A review. *Tropical Medicine & International Health, 11*(11), 1749–1758. doi:10.1111/j.1365-3156.2006.01734.x PMID:17054756

Ilesanmi, O. S., Akosile, P. O., Afolabi, A. A., & Ukwenya, V. O. (2023). Handling distrust on risk communication in Nigeria: A strategy to strengthening the COVID-19 outbreak response. *Disaster Medicine and Public Health Preparedness, 17*, e27. PMID:34308825

Kott, A., & Limaye, R. J. (2016). Delivering risk information in a dynamic information environment: framing authoritative voice in centres of disease control (CDC) and Prime time broadcast news 211

Lucas, J. M., Targema, T. S., Jibril, A., Sambo, E. O., & Istifanus, B. A. (2020). Combating COVID-19 infodemic in Nigerian rural communities: The imperatives of Traditional Communication Systems. *ASEAN Journal of Community Engagement*, *4*(2), 360–385. doi:10.7454/ajce.v4i2.1102

Manno, F. A. M. III, Lively, M. B., Manno, S. H. C., Cheng, S. H., & Lau, C. (2018). Health risk communication message comprehension is influenced by image inclusion. *Journal of Visual Communication in Medicine*, *41*(4), 157–165. doi:10.1080/17453054.2018.1480321 PMID:29987960

Naffi, N., Davidson, A., & Jawhar, H. (2023). (5). ways to help stop the "infodemic," the increasing misinformation about coronavirus. *Retrieved*, (August), 21.

Obiorah, K. E. (2021). The role of Nigerian indigenous languages in COVID-19 discourse. *Journal of Language and Health*, *2*(2), 43–52. doi:10.37287/jlh.v2i2.514

Obukadeta, F. M. (2019). *Language Policy and Planning in the Broadcast Media of a Multilingual Context: A Case Study of Kogi State, Nigeria* (Doctoral dissertation, University of Sheffield).

Olaoye, A. A. (2013). The role of indigenous languages in national development: A case study of Nigerian linguistic situation. *International Journal of Applied Linguistics and English Literature*, *2*(3), 29–34. doi:10.7575/aiac.ijalel.v.2n.3p.29

Prezi, G. O. (2022). Language Attitudes of the Igbo: A Threat to the Igbo Language. *Styles of Communication, 14*(1).

Salawu, A. (2015). A political economy of sub-Saharan African language press: The case of Nigeria and South Africa. *Review of African Political Economy*, *42*(144), 299–313. doi:10.1080/03056244.2014.988695

Salawu, A. (2022). Toward a Model of Indigenous Language for Development Communication. *Indigenous Language for Development Communication in the Global South*, 13.

Tambo, E., Djuikoue, I. C., Tazemda, G. K., Fotsing, M. F., & Zhou, X. N. (2021). Early-stage risk communication and community engagement (RCCE) strategies and measures against the coronavirus disease 2019 (COVID-19) pandemic crisis. *Global Health Journal (Amsterdam, Netherlands)*, *5*(1), 44–50. doi:10.1016/j.glohj.2021.02.009 PMID:33850632

Thompson, R. G., Nutor, J. J., & Johnson, J. K. (2021). Communicating awareness about COVID-19 through songs: An example from Ghana. *Frontiers in Public Health*, *8*, 607830. doi:10.3389/fpubh.2020.607830 PMID:33537281

Ude-Akpeh, C. E., & Onyima, T. (2020). Influence of Indigenous Language and authority figures in broadcast of COVID-19 Pandemic messages among rural dwellers in south East Nigeria. *Nnamdi Azikiwe University Journal of Communication and Media Studies, 1*(2).

Ugande, G. B. (2008). An evaluation of radio Benue's role in HIV/AIDS awareness creation in Vandiekya Local Government Area of Benue State. *The Nigerian Journal of Communication*, *6*, 122–140.

Uwom, O. O., Ajaegbu, C., Oloyede, D. B., & Sowemimo-Coker, S. (2014). Prospects of Internet technology in news production: A study of Voice of Nigeria and Nigeria television authority. *Global Journal of Arts Humanities and Social Sciences*, *2*(1), 56–66.

Wakefield, M. A., Loken, B., & Hornik, R. C. (2010). Use of mass media campaigns to change health behaviour. *Lancet*, *376*(9748), 1261–1271. doi:10.1016/S0140-6736(10)60809-4 PMID:20933263

Winograd, D. M., Fresquez, C. L., Egli, M., Peterson, E. K., Lombardi, A. R., Megale, A., Tineo, Y. A. C., Verile, M. G., Phillips, A. L., Breland, J. Y., Santos, S., & McAndrew, L. M. (2021). Rapid review of virus risk communication interventions: Directions for COVID-19. *Patient Education and Counseling*, *104*(8), 1834–1859. doi:10.1016/j.pec.2021.01.024 PMID:33583651

World Health Organization. (2017). Communicating risk in public health emergencies. A WHO guideline for emergency risk communication (ERC) policy and practice. Retrieved from https://apps.who.int/iris/bitstream/handle/10665/259807/9789241550208-eng.pdf?sequence=2

Chapter 4
Kiswahili Video Messaging on COVID-19 Awareness in Kenya:
The Peaks and Valleys

Wendo Nabea
Laikipia University, Kenya

ABSTRACT

The first cases of Covid-19 in the world can be traced to 2019. However, in Kenya and a number of other East African countries, the first cases of the disease were documented in March 2020. As the day went on, the spread of the virus gained momentum causing panic in the country. Awareness messaging on Covid-19 led by the government and supported by health agencies became regular on the Kenyan media, especially on the radio, television, and mainstream newspapers. Messaging was mainly done in English, Kiswahili, and mother tongue with the earlier enjoying a skewed advantage. A portion of this messaging was done via video, composed locally and internationally. The objective of the study was to examine the strategies employed in this video communication to create awareness of Covid-19. The results demonstrate that in a substantial number of cases, the dissemination was hampered by wanting grammar, English to Kiswahili translational flaws, and unsuitable animatronics. The chapter contends that the Kiswahili video messaging mainly failed the test of communicative value.

In 2019, the world experienced the first cases of Covid-19. These were reported in Asian countries, followed by countries in Europe. The scourge was dreaded for the fact that it was said to be deadly while its spread was rapid, yet it did not have a cure. The disease was reported in African countries in early 2020, and for Kenya, the first case was confirmed on March 13, 2020. The pronouncement was received with ambivalence since many people did not have much information about the disease. Weeks later, there was a lockdown in the country whereby all public facilities such as schools, churches, mosques, sporting, wedding and burials involving many people were banned. There was also closure of entertainment places and eateries, while a dusk to dawn curfew was imposed in the country to check the robust nightlife especially in towns. The government also came up with protocols to observe as a measure to prevent further infections from the pandemic. Amid all this, the Kenyan government alongside other

DOI: 10.4018/979-8-3693-0624-6.ch004

agencies started releasing information on the pandemic especially on how to keep it a bay. This effort was in line with what many other governments were doing the world over (Ji and Liu 2022, Maarek 2022, Steinbuka 2022). In Kenya, various methods were used to carry out the dissemination. These included radio and television programmes and adverts, Covid-19 awareness posters, word of mouth and social media messaging.

However, it is Kenya's Ministry of Health daily to regular media briefings that became notable and memorable sites for Covid-19 updates in the country. The briefings were mainly done by the Health Minister, the Director General in the Ministry and the Cabinet Assistant Secretary of Health. The briefings entailed bringing the public update on the status of coronavirus in the country before the glare of television and radio channels, in a language of choice by the officials. This is because Kenya is a multilingual country and therefore there were videos in English, Kiswahili and mother tongue. English and Kiswahili are the official languages, while Kiswahili is the national language. This paper concentrated on Kiswahili video instruction on Covid-19 in three phases: Information on it, preventive measures and the treatment of those who had contracted the virus. Language alone cannot be used adequately in transmission of important information and it for this reason that other necessary devices are called into play as reinforcement (Martin 2014). Among these are semiotic configurations which are packaged in a variety of ways. However, semiotic signs ought to be used tactfully to remain in sync with the type of audience that semiology targets are.

Data was collected from Kiswahili video messaging on Covid-19. From a total of 29 videos, 8 videos were selected for analysis since they were in line with objectives of the study. The video messaging data was transcribed and coded in view of three themes of Covid-19 awareness campaign. These were; preventive measures, vaccination and management of the sick. Data was coded as follows: CAVPI would stand for Covid-19 Awareness Video on Prevention Number 1, while AVCT1 denotes Awareness Video on Covid-19 Testing Number 1, while CAVV2 represent Covid-19 Awareness Video on Vaccine Number 2. The data used in the paper was not edited for the purpose of language analysis in its natural manner.

AWARENESS ON PREVENTION OF COVID-19

Awareness of Covid-19 prevention was done using audio-visual materials. In CAVP1 there is a Kiswahili dissemination which is delivered in a form of drama. A well-known Kenyan medical doctor who was common in the media as a regular campaigner against the spread of the coronavirus is holding a dialogue with children who are seated outside a house. In the excerpt below, D stands for Doctor while C stands for Child as follows:

D: *Sasa? Mjanua Corona ni nini?* Do you know what Corona is?

C1: *Mtu asichukue kitu ambacho kimekuwa kwa mdomo wa mtu mwingine.* Let nobody eat anything that has been another person's mouth

C2: *Usisalimiane kwa mguu.* Do not 'greet' people by the leg (laughter from Doctor as Child 3 refuses leg contact from him)

D: *Ni nini nyingine unajua kuhusu Corona*? What else do you know about Corona?

C3: *Usikule uchafu.* Do not ingest dirt.

D: *Ehe .. usikule uchafu? Nini nyingine?* Ehe, don't ingest dirt, what else do you know?

C2: *Ukishika mchanga, usinyonye mkono.* If you touch the soil, don't suck the hand [finger]

D: *Ukishika mchanga, usiyonye mkono, si ndiyo? Hii ugonjwa ndiyo iko kwa watu. Inaweza kukushika kwa kuambukizana … unaweza kuambukizwa na mtu mwingine, na kama mtu anataka kukushake mkono unafanya nini?* If you touch the soil, don't suck the hand, isn't it? This is the disease that has affected people. You can contract it … you can contract it from another person, and if a person wants to shake your hand what do you do?

C2: *Ninamwambia hapana.* I tell him/her no.

D *Unamwambia hapana. Unamsalimia hivi [igizo]. Ama unampatia mguu ee hivyo …* You tell him/her no. You greet him/her like this [a demo] or you give him/her the leg, ee that way …

The Covid-19 awareness appearing on CAVP1 is based on a conversation which is rendered in Kiswahili. Some words are nevertheless grammatically incorrect, but this does not distort the message at hand. There is also use of Sheng in the verb *kukushake*, to shake your hand. Sheng is a popular argot in Kenya deriving from Swahili and English, and based on Kiswahili and Bantu languages morphosyntactic structure (Ogechi 2005; Nabea 2009). The choice of Kiswahili in this awareness video is important considering the children paint a humble background, a matter that may also suggest that they may not be very comfortable to use English, which they might have just started learning in school. However, in many households especially in urban centres, Kiswahili could be the first language for the children, hence the ease with which to use it.

There are English translation chyrons on the lower side of the video. The foregoing begs the question as to who the audience should be for such English translation. In view of the Kenyan audience, it follows that a large number of people who understand English also understand Kiswahili, but the same cannot be said about users of Kiswahili, the national language. In this case, the choice to translate Kiswahili conversation into English is dumbfounding since it does not have a lot of import to the audience. However, if English was translated into Kiswahili, one would be sure of a higher viewership. The scenario suggests that the crafters of the Covid-19 awareness videos in Kenya might not have been very clear regarding the linguistic landscape in the country, and therefore their objective of translating Kiswahili conversation to English, was somewhat warped. Translation has a variety of benefits chief among them to transfer source language to target language so that those who do not understand source language can understand through the translated version (Mwansoko 2006).

In the video, the doctor starts by asking children whether they know the coronavirus to which they respond in the affirmative. The interrogative in CAVP 1 is simulates a teacher – student relationship whereby the teacher is asking pupils questions, to which they respond. There is humour when C2 states that another preventive measure of Covid-19 is to shun kicking legs as a form of greeting. One of the children indeed refuses to accept the doctor's kick for fear of infection. The child's fears and response are crucial in that they show the extent to which the children's knowledge on preventive measures of coronavirus is concerned. However, the doctor comes in handy to correct the misconception that leg contacts can spread Covid-19. The introduction of leg contacts as a form of greeting is however interesting. Worldwide greetings can be done in a variety of ways such handshaking, verbal salutations, gestures, touching on the head and other kinetic signs. However, leg kicking as a greeting issues from Covid-19 preventive measures, and therefore an important addition to the greetings repertoire.

In a like vein, the choice to use a video which could easily be transmitted on any audio-visual media including the television and social media is welcome because the audio message is reinforced by the visual portion. Nonetheless, there is a concern regarding the choice of the video. It is acknowledged that there are over 63 million mobile connections in Kenya (Communication Authority of Kenya 2023), from which they can access such video messaging on their social media platforms, besides the radio and television. However, ownership of mobile phones is one thing, and having bundles to access the social media content is another. In addition, there are Kenyans who own mobile phones for the purpose of communication – either to make or receive calls and nothing more. In view of the foregoing, it is apparent that the messaging on CAVP1 fell short of its objective in a sense in view of the fact that the choice of the video to send message in the final analysis served only a fraction of Kenyans. However, if the same messaging was relayed on television or radio stations which have a wider audience, its reach would have been remarkable. This points out to the fact that while there was composition of sound messages to create awareness on Covid-19 in Kenya, the choice of the platform for the purpose was not well thought of.

Further Covid-19 preventive measures awareness appears on CAVP2. In this video, there is an Asian medical doctor who introduces himself in English before inviting an African woman by the name of Debra to present the message. In the extract, Dr stands for Doctor while Deb stands for Debra.

Dr: Hi. My name is Dr. Michael Do, a pediatrician with Valleywise Health. Today I'm here to share an important message with you about Covid-19 also known as the coronavirus infection. To tell you more about that, we have Debra.

DEB: *Covid ya kumi na taisa inayojulikana kama koronavirusi ni ugonjwa ya kupumua ambayo umewaathiri watu katika nchi mia na sabini na nane duniani kote na sasa ni katika kila hali nchini kote Marekani, Virisi hivi ni wazo la kuenea kwa mtu hadi mtu aliyeambukizwa kikohozi au kutoa chafya. Inaweza kuwa ya kuambukiza sana na kwa sasa hakuna chanzo ya kuzia. Bado sasa tunajifunza kuhusu jinsi maambukizo haya yalikuwa na nguvu...*

Covid-19 which is known as coronavirus is a viral disease that has affected many people in one hundred seventy eight countries in the world and now everywhere in America. The viruses are an idea of spreading from one person to a person who is suffering from coughing or sneezing. It can be of spreading very fast and as of now there is no vaccine. Right now we are learning how the disease became very strong ...

In CAVP2, there is an instance of turn taking in presentation whereby the doctor spells out that he is out to share some crucial information on Covid-19. He does the introduction before distributing his chance to Debra who delivers the message in Kiswahili. The choice of the doctor is important for the information being disseminated is given credence. Doctors are knowledgeable in the medical sphere and therefore, the message that is being put across appears genuine and can easily be believed by viewers. However considering that the doctor speaks English unlike the deliverer of the message, there is a point of concern. It is not clear why the doctor is of Asian origin, yet the Kiswahili speaking countries have enough medical doctors who can ably express themselves in the language.

The lady who comes to deliver the message in Kiswahili does not help matters either. She appears to read the message on possibly an autocue using broken Kiswahili. She is inarticulate, fumbles and her accent does not resonate with that of Kiswahili speakers especially in the Eastern African region. It is not clear why she was identified for the task considering that there are many people who can read and express themselves in Kiswahili with a lot of ease. Her struggle in reading Kiswahili does not endear her to the viewer or listener, and worse still, she is unconvincing. She mispronounces the Kiswahili word *tisa* (nine) as *taisa*, and wrongly refers to *virusi vya korona,* Coronavirus as *virusikorona*. This is a breach of Kiswahili sentence structure, a matter that presents her as a quack in the messaging. The message is opaque owing to wanting vocabulary and poorly constructed sentences. A good example would be the sentence: *sasa ni katika kila hali nchini kote Marekanini, Virisi hivi ni wazo la kuenea kwa mtu hadi mtu aliyeambukizwa kikohozi au kutoa chafya,* whose translation reads as, "now it is in every situation in the whole American country, these viruses are an idea of spreading from one person to a person who has contracted coughing or sneezing." The obscure messaging is outrageous and a disservice to the consumers of intended message on Covid-19. There is also mispronunciation of *virusi*, virus as *virisi*, which further blurs the message.

The message is also rendered murky as a result of failure to adhere to the Kiswahili or Bantu Class concordial agreement. Other grammatical mistakes which smudge the message include *wagonjwa* for *ugonjwa* disease, *kuzia* instead of *kuzuia* to stop or t*afazali* instead of *tafadhali* please. The mistakes appearing in the above excerpt are many and shameful. It is disconcerting to learn that the sponsor would allow Covid-19 awareness messaging that is replete with grammatical mistakes that blur the lesson being put across. The pandemic was a serious illness that required crystal clear dissemination in order for the people to keep it at bay. However, failure to use Kiswahili language appropriately clouded the message, and in the final analysis, it is doubtful as to whether it benefited anybody. Ironically, it is arguable that a lot of investment went into the crafting of the message, but it is surprising that the sponsor did not care to crosscheck whether it had any communicative value. It is doubtful whether any Kiswahili radio or television station allowed the blotted messaging in their stations.

In CAVP3, there is further awareness on ways to prevent Covid-19. The video, which is composed in Kiswahili, uses animation unlike other videos that use people such as doctors or lay people. It says:

Covid-19 ni ugonjwa wa kupumua unaosababishwa na virusi. Mtu yeyote anaweza kuambukizwa. Virusi husambazwa wakati mgonjwa anakohoa, kupiga chafya, kuongea au kupumua akiwa karibu na mtu, kuvuta pumzi au matone. Dalili ni kikohozi kavu, joto jingi mwilini, kupumua kwa kishindo, koo kuwasha, homa ya mafua, unyonge, kupoteza ladha ya chakula na harufu. Ukiwa na dalili kama hizi, jitenge nyumbani na uwasiliane na msimamzi wako kazini na kisha ufuate ushauri wa daktari. .

Covid 19 is a viral disease. Anybody can contract the disease. The virus is spread when the patient is coughing, sneezing, talking or breathing. The symptoms are a dry cough, fevering, laboured breathing, itchy throat, flu, weakness, losing the senses of taste and smell. If you have such symptoms, quarantine yourself in the house and call your supervisor at work and thereafter, seek the doctor's advice...

The messaging in CAVP3 can be viewed in contradistinction to the crappy one in CAPV2. The message is delivered in good Kiswahili and the speaker sounds confident. The sentences are short and simple and therefore easy to follow. The instruction is packaged in four important phases. The first one dwells on what Covid-19 is, the second is the symptoms of the disease, the third is the preventive measures and fourth is an exhortation to viewers on the need to protect not only themselves, but other people.

In regard to the explanation as to what Covid-19 is, the video is richly successful. It illustrates the virus in red, round, circular objects. On the edges of the configuration are spindles which could be deemed as the legs of the virus. One image of the virus is foregrounded, while the rest of the images are much smaller. It is evident that the virus is widely spread in view of the fact that it occupies almost every space in the particular episode of the video. The choice to use images is good because the viewer is able to conjure the impression of the virus though it cannot be seen through unassisted vision. The crafter of the images has done a suave job for making the virus appear scaring not only in terms of colour and the pigments, but also because of the tick-like appearances that he has accorded it. The movement of the virus is illustrated as terrific and no wonder the disease is said to spread very fast.

The animation demonstrates how the virus is spread from one person to another. It is seen spreading from the mouth and nose of one person to another. The simulation further shows the symptoms of the disease as coughing, fevering as appears on the thermometer readings, laboured breathing, loss of the senses of taste and smell which are highlighted by pointing to the tongue and nose respectively. More animatronics are employed to demonstrate the preventive protocols against coronavirus. These include mask wearing, hand washing, keeping distance of 1.5 meters between people, avoiding crowded places and handshakes. The animation also emphasizes the need to clean house articles, keeping houses well-aerated and avoiding touching the mouth and nose. The video ends by demonstrating a united people who have kept the virus at bay as a result of observing the Covid-19 preventive measures.

The video enjoys rich communicative value as a result of the audio-visual messaging. It is apparent that the aural message could easily be used on a variety of audio channels including the radio. CAVP3 could also be adequately used on different audio-visual channels including the television. It is different from CAVP1 and CAVP2 for it does not use any noticeable human agency to convey the message. The messaging is borne of animation and a voice-over and therefore, it cannot be ascribed to any particular individual. While CAVP1 and CAVP2 are enacted by people that are seen, the message reader on CAVP3 remains unknown for his physiology does not appear anywhere.

Granted, the use of medical doctors in CAVP1 and CAVP2 could reinforce the messaging at hand, but the messaging on CAVP3 is interesting because it detaches itself from any known person hence dis-engaging any human agency. This is partly an effort in demonstrating neutrality of the massage that is being put across rather than staking an ascription to a particular agent. While well-known human agents could reinforce dissemination of Covid-19 to particular locales and contexts, in CAVP3, the message is equally sound despite the lack of any physical person to articulate it. Covid-19 was a global pandemic and therefore to present the message in a general aura is welcome for it is bound to fit a cross-section of Kiswahili speakers around the globe and not necessarily those are in specific contexts such as Kenya or East Africa. What counts regarding CAVP3 is that at the end of the day, there is a message that is delivered on Covid-19 by use of good and clear Kiswahili and with no particularized audience. It is only at the end of the video that a viewer is able to see that the video has been sponsored by a variety of organisations.

In CAVP4 is a song is used to disseminate information on Covid-19. The message is delivered by a guitarist who is singing. The title is "SAWBO coronavirus song" and the gist of the message is self-protection from the disease. Before the lyrics are delivered, there is a map of different continents in the world. Overlapping the maps is a monstrous image of the coronavirus with similar configuration to the one that appears on CAVP3. The singer states:

Janga hili limetupata, janga kuu la korona
nawasihi mjitie moyo, msibabaike tutashinda
Tufuate maagizo ya wizara ya afya
Tusafishe mikono mara kwa mara
Tuepuke kukaa kwa vikundi
Hili janga tutashinda
Korona, korona, korona, korona
Tuepuke hili janga
Ni jukumu letu kukarantini x2

This scourge has caught us, the scourge of coronavirus
I exhort you to gain courage, don't worry we'll win
Let's follow the guidelines of the Ministry of Health
We wash our hands regularly
We avoid crowding
We will defeat this scourge
Corona, corona, corona, corona
Let's avoid this scourge
It is our responsibility to observe distancex2

The message is wrought in simple and straightforward Kiswahili. The artist acknowledges that the coronavirus pandemic has affected people in Kenya. The use of the independent possessive pronoun 'our' is crucial in the messaging. It shows that the artist is part and parcel of the people who have been affected by Covid-19. Unlike in the messages that simply play an instructive role from a detached position, the artist presents himself as part and parcel of those that have been affected by the pandemic. He encourages his audience to remain bold for finally they will all win. In this case, the choice of pronoun *tu,* we, in the word *tutashinda*, we will win, further emphasizes the fact that the singer is in an elemental connection with the people who have been affected by the illness. He goes on to use the same pronoun to advise his audience to follow the guidelines of the Ministry of Health, hence to clean hands regularly while avoiding crowding. The refrain emphasizes the need to defeat the scourge while asserting that it is the responsibility of everybody to observe the protocol of keeping distance.

After the first refrain, the artist is joined by a female artist who relays further information on how people should protect themselves against Covid-19. She states that there are many people who have contracted the virus for failure to adhere to the preventive guidelines. The male artist takes another turn to sing and advises people to report any suspicious incidents of covid-19 to health officials. He outlines these as frequent coughing, laboured breathing, dry throats and fevering. He adds that the World Health Organisation urges people to stay in their homes, hand-wash regularly using *kitakasa,* one of the translations for sanitizer, avoid touching eyes, mouth and nostrils and keeping their surroundings clean.

After the song, the ending picture on the video has some information which is printed in English without any Kiswahili translation. It states:

Because COVID-19 is so contagious, social distancing is absolutely necessary to protect your health and the health of others. Do post this video on public websites with the request that it will be forwarded via WhatsApp or similar applications to as many recipients as possible. Do send this video yourself to others via WhatsApp and similar applications. DO NOT hold meetings to share this video, DO NOT share this video via Bluetooth in close proximity to others, DO NOT stand in close proximity to anyone to show them how to share this video.

Failure to translate the foregoing message in Kiswahili is a matter of concern considering that the advisory in the song is in Kiswahili, but the concluding printed message has solely been rendered in English. This is especially worrisome considering that the instruction in question is crucial in preventing the spread of coronavirus. The choice of English to create awareness in CAVP4 is interesting though anomalous in view of the wider Kenyan population. According to Nabea (2009) and Ogechi (2002) English is barely understood by 25 percent of the Kenyan population, yet it is the one that campaigners elected to use to create awareness on Covid-19 prevention. Considering that Kiswahili is not only Kenya's national language, but also a notable linguafranca in East Africa, why did the advocates against the spread of coronavirus chose English for the foregoing dissemination?

Ogola (2003) observes that the sociolinguistic situation in Kenya is triglossic with English at the top, Kiswahili in the middle and the mother tongue at the base. The inclination to use English language for national purposes such as creating awareness on the preventive measures against Covid-19 was therefore a great disservice for the approximately two-thirds of the Kenyan population that does not understand it well. The essence of every communication is to put a message across for its consumption. However, it is arguable that the message on CAVP4 might have benefited only a small section of the Kenyan population, unlike the impact of the same message if it were conveyed Kiswahili. The lack of translation is arguably lethargy on the part of the sponsor since the target audience is Kiswahili speakers going by the medium chosen for the song. The sponsor can be indicted for offering the message on the prevention of Covid-19 in a lopsided manner, whereby a portion of the message is delivered well, unlike the other bit.

Lack of the Kiswahili version of the message aside, the printed English information is fundamental in some perspectives unlike most of the messages that have been treated on the videos. The DO NOT messaging is cautionary that the video material dissemination can also be an agent of spreading the coronavirus if it is not handled well. There is caution against sharing of the video in meetings, which point to a crowded place and therefore could militate against the very message of preventing Covid-19. There is also a caveat against sharing the video via Bluetooth in close quarters, a matter that can breach the Covid-19 protocol of observing the distance of 1.5 meters between people, thereby spreading the disease. There is also an alert regarding standing in close proximity with people to show them the video, a matter that would also breach the keep-distance preventive measure.

The printed messaging engenders the question of inequality in the technological messaging of Covid-19. The message is tailored to people who are not only owners of high-tech gadgetry such as computers, laptops and mobile phones, but also those who are savvy in the technology. While part of the message is delivered in melodious Kiswahili lyrics, it may not be accessible to many Kiswahili speakers who have inadequacies in technological gadgetry. The inequality divide is similar to the digital divide that Stout and McGlynn (2022) address with respect to Covid-19 or the racial divide that Gordon-Brilla et al. (2022) address regarding the same pandemic. Suffice to state that the song could still pass the message through the radio and a variety of television channels which have wider reception, but it is not clear whether the Kenyan the stations ever played it.

AWARENESS ON COVID-19 TESTING

In AVCT1, there is information on Coronavirus testing. The deliverer of the message is disengaged as was seen in CAVP3, while the message is passed through animation and voicing in Kiswahili. There is simulation of the virus in colourful images as was noted about CAVP3. However, in AVCT1, the virus is represented in both red and yellow. The cartoons involved in illustrations are representative of people of a variety of descents in the world. The choice of these images is crucial in that it shows that Covid-19 affecting the human race around the globe. But for Kiswahili language, it is arguable that the message in the video resonates with a global audience rather than a localized context as seen in CAVP1. The animation also entails a cross-section of people from the young to the old as well as the healthy and the indisposed. Though the video starts by explaining what Covid-19 is as well as the disease's symptoms, the gist of its advisory is what a patient ought to or not to do. It states:

Ikiwa unaumwa, baki nyumbani mpaka upone. Inapimaje ugonjwa wa Covid-19? Ukiwa na dalili za ugonjwa wa Covid-19, hata dalili zisizo kali, nenda kupimwa. Mtu yeyote anaweza kupimwa na hakuna kujisikia aibu. Ni haraka, salama na safi. Kipimo cha Covid-19 ni bure katika kliniki za SA Health Covid-19 Clinics kwa wote hata ikiwa ni wakaazi wa ng'ambo. Hauhitaji Mediare wala bima ya kusafiri.

If you are sick, stay at home until you get well. How do you test Covid-19? If you have symptoms of Covid-19, even mild symptoms, go and get tested. Anybody can be tested and there is no cause for embarrassment. It is quick, safe and clean. Testing of Covid-19 is free in SA Health Covid-19 Clinics even for foreigners. You don't require Medicare or travel insurance.

The Kiswahili used in the advisory is simple and understandable. There are a number of English translation cutlines as the message unfolds. However, there is a grammatical error in *inapimaje*, instead of *unapimaje?* how do you test? However, the mistake is inconsequential because it does not distort the message unlike the observation made on CAVP3. The simulated house in the animation depicting where a patient should remain in order not to interact with other people might nonetheless lack resonance with most of the target audience. This is because the house that is used to exemplify the message is exotic in design. The building fails to resonate with majority of lay people who live either in middle class or below middle class levels. This implies that while there are many Kenyans who can easily identify with the messaging conveyed in Kiswahili, the illustration of the house might cause a disconnect. It somewhat suggests that the message is tailored to people living in such alien houses, and not those who live in typical Kenyan houses.

However, it is apparent that the messaging was not necessarily meant for the Kiswahili polity especially in East Africa. It has already been observed that going by the visual illustrations on the video, the message could be tailored to a variety of people in the world hence the message is not necessarily designed for a particular audience. However, this is a weakness because the message crafters should have made some effort to ensure that the illustrations that they employed were specific to contexts, just as one can infer regarding the use of Kiswahili. Considering that the Kiswahili instruction is not contextually in tandem with the various illustrations, it follows that the viewer of the video may fail to appreciate the messaging fully as a result of the disconnect between content and the visual illusions.

The message is persuasive in regard to taking tests for Covid-19. It states that any person can be tested and therefore there is no need to be embarrassed. Embarrassment might be the wrong word in connection to testing of people for coronavirus in Kenya. Instead, people shunned Covid-19 testing for stigma and possible isolation, in case they turned positive, and got incarceration which was feared as a death sentence. The test is touted as quick, safe and clean and that there is no payment for the task in SA Health Clinics. The invocation of SA Health Clinics causes a further lapse in the messaging because there are no such clinics in Kenya let alone in the rest of the East African region. An investigation reveals that SA Health is Southern Adeilaide Local Health Network (SALHN) in Australia. It is therefore ridiculous to advise a Kenyan, Ugandan, Tanzanian or many other Africans to seek health assistance in clinics that are domiciled in Australia.

It is arguable that the Covid-19 messaging in AVCT1 was initially done targeting Australians. It is possible that when Australia realised that their vaccine was one of the most sought in the world, they decided to translate the message into other languages including Kiswahili. However, in the course of this translation, there was failure to anchor some important snippets in their rightful contexts. For example, the translation would have made sense to ask Kenyans to go to different health clinics in their counties, a message that would bode well by invoking similar contexts for people in Uganda or Tanzania. The Covid-19 Kiswahili messaging on AVCT1 is therefore undermined by failure to contextualize crucial information especially as regards the names of health institutions. It is inferable that just as observed in CAVP3, the message translator from English to Kiswahili adopted a wanting translation approach which ignored context.

It is shameful to render such messaging only to be asked where the SALHN clinics are, only to get a response that they are in Australia. It is understandable that Covid-19 struck the world suddenly and many people and nations were caught pants down. However, that should not be an excuse for providing flawed translations on testing of the disease in whichever language. The translation actually breaches a cardinal rule of translation whereby showing fidelity to the source and target languages is important (Pym 2012). Similar contextual information that may not be palatable to most of the Kiswahili audience appears in the suggestion that for people to be tested for the coronavirus, they do not require any Medicare. Research shows that Medicare in Australia is a universal health insurance scheme that caters for Australians and visitors to the country in health and hospital services at low or zero costs. To suggest to a Kenyan or any other person in the East African region where Kiswahili is predominantly used that they do not require Medicare to get the coronavirus test is ludicrous for the insurance does not exist in their countries and further, they do not know it. Such lapses hamper the message's communicative value because part of the information provided is not helpful at all.

The messaging continues to urge people to wash their hands regularly using water, and if they want to avoid water, they use *kitakasamikono,* loosely translatable as a hand-washing apparatus. However, the illustration of the so-called *kitakasamikono* points to a sanitizer, which is known as *kieuzi* in Kiswahili. Usage of k*ieuzi* gained currency in the wake of Covid-19, and therefore a translator can be forgiven for naming a sanitizer differently. However, the translation may confuse the viewers for *kitakasamikono* suggests a variety of gizmos for washing hands.

COVID-19 AWARENESS VIDEO ON VACCINE

There is direction on the Covid-19 vaccine as appears on CAVV1. It highlights what to expect when receiving the vaccine as follows:

Ikiwa unapokea au unanuia kupokea chanjo ya Covid-19, unapaswa kujua yafuatayo kabla ya kupokea chanjo. Chanjo hii ni salama na itasaidia kukulinda dhidi ya Covid-19. Huwezi kuambukizwa Covid-19 kutoka kwa chanjo. Chanjo haina kemikali ya kuizuia kuharibika. Unaweza kutembelea Tovuti ya Afya ya Minnesota upate maelezo zaidi kuhusu viungo vya chanjo. Kila mmoja atapokea chanjo bila malipo yoyote. Hatutazingatia malipo yako ya bima na uhamiaji.

If you are receiving or intend to receive the Covid-19 vaccine, you need to know the following before the vaccination. The vaccination is safe and will protect you against Covid-19. You cannot contract Covid-19 from the vaccine. The vaccine has no chemicals to deter it from expiry. You may go to the Minnesota

Health Website for more information regarding the contents of the vaccine. Everybody will receive the vaccine for free. We will not ask for your insurance or immigration status.

The message is conveyed in good, simple and flawless Kiswahili. This makes it enjoyable to listen. The video starts by highlighting what recipients of Covid-19 vaccine ought to know prior to the receiving the jab. It is stated that the vaccine is safe and protects against the coronavirus infection. There is important information that the vaccine cannot spread the virus. The information is crucial considering that injections are said to spread diseases like HIV/AIDS, and therefore people are always wary of jabs. The message therefore allays fears that some people could be habouring about the vaccine in view of spreading the virus. There is also essential information that the vaccine has a lifespan and thereafter, it can expire. This gen is critical because it demonstrates the fidelity of the message disseminator contrary to instances where people buy and use drugs that have expired. The message is therefore cautionary to the possible vaccine recipients that they should be wary of vaccines that have outlived their lifespan and which could be unhealthy for use.

However, things come to a head when the listener is advised to go to the website of Minnesota to get further information of the contents of the vaccine. The mention of Minnesota somewhat throws spanner in the works of the message. The Kiswahili message on the video definitely targets Kiswahili speakers especially in East Africa where the language is widely used. It can further be argued that viewers easily identify with Kiswahili language since it is homegrown. However, Minnesota is a state in the United States of America, and a viewer finds a gnawing hiatus between the message and website given. The choice of the Minnesota website renders the good message shaky for the context is alien and therefore the audience is not able to identify with it. Considering that there were websites articulating Covid-19 messaging in the East African region, the deliverer of the message should have considered the context and cited the appropriate stations. Else to convey the message in Kiswahili and refer viewers to a Minnesota website which is designed in English is anomalous not only because viewers cannot identify with the city, but because the use of English language screens out most of them.

The rest of the information that follows in the messaging is suspect owing to Minnesota as the origin of the information. It is said that the vaccine is offered for free and recipients do not require any insurance or evidence of immigration documents. It is elaborate that the information was initially targeted to people in the United States and not those living in regions where Kiswahili is predominantly used. It is arguable the message was translated from English to Kiswahili but the translator failed to reflect on context to package the message appropriately. This is further evidence of translational flaws whereby context is overlooked resulting in the creation of doubts in the messaging. The blemish undermines the rest information on the video which borders on what to expect prior to receiving the vaccine, its effects and the importance of adhering to coronavirus preventive measures even after even after the jab.

In CAVV2, the video does not only create awareness on the Covid-19 vaccine but briefly disseminates information to people who fall ill as a result of the pandemic. This is a departure from the rest of the messages so far seen which banked on creation of awareness on the pandemic, testing and vaccines. This is an important development considering that besides people who were not affected by the disease, there were those affected. In CAVV2, the video starts with some background music and an image of the coronavirus. It states:

Watu wengi walio na Covid-19 wanapata nafuu. Lakini wakati mwingine, inaweza kusababisha ugonjwa kali na wakati mwingine kifo. Chanjo zinaweza kusaidia kinga za asili za mwili wetu kupambana na Covid-19 ... Miili yetu inachukua hatua ya kutengeneza seli maalumu za kupambana na virusi hivi.

Many people who have Covid-19 are getting cured. However, there are times it can cause severe illness and death. Vaccines can help to protect against Covid-19. ... Our bodies prepare special cells to fight the viruses.

The narrator has instances of wanting Kiswahili grammar such as *mwili yetu* instead of *miili yetu,* our bodies, or *virusi hizi* instead of *virusi hivi,* these viruses. However, unlike what was observed regarding CAVP3, the wanting grammar does not distort the message. There is an encouraging instruction that there are many people who have recovered after suffering from Covid-19, allaying fears that the acquisition of the disease is simply a death sentence. The video also spells out that Covid-19 was spreading fast because the strain was new and people's bodies have no memory or information on how to identify it in order to fight it. It adds that people's bodies have never produced antibodies to counter the disease that is new, hence the difficulties in fighting it. The educative message spells out that vaccines are prepared to introduce combative cells to the coronavirus. It is for this reason that a person whose body has received the vaccine and happens to contract the disease is able to fight back for the body has the necessary combative cells thanks to the vaccine. The lesson indicates that vaccines have been used to treat diseases like smallpox, measles and polio previously. The video ends by advising those who have been vaccinated to continue observing coronavirus preventive measures. The reference of the foregoing diseases gives hope that the Covid-19 vaccine is bound to eradicate the scourge.

CONCLUDING REMARKS

This paper has presented results of a study on Kiswahili video messaging of Covid-19 in Kenya. The objective of the study was to examine the themes and strategies employed in this video communication to create awareness on Covid-19. Results have shown that the videos were themed on Covid-19 awareness in connection to what the pandemic was, the preventive measures and the vaccine to fight the virus. The paper has demonstrated that Covid-19 messaging was in a number of cases hampered by poor grammar, English to Kiswahili translational flaws and wanting animation. It is for this reason that the paper has argued that the Covid-19 video messaging fell short of the communicative value. The paper indicts the sponsors of such dissemination for failure to communicate effectively in the face of the deadly Covid-19.

REFERENCES

Communication Authority of Kenya. (2023). Mobile Subscription Hit 66m as at March 2023. https://www.ca.go.ke/mobile-subscriptions-hit-66m-march-2023

Gordon-Brilla, S., & Rogers, D., *Higginbottom, J. Ensha, L., & Sutherland, R. (n.d.). The Colour of Covid-19. The Racial Inequality of Marginalised Communities.* Routledge.

Ji, D., & Liu, L. (2022). Fighting Covid-19 by National Mobilization: A Communicative Analysis of the Roles of the Chinese Government. In Manufacturing Government Communication on Covid-19. A Comparative Perspective. Paris: Springer. doi:10.1007/978-3-031-09230-5_3

Maarek, P. (2022). Similar and Dissimilar Patterns of Government Communication on Covid-19. In Manufacturing Government Communication on Covid-19. A Comparative Perspective. Springer. doi:10.1007/978-3-031-09230-5_1

Martin, B. (2014). Semiotics and the Media. In R. S. Fortner & P. M. Fackler (Eds.), *The Handbook of Media and Mass Communication Theory* (pp. 56–73). Wiley Blackwell. doi:10.1002/9781118591178.ch4

Mwansoko, H. J. M. (2006). Kitangulizi cha Tafsiri: Nadharia na Mbinu. Dar es Salaam: TUKI.

Nabea, W. (2007). Language Policy in Kenya: Negotiation with Hegemony. *The Journal of Pan African Studies*, *1*(3), 121–138.

Najafi, S., Tofigh, S., & Sobczyk. (2023). Covid 19: Virology. In Corona Virus Disease 2019 (Covid-19). A Clinical Guide. Wiley Blackwell.

Ogechi, N. (2002). The Reality and Challenges of Publishing in Kiswahili in Kenya. In Utafiti wa Kiswahili,. Eldoret: Moi University Press.

Ogechi, N. (2005). On Lexicalization in Sheng. *Nordic Journal of African Studies*, *3*(14), 334–335.

Ogola, O. (2003). The National Language Policy Implementation and Experience: The Case of Kiswahili in the Parliament of Kenya. Dissertation Zur Erlangung des Doktorgrades der Philosophie, Universitat Wien.

Pym, A. (2012). *On Translator Ethics. Principles for Mediation Between Cultures* (Revised Edition). John Benjamins Publishing Company. doi:10.1075/btl.104

Steinbuka, I. (2022). Pros and Cons of the EU Response and Communication during Covid-19 Crisis. In Manufacturing Government Communication on Covid-19. A Comparative Perspective. Paris: Springer. doi:10.1007/978-3-031-09230-5_2

Stout, C., & McGlynn, A. (2020). Necessity as the Mother of Invention: Attempts to Overcome the Digital Divide During the Covid-19 Pandemic. In S. Navarro & S. Hernandez (Eds.), *The Colour of Covid-19. The Racial Inequality of Marginalised Communities* (pp. 29–45). Routledge.

Chapter 5
The Role of Language in Social Media During the COVID-19 Pandemic

Billy James
https://orcid.org/0009-0003-6618-8560
University of Limpopo, South Africa

Wilfred W. Wilfred
University of Limpopo, South Africa

ABSTRACT

The COVID-19 pandemic brought about unprecedented challenges to societies worldwide, compelling individuals and institutions to adapt rapidly to a new reality dominated by digital communication. Social media platforms emerged as essential channels for information dissemination, community building, and emotional expression during this global crisis. Language played a pivotal role in shaping these interactions, influencing the spread of information, the formation of online communities, and the impact of public health campaigns. This chapter explores the multifaceted role of language in social media during the COVID-19 pandemic. Firstly, it highlights the significance of language as a medium for facilitating real-time updates and news dissemination. Governments, health organizations, and news outlets utilized language to convey critical information, ranging from infection rates and safety measures to vaccination updates, reaching a diverse and vast audience worldwide. This chapter will examine how language served as a crucial tool in combating misinformation.

1. INTRODUCTION

This chapter examines the emergence of new COVID-19-related vocabulary and language evolution during the pandemic. Neologisms and linguistic trends on social media reflected the social and cultural impact of the crisis, shaping online discourse and communication patterns. The chapter reflects on various roles played by language during the 2019 Covid pandemic in disseminating information to the community.

DOI: 10.4018/979-8-3693-0624-6.ch005

1.1 Facilitating Information Sharing and Dissemination

The role of language in social media during the COVID-19 pandemic was instrumental in facilitating information sharing and dissemination. Social media platforms served as crucial channels for the rapid spread of information related to the pandemic. According to Chinelli et al (2020), to distribute information fast and reach a large audience, platforms were also utilized by political groups, national and state level health organizations, and politicians. This has led to the following subheadings on how language played a significant role in this process.

i. Real-Time Updates and News Dissemination

Language was the primary means of conveying real-time updates, news, and developments related to COVID-19. Government agencies, health organizations, and news outlets utilized language to share critical information about infection rates, safety measures, travel restrictions, and vaccination updates. Through posts, tweets, and articles, this information reached a wide audience quickly. Infographics, images, and videos shared on social media platforms often contained vital information about COVID-19. Language, in the form of captions and text overlays, accompanied these visuals, enhancing their impact and ensuring that the intended messages were effectively communicated.

ii. Hashtags and Keywords

According to Cardoso et al. (2019:58), a given subject may be addressed by different hashtags, the topics of discussion in the platform are automatically obtained by community detection in the semantic network and we consider that each community constitutes a topic of discussion in the platform. This means that the idea of using hashtags for Twitter and keywords allows for a global comparison of the dynamics of the discussion in both media. Language played a key role in organizing and categorizing COVID-19 content using hashtags and keywords. Trending hashtags such as #COVID19, #coronavirus, and #pandemic helped aggregate information and discussions related to the virus, making it easier for users to find relevant content. Social media provided a platform for information to be shared in multiple languages, catering to diverse audiences around the world. Government agencies, healthcare organizations, and influencers used various languages to reach non-English-speaking communities and promote inclusivity. Language was crucial in the efforts to combat misinformation and fake news. Social media users, fact-checking organizations, and health experts used language to identify, analyse, and debunk false information, ensuring that accurate and reliable information prevailed.

iii. Amplification of Public Health Campaigns

It was found that during Covid-19 pandemic, people engaged with an imperfect assortment of local news media, epidemiological specialists, political pundits, public health officials, and financially motivated opportunists online, they collectively amplify a small set of disproportionately influential COVID-19 information sources, or crowdsourced elites. This led to the governments and health authorities to employ language strategically to promote public health campaigns and COVID-19 safety measures. By crafting clear and compelling messages, these campaigns gained traction on social media, encouraging people to adopt preventive measures and follow health guidelines. Language facilitated interactive communication between healthcare professionals, experts, and the public. Social media platforms hosted live questions and answer sessions, webinars, and town hall meetings where experts used language to engage with the audience and address their concerns directly. Social media users themselves became sources of valuable information. Individuals shared their personal experiences, coping strategies, and pandemic-related knowledge through language, creating a sense of community and support during challenging times.

iv. Rapid Information Dissemination

Rubin et al. (2019) highlighted that journal published case reports quickly, through expediated review, and made them freely available, while simultaneously encouraging preprint publication as a means in which to bring data to a wide audience expeditiously. This was done to permit the lay press and public health authorities to get an early look at the range of clinical manifestations and the basic epidemiology of COVID-19. The above information is supported by Rothe et al. (2019), who indicated that publishing timeframes had also became increasing tight, as illustrated in a paper by Rothe et al. (2020). The speed of information sharing on social media allowed critical updates and warnings to spread rapidly, helping people stay informed about the evolving situation. Language played a central role in the efficiency and effectiveness of this dissemination process. Overall, the role of language in social media during the COVID-19 pandemic was essential in ensuring that accurate information reached a vast audience quickly. It enabled effective communication, raised awareness, and empowered individuals to make informed decisions during a time of global uncertainty. However, it also posed challenges, as misinformation and misinterpretation could spread just as quickly, highlighting the need for responsible language use and critical evaluation of online content.

2. MISINFORMATION AND FAKE NEWS

According to Wardle and Derakhshan (2020:76), there was an increase in false information which was shared unconsciously (not knowing that the information is whether correct or not) and without any purpose to make harm to anyone. This is called misinformation; on the other side, disinformation is false information and shared consciously to make harm intentionally. The COVID-19 pandemic saw an explosion of misinformation and fake news on social media platforms, contributing to what was termed an "infodemic." Misinformation and fake news were highlighted by Moscadelli et al. (2020); Apuke and Omar (2021) where they indicated that there was interference in the behaviour and health of people, generating social unrest associated with violence, distrust, social disturbances, and attacks on health professionals. People of different nationalities were affected by sharing unverified information. According to Lin et al. (2020), people feel anxious, depressed, or emotionally exhausted, and these expressive health effects are directly associated with the spread of this information. This has led researchers to analyse the rapid spread of false information and its impact on public health responses. This led to social media and misinformation where studies focused on the role of social media platforms in amplifying misinformation and the challenges faced by tech companies in combating fake news during the pandemic. Research delved into identifying the sources and origins of COVID-19 misinformation, such as conspiracy theories, political interests, and pseudoscientific claims. Scholars investigated how exposure to COVID-19 misinformation influenced public behaviour, including adherence to preventive measures and vaccine hesitancy. Some studies focused on deliberate disinformation campaigns and their potential consequences during the pandemic. Misinformation and fake news were significant challenges in the role of language on social media during the COVID-19 pandemic. The rapid and widespread dissemination of false information exacerbated the impact of the crisis, leading to confusion, panic, and even potential harm to public health. Several factors contributed to the spread of misinformation, and language played a crucial role in this process.

2.1 Amplification Through Language

Macintyre et al., (2020) highlighted that language teachers and learners had to rapidly shift to unfamiliar learning methods and environments, while coping with the individual and societal effects of the pandemic on their daily lives and well-being. This indicated that the effects of the COVID-19 pandemic on language teaching (LT) have become an area of intense interest within the research community. Social media platforms provided a fertile ground for the amplification of misinformation. Language, when used sensationally or provocatively, tended to attract more attention and engagement, leading to the rapid dissemination of false or misleading content. Misleading headlines, clickbait phrases, and emotionally charged language often accompanied misinformation, making it more shareable. Misinformation often played on people's emotions and existing beliefs, reinforcing confirmation bias. Language was carefully crafted to appeal to certain groups, exploiting their preconceived notions and ideologies. This created echo chambers where false information could circulate unchecked. Some individuals and groups, often with no credible expertise, used language to present themselves as experts or authorities on COVID-19. Their misinformation, wrapped in seemingly technical or scientific language, misled the public and eroded trust in legitimate sources. Social media's speed and reach allowed misinformation to spread rapidly across networks. Language played a key role in how information was framed and presented, influencing its virality. Misinformation, once it gained traction, could quickly become a viral "infodemic."

2.2 Language Barriers and Cultural Context

According to Singer (2016), culture, which is defined as the beliefs, attitudes, practices, and explanations used to create behavioural norms in a group, can play a key role in the adoption of protective behaviours during the COVID-19 pandemic. On the other hand, language barriers were the most contributing factor in the role of language during Covid-19 pandemic and this was evident on misinformation which was not limited to a specific language or culture. Language barriers made it challenging to combat misinformation on a global scale. The lack of accurate translations and cultural context could lead to misinterpretations of information. Social media algorithms were designed to maximize engagement, inadvertently amplified misinformation. Language-based engagement patterns, such as likes, shares, and comments, contributed to the algorithm's recommendation of content, regardless of its accuracy.

2.3 Lack of Fact-Checking and Source Verification

Fact-checking is one of the essential elements of journalism and it is an indispensable dimension shared by all journalism professionals throughout its modern history. This was done because some information was correct and some not. The speed of social media often outpaced fact-checking efforts, allowing misinformation to circulate unchecked. Language played a role in disguising false information as credible news, making it difficult for users to discern its authenticity. Automated bots and fake accounts were used to propagate misinformation on social media. These accounts used language patterns to mimic human behaviour, contributing to the illusion of widespread support for false narratives. To address the challenges posed by misinformation and fake news during the COVID-19 pandemic, several strategies were employed. Fact-checking organizations and social media platforms implemented measures to identify and label false information. Additionally, promoting media literacy and critical thinking skills among social media users became essential to empower individuals to identify and question dubious content.

3. COMMUNITY BUILDING AND ONLINE ACTIVISM

Community engagement within health is crucial to achieve primary healthcare and promote people-centred services. This led to the formation of virtual communities. Virtual communities were formed and strengthened during the pandemic, emphasizing the role of social media and online platforms in connecting people despite physical distancing measures. Community engagements is used as a parent notion with terms like communication, social mobilisation, community participation, community action and empowerment. On the same note, several measures to engage communities were undertaken, including building partnerships with local and religious leaders and working with the community to develop and adjust key messages for behavioural change. Online activism and advocacy were used to raise awareness about various issues related to the pandemic, such as healthcare disparities and public health measures. Virtual events and campaigns explored the effectiveness of virtual events and campaigns in mobilising communities and promoting collective action during Covid-19. Digital storytelling and online narratives were utilized to raise awareness about the experiences and challenges faced by various communities during the pandemic. Online platforms fostered collective resilience and providing mutual support among individuals and communities affected by the pandemic.

3.1 Language Barriers and Inclusivity

Language barriers and inclusivity were significant issues during the COVID-19 pandemic. The pandemic exacerbated existing disparities and created new challenges for individuals who did not speak the dominant language of their region or country. During Covid-19 pandemic, linguistic barriers are a significant contributor to COVID-19-related health disparities in racial/ethnic minority communities whose health communication needs cannot be adequately met in English. In the early stages of the pandemic, vital information about COVID-19, such as prevention measures, testing sites, and vaccination information, was often communicated in the official language(s) of a region or country. This left non-native speakers with limited access to critical information, making it difficult for them to protect themselves and their communities. Language barriers made it challenging for individuals to communicate their symptoms or medical history effectively. This hindered healthcare providers' ability to diagnose and treat COVID-19 patients accurately. Additionally, testing sites and healthcare facilities often lacked interpreters or materials in multiple languages, further exacerbating disparities in healthcare access.

3.2 Vaccine Distribution

The distribution of COVID-19 vaccines has been a critical issue during the pandemic. Vaccine allocation and distribution have been reviewed in the context of the COVID-19 pandemic. As vaccines became available, governments and healthcare providers faced challenges in ensuring equitable vaccine distribution. This included reaching out to linguistically diverse communities and addressing vaccine hesitancy. Many countries, especially developing countries, often encounter a shortage of vaccines. It was believed that the shortage of vaccines was the production monopoly, complex production processes, increased oversight of manufacturing facilities, unforeseen fluctuations in demand, and reduced producers are the most frequently cited reasons for vaccine shortage. This chapter discusses the implications of vaccine distribution and allocation and suggests future research. Disparities in vaccine distribution across counties have been studied using geographic information systems. The study found that the association between vaccine distribution and sociodemographic of the population served by facilities could have changed over time. Vaccine nationalism has led to vaccine inequity during the pandemic, creating a considerable barrier to attaining global immunity. This can disturb all efforts in ending the COVID-19 mortalities and intervene in economic recovery, which collapsed drastically during the pandemic. Vaccine acceptance reflects the overall perception of disease risk, vaccine attitudes, and demand within the general population, which is critical for the success of vaccination programs. Governments play a crucial role in promoting confidence in the effectiveness and safety of vaccines through effective communication. The COVID-19 pandemic has reinforced existing challenges in national health systems, including disruptions to existing national immunization programs against diseases such as diphtheria, measles, and polio. Principles for vaccine distribution within countries have been proposed, such as prioritization of health workforce and older people.

3.3 Education

During Covid-19 pandemic education has been shown to create more student-tutor and student-student interaction, which can promote better engagement. As time goes on things changed where formal and informal learning have ceased and professional courses have been required to move to exclusive delivery through online education remote learning became the norm for many students during the pandemic. Language barriers created disparities in educational access, particularly for students who did not have access to materials in their native language or struggled to navigate online learning platforms in a language they were not proficient in. Many essential workers faced language barriers in their workplaces, making it difficult to communicate safety protocols, understand health guidelines, and advocate for their rights. This posed additional risks to their health and well-being. Community organizations and public health agencies had to adapt their outreach strategies to reach linguistically diverse populations. This involved translating materials, utilizing interpreters, and collaborating with community leaders who could bridge the language gap.

3.4 Inclusivity Measures

To address these challenges, governments, organizations, and communities implemented various inclusivity measures. These included translating materials into multiple languages, providing interpreters at testing and vaccination sites, and offering culturally sensitive information to build trust and address vaccine hesitancy. How to prevent the spread of the virus and high infection rates, governments around the world imposed strict school closure measures which required a rapid and hasty transition into online teaching formats. Students, on the other hand, had to learn from home in a more autonomous way compared to regular classes and without having face-to-face contact with their teachers and classmates.

Improving digital inclusion and accessibility became a priority, as much of the information and services shifted online. Efforts were made to ensure that online resources were available in multiple languages and that technology was accessible to everyone. The experiences of language barriers during the pandemic underscored the importance of inclusivity and equitable access to information and services. Many organizations and governments are now working to ensure that these lessons are applied in future emergency preparedness and response efforts. Lastly, language barriers posed significant challenges during the COVID-19 pandemic, affecting access to information, healthcare, education, and social inclusion. Addressing these barriers through inclusive measures is crucial for ensuring the well-being of linguistically diverse communities during public health crises and beyond.

3.5 Public Health Campaigns and Communication

Public health campaigns and communication during the COVID-19 pandemic have played a critical role in controlling the spread of the virus, providing accurate information to the public, and encouraging behaviour that reduces transmission risk. According to WHO (2021), most developed counties have achieved high levels of vaccination, campaigns have proven highly effective in limiting disease impacts while allowing the relaxation of restrictions and a return to pre-pandemic-like behaviour. Effective communication has been essential in promoting public awareness, fostering trust, and facilitating adherence to recommended guidelines. There are key elements and strategies used in public health campaigns and communication during the COVID-19 pandemic:

i. Clear and Timely Information Sharing

Information sharing played a significant role during Covid-19 pandemic where separate studies have shown that a high proportion of tweets are informative, meaning they seek to share information or updates. Tweets play a significant role in sharing information to the whole world. Governments and health organizations have provided regular updates on the status of the pandemic, including case numbers, testing and treatment information, and safety guidelines. Timely and transparent reporting of information has been crucial to keep the public informed and to prevent the spread of misinformation. There were short and easily digestible PSAs in various media formats (TV, radio, social media, etc.) were used to convey key messages, such as mask-wearing, hand hygiene, and social distancing. In the same vein, authorities have consistently relied on experts from the fields of epidemiology and infectious diseases to deliver information.

ii. Multilingual and Accessible Communication

Li et al. (2020), speak of National Emergency Language Competence (NELC) as the capacity to use language to cope with domestic and international public emergencies. They further indicated that they observe that most of the measures implemented to address multilingualism during the COVID-19 crisis were not “conscious actions”, as they were not part of a previously developed long-standing emergency plan, but rather hasty measures adopted to face an unexpected crisis. Any efforts have been made to reach diverse populations by providing information in multiple languages and ensuring accessibility for individuals with disabilities. This means that information from the government to the citizens does not only flow through official documents but by television, internet etc. Public health campaigns have not only informed people about the virus but have also provided practical advice on how to reduce transmission risk, such as wearing masks, maintaining physical distance, and getting vaccinated. It was noted that vaccination campaigns have been a major focus, with communication emphasizing the safety and efficacy of vaccines and encouraging widespread vaccination. The government was not alone in conveying the message to the community where engagement with local communities and leaders has been essential to gain support and compliance with public health measures.

iii. Continual Evaluation and Adaptation

During Covid-19 pandemic schools adapted their learning where UNESCO implemented strategies and measures to reduce the impact of school closures on students with disabilities. The reason was because the COVID-19 pandemic has an uneven impact on students with disabilities as they face a lack of accessible public health information, obstacles to implementing necessary hygiene measures, inaccessible health facilities, even they face a greater risk of domestic violence. Campaigns and communication strategies have been adjusted based on changing circumstances, scientific knowledge, and the evolving needs of the population. Effective communication and public health campaigns have been instrumental in navigating the challenges posed by the COVID-19 pandemic. They have not only provided information but have also influenced behaviour, fostered a sense of shared responsibility, and contributed to the global effort to control the spread of the virus.

4. ONLINE DISINFORMATION DETECTION AND MODERATION

Detecting and moderating online disinformation during the COVID-19 pandemic has been a significant challenge due to the rapid spread of false information on various digital platforms. Effective strategies have been implemented by governments, social media platforms, and fact-checking organizations to identify and mitigate the impact of disinformation.

5. LINGUISTIC ANALYSIS FOR EPIDEMIOLOGY

Linguistic analysis has played a crucial role in epidemiology during the COVID-19 pandemic. It involves the study of language patterns, textual data, and communication to gain insights into the spread of the virus, public sentiment, and behaviour. Sentiment analysis tools have been used to assess public sentiment towards COVID-19-related topics. Understanding public sentiment can help health authorities gauge public compliance with measures and identify areas where more information or support is needed. Linguistic analysis of social media posts and comments has provided real-time data on public concerns, misinformation, and compliance with health guidelines. Trends in social media conversations have been used to anticipate outbreaks and public reactions. This has led to the identification of misinformation where linguistic analysis helps in identifying false or misleading information related to COVID-19. Natural Language Processing (NLP) techniques are used to detect and categorize misinformation, allowing for timely debunking and mitigation. Contact tracing efforts have utilized text messages to trace the movements and interactions of infected individuals. Linguistic analysis of text messages and mobile app data helps identify potential contacts and transmission routes. Psychological and Emotional Insights were noticed amongst people and communities. Linguistic analysis of text data has been used to gain insights into the emotional and psychological impact of the pandemic on individuals and communities. Linguistic analysis has been a valuable tool in epidemiology during the COVID-19 pandemic, helping researchers and health authorities understand the evolving dynamics of the virus, public reactions, and the effectiveness of interventions. It has also played a critical role in managing the infodemic and ensuring that accurate information is accessible to the public.

6. LANGUAGE ADAPTATION AND NEOLOGISMS

The COVID-19 pandemic has led to the emergence of new words and phrases, as well as changes in language use. The pandemic has given rise to new words and phrases, including neologisms, which have spread almost as fast as the virus itself. Neologisms are newly coined words or phrases that have not yet entered common usage. Neologisms related to COVID-19 have been studied from the perspective of comparing the features of semantically related neologisms. The study found that neologisms can have a significant impact on the metaphoric language of socio-political discourse. The use of neologisms during the pandemic has been found to have a trending role. A study found that the use of neologisms in English language teaching can be beneficial for EFL students. Many new and newly common unusual words have come into use because of the COVID-19 pandemic. The pandemic has led to the emergence of new words and phrases related to the virus, such as "social distancing" and "flatten the curve." The pandemic has had an impact on language use, with some university students in Greece reporting neuropsychological mechanisms that induce the adaptation of spoken languages, including neologisms, poor vocabulary, misspelling, syntactic and vocabulary. The COVID-19 Multilingual Project has been launched to help languages adapt to the sudden influx of neologisms and scientific terminology during the pandemic. The project aims to provide resources and support for language adaptation during the pandemic.

7. COVID-19 TERMINOLOGY

The pandemic led to the widespread use of terms like "COVID-19," "coronavirus," and "SARS-CoV-2" to describe the virus and the disease it causes. Acronyms like PPE (Personal Protective Equipment), ICU (Intensive Care Unit), and WFH (Work from Home) became common.

7.1 Social Distancing

Social distancing is a term that has become widely used during the COVID-19 pandemic. Social distancing is a practice that involves staying at least 6 feet away from others to avoid catching a disease such as COVID-19. It is also known as physical distancing. The goal of social distancing during the pandemic is to slow down the outbreak and reduce the chance of infection among high-risk individuals. This can help to lower the pace and extent of the spread of COVID-19 in any given city or community. Social distancing involves avoiding contact with people who have COVID-19, whether they feel sick, to reduce the risk of catching the virus from them. If possible, individuals should avoid being around a person who has COVID-19 until they can safely end home isolation. The Centres for Disease Control and Prevention (CDC) recommends social distancing measures, such as remaining out of congregate settings, avoiding mass gatherings, and maintaining distance (approximately 6 feet or 2 meters) from others when possible. This means no hugs or handshakes. Social distancing can help to limit the spread of COVID-19 and reduce strain on healthcare systems. Limiting gatherings with people outside of one's household, like group activities and religious events, can also reduce the spread of COVID-19.

7.2. Flattening the Curve

Flattening the curve is a term that has been widely used during the COVID-19 pandemic. Flattening the curve refers to the practice of slowing down the spread of a disease, such as COVID-19, to avoid overwhelming healthcare systems. The goal is to reduce the number of cases that occur at any given time, which can help to ensure that healthcare resources are available to those who need them. Flattening the curve involves implementing social distancing measures, such as staying at home, avoiding large gatherings, and maintaining physical distance from others. These measures can help to slow the spread of the virus and reduce the number of cases that occur at any given time. Flattening the curve is a complex concept that involves multiple components, including the shape of the epidemic curve, social distancing measures, and the reproduction number R0. Each component has its own history and plays a different role in controlling the spread of COVID-19. There are some common misconceptions about flattening the curve, such as the idea that the curve has a single peak or that flattening the curve is the only strategy needed to defeat COVID-19. Empirical evidence suggests that non-pharmaceutical interventions, including social distancing measures, have been effective in flattening the curve during the COVID-19 pandemic. These interventions have helped to reduce the spread of the virus and prevent healthcare systems from becoming overwhelmed.

7.3 Lockdown and Shelter-in-Place

Lockdowns and shelter-in-place orders have been implemented in many countries during the COVID-19 pandemic. Shelter-in-place orders have been controversial, but studies have shown that they can be effective in reducing the spread of COVID-19. These policies involve requiring people to stay at home and avoid non-essential activities and travel. Shelter-in-place orders can have negative effects on mental health and wellbeing, including increased anxiety and depression. These orders can also lead to economic hardship, particularly for low-income individuals and small businesses. The impact of shelter-in-place orders on human rights has been a topic of discussion, with some arguing that these policies can infringe on individual liberties. It is important to ensure that human rights protections are in place for those who are subject to quarantine or shelter-in-place orders. Shelter-in-place orders can be effective in reducing the spread of COVID-19, but their effectiveness depends on compliance and enforcement. It is important to communicate the rationale for these policies and provide support for those who are affected by them.

7.3.1 Life Under Lockdown

Life under lockdown can be challenging, particularly for those who live alone or have limited social support. The pandemic has highlighted the importance of social connections and the need for creative solutions to maintain these connections during lockdowns. Lockdowns can have different effects on different communities, with some groups being disproportionately affected by these policies. It is important to consider the needs of vulnerable populations when implementing lockdowns and shelter-in-place orders. The impact of lockdowns on mental health and wellbeing is an important consideration, and support services should be made available to those who need them. This can include telehealth services and online support groups.

7.4 Essential Worker

Essential workers are individuals who perform critical jobs that cannot be done remotely and are necessary to maintain the basic functions of society during the COVID-19 pandemic. These workers have been on the front lines of the pandemic, putting themselves at risk to provide essential services to the public. The following are some examples of essential workers:

7.4.1 Healthcare Workers

All paid and unpaid persons serving in healthcare settings who have the potential for direct or indirect exposure to patients or infectious materials, including those not directly involved in patient care but potentially exposed to infectious agents while working in a healthcare setting.

7.4.2 Frontline Essential Worker

This subset of essential workers is likely at the highest risk for work-related exposure to SARS-CoV-2, the virus that causes COVID-19, because their work-related duties must be performed on-site and involve being in proximity (<6 feet) to the public or to coworkers.

7.5 Other Essential Workers

This category includes essential workers not included in Phase 1a or 1b, such as those who maintain critical infrastructure and continue critical services and functions.

7.5.1 Grocery Store Workers

Workers in grocery stores, health care, delivery services, retail establishments, agriculture, and other essential industries have remained on the job despite the pandemic.

7.5.2 Low-Wage Essential Workers

These workers generally include racially diverse, low-wage workers whose jobs require close interaction with the public and/or proximity to their coworkers, placing them at increased risk of infection.

7.6 Contact Tracing

The practice of tracking and tracing individuals who may have been exposed to the virus led to the increased use of this term.

7.7 Zoom Bombing

With the rise of virtual meetings and classes, the term "Zoom bombing" emerged to describe the intrusion of uninvited individuals into online sessions.

7.8 Infodemic

This term refers to the rapid spread of misinformation and disinformation during the pandemic.

7.9 Covidiot

A derogatory term emerged to describe individuals who blatantly ignored safety guidelines or engaged in risky behaviour during the pandemic.

7.10. Pandemic Pod

This term described a small, controlled group of people who chose to interact exclusively with one another to minimize the risk of virus transmission.

7.11 WFH (Work From Home)

The acronym Work from Home "WFH" gained popularity as millions of people transitioned to remote work setups.

7.12 Asymptomatic and Pre-symptomatic

These terms became essential in describing individuals who carry the virus but do not display symptoms.

7.13 Long COVID

A term used to describe persistent symptoms in individuals who have recovered from the acute phase of the disease.

7.14 Vaccine Hesitancy

With the development of COVID-19 vaccines, this term came to represent the reluctance of some individuals to get vaccinated.

7.15 Variants of Concern

Terms like "Alpha," "Beta," "Delta," etc., were used to identify and categorize different strains of the virus.

7.16 Vaccine Passport

A vaccine passport is a digital or paper document that shows proof of vaccination against COVID-19. It is typically issued by a government or health authority and may include a scannable QR code. Vaccine passports have been implemented in some countries and jurisdictions as part of efforts to control the COVID-19 pandemic via vaccination. The use of vaccine passports is based on the general presumption that a vaccinated individual would be less likely to transmit SARS-CoV-2 to others and less likely to experience a severe outcome if they were to be infected. Vaccine passports can be used to gain access to certain establishments, activities, and events, and may be required for international travel. The availability of vaccines during the height of the COVID-19 pandemic prompted the idea of implementing a vaccine passport system. The concept was that an official registry of who was vaccinated would allow companies to fully open for business to anyone who shows proof of vaccination, thus helping to boost economies while limiting the spread of the disease. For years, people who have travelled to certain areas of the world have needed to show papers or a medical passport called a yellow card, created by the World Health Organization (WHO), to prove that they have gotten vaccines against diseases like yellow fever. While vaccine passports can be useful in controlling the spread of COVID-19, there are concerns about their potential impact on equality and individual liberties. In addition, vaccine passports may not be accessible to everyone, particularly those who cannot get vaccinated due to medical reasons or those who do not have access to the technology needed to obtain a vaccine passport.

7.17 Hybrid Learning

Hybrid learning, which combines elements of face-to-face and online learning, has become increasingly popular during the COVID-19 pandemic. Hybrid learning has been found to be effective in mastering course outcomes and achieving success in higher education institutions during the pandemic. The study suggests that a specific type of hybrid learning model was the most effective in achieving these outcomes. Teachers faced challenges in adapting their classroom pedagogical practices to online teaching during the pandemic. However, hybrid teaching has allowed educators to incorporate elements of conventional face-to-face learning methods with structured online schemes. Hybrid learning was found to be a more effective learning modality than remote learning alone, despite lower satisfaction levels in online courses. However, remote classrooms have lower attendance and interest than on-site classes. Hybrid learning has been associated with child behaviour and sleep concerns during the pandemic. However, the prevalence of these concerns was not significantly different between remote and hybrid schooling. Students have reported being less attentive and motivated during remote learning compared to before the pandemic. However, hybrid learning has been found to be effective in maintaining student engagement and motivation. Adaptations to hybrid teaching and learning made during the COVID-19 pandemic may become standard in the workplace. This highlights the potential long-term impact of hybrid learning on education and training.

7.18 Zoom Fatigue

Zoom fatigue, also known as videoconferencing fatigue, is a phenomenon that has emerged during the COVID-19 pandemic because of increased use of video conferencing platforms for work, education, and social interactions. The technostress model is used to explain the factors contributing to Zoom fatigue, including the increased cognitive load, constant self-evaluation, and reduced nonverbal cues in videoconferencing interactions. Zoom fatigue is characterized by feelings of exhaustion, burnout, and decreased motivation after participating in videoconferencing activities. Factors such as the length and frequency of videoconferencing sessions, the number of participants, and the nature of the tasks being performed can contribute to the development of Zoom fatigue. Strategies for reducing Zoom fatigue include taking regular breaks, practicing self-care, and implementing effective meeting management techniques. While some studies suggest that Zoom fatigue is a real and significant issue during the pandemic. Others argue that it may be influenced by individual differences and other factors, and further research is needed to fully understand the phenomenon.

7.19 Quarantine 15

The term "Quarantine 15" refers to the weight gain that many people experienced during the COVID-19 pandemic while staying at home and facing disruptions to their daily routines. The pandemic created a perfect storm for weight gain, with gym and park closures disrupting exercise routines and increased stress levels for parents who had to work from home while also teaching their children. Some of the specific challenges that contributed to weight gain during the pandemic include:

8. LIMITED ACCESS TO PHYSICAL ACTIVITY

Gym and park closures, as well as restrictions on outdoor activities, made it difficult for people to maintain their regular exercise routines.

8.1 Increased Stress Levels

The pandemic brought about significant stress for many individuals, which can lead to increased cortisol levels and a higher intake of hyperpalatable foods (foods high in salt, fat, or both).

8.2 Changes in Eating Habits

With more time spent at home, people may have turned to comfort foods or engaged in stress eating, leading to an increase in calorie intake.

8.3 Lack of Structure and Routine

The disruption to daily schedules and the blurring of boundaries between work and home life may have contributed to unhealthy eating habits and a lack of portion control.

8.4 Emotional Eating

The uncertainty and anxiety surrounding the pandemic may have caused some individuals to turn to food for comfort, leading to weight gain.

8.5 Remote Socializing

Remote socializing has become increasingly important during the COVID-19 pandemic to combat social isolation and maintain social connections.

8.6 Tips for Remote Socializing

Use video chat, conference calling, and text chat to connect with others outside of isolation. Create a sense of belonging while working remotely by engaging in physical interaction, such as stepping out of your home to work with friends. Make time for socializing during the workday, such as virtual coffee breaks or happy hours. Participate in online communities or groups related to your interests or hobbies. Be intentional about maintaining social connections, such as scheduling regular virtual hangouts with friends and family. Take advantage of workplace socialization opportunities, such as virtual team-building activities.

8.7 Findings on Remote Socializing

Social isolation can become one of the biggest pitfalls faced by remote workers. It is important to create a sense of proximity and belonging while working remotely. Remote work can increase the amount of control that people have over their level of social interaction. For some, this may mean less social interaction, while for others, it may mean more. The COVID-19 pandemic has made remote work and socialization important topics of concern for businesses. Companies may need to provide more opportunities for socialization as remote work becomes more common. Studies have shown that virtual teams can effectively manage technology-enabled social interaction with colleagues at a distance. This can help to maintain social connections and reduce social isolation.

9. CONCLUSION

In conclusion, the role of language during the COVID-19 pandemic has been multifaceted and central to how individuals, communities, and governments have navigated the crisis. Language has served as a critical tool for communication, information dissemination, and sense-making in the face of unprecedented challenges. In essence, language has been both a tool and a reflection of the challenges and responses during the COVID-19 pandemic. It has underscored the importance of clear, transparent, and trustworthy communication in public health crises, while also highlighting the capacity of individuals and societies to adapt and come together in times of adversity. As the pandemic continues to evolve, the role of language in shaping our understanding and response remains as critical as ever.

REFERENCES

Cardoso, F. M., Meloni, S., Santanchè, A., & Moreno, Y. (2019). Topical alignment in online social systems. *Frontiers in Physics (Lausanne)*, *7*, 58. doi:10.3389/fphy.2019.00058

Cinelli, M., Quattrociocchi, W., Galeazzi, A., Valensise, C. M., Brugnoli, E., Schmidt, A. L., Zola, P., Zollo, F., & Scala, A. (2020). The COVID-19 social media infodemic. *Scientific Reports*, *10*(1), 1–10. doi:10.1038/s41598-020-73510-5 PMID:33024152

Derakhshan, A, (2020). Information Disorder: Toward an Interdisciplinary Framework for Research and Policymaking. Council of Europe.

Haug, N., Geyrhofer, L., Londei, A., Dervic, E., Desvars-Larrive, A., & Loreto, V. (2020). Ranking the effectiveness of worldwide COVID-19 government interventions. Academic Press.

Li, S., Wang, Y., Xue, J., Zhao, N., & Zhu, T. (2020). The Impact of COVID-19 Epidemic Declaration on Psychological Consequences: A Study on Active Weibo Users. *International Journal of Environmental Research and Public Health*, *17*(6), 2032. doi:10.3390/ijerph17062032 PMID:32204411

Moscadelli, A., Albora, G., Biamonte, M. A., Giorgetti, D., Innocenzio, M., Paoli, S., Lorini, C., Bonanni, P., & Bonaccorsi, G. (2020). Fake news and Covid-19 in Italy: Results of a quantitative observational study. *International Journal of Environmental Research and Public Health*, *17*(16), 5850. doi:10.3390/ijerph17165850 PMID:32806772

Rothe, C., Schunk, M., Sothmann, P., Bretzel, G., Froeschl, G., Wallrauch, C., Zimmer, T., Thiel, V., Janke, C., Guggemos, W., Seilmaier, M., Drosten, C., Vollmar, P., Zwirglmaier, K., Zange, S., Wölfel, R., & Hoelscher, M. (2020). Transmission of 2019-nCoV infection from an asymptomatic contact in Germany. *The New England Journal of Medicine*, *382*(10), 970–971. doi:10.1056/NEJMc2001468 PMID:32003551

Rubin, E. J., Baden, L. R., Morrissey, S., & Campion, E. W. (2020). Medical journals and the 2019-nCoV outbreak. *The New England Journal of Medicine*, *382*(9), 866. doi:10.1056/NEJMe2001329 PMID:31986242

Singer, M. K., Dressler, W., & George, S. (2016). Culture: The missing link in health research. *Social Science & Medicine*, *170*, 237–246. doi:10.1016/j.socscimed.2016.07.015 PMID:27542574

World Health Organization. (2021). Weekly epidemiological update on COVID-19—14 September 2021. https://www.who.int/publications/m/item/weekly-epidemiological-update-on-covid-19---14-september-2021

Chapter 6
Cultural Perspectives on Health Communication:
The Case of Katkari Tribals in Western Maharashtra, India

Manisha Nitin Gore
Symbiosis International University (Deemed), India

Reshma Patil
Symbiosis Medical College for Women (Deemed), India

Revati Pathak
Symbiosis International University (Deemed), India

ABSTRACT

Communication is a fundamental aspect of human existence, serving as a platform for sharing information and conveying symbolic meaning. Public health communication is crucial for disease prevention, health promotion, emergency preparedness, and vaccine advocacy. A qualitative study applied the framework of 'Communication Anthropology' to understand cultural sensitivity, contextual nuances, recommendations within a specific tribal community in western Maharashtra, India. Themes "Uncovering the Sources of Health Communication Dynamics in a Tribal Community," "Impact of Media and Technology on Tribal Community Health and Lifestyle," and "Cultural Influences on Tribal Health Behavior" emerged from the study. Enhancing health communication for India's tribal populations requires culturally tailored strategies. Involving local communities is recommended, leveraging traditional art and local artists to convey health messages effectively. Integrating multimedia such as radio jingles and videos, incentivizing healthcare workers, and utilizing visual aids with simplified language can further enhance health communication.

DOI: 10.4018/979-8-3693-0624-6.ch006

COMMUNICATION AND PUBLIC HEALTH COMMUNICATION

Communication lies at the core of our human existence, an essential aspect of our identity. It aids as our platform of sharing information and echoes our symbolic prowess. These dual functions align with James Carey's distinction between the transmission and ritual perspectives of communication. Carey acknowledged that communication not only plays an instrumental role, such as facilitating knowledge acquisition but also fulfils a ritualistic function, emphasizing our role as participants in a social community (Rimal and Lapinski, 2009). Consequently, we can define communication as the symbolic exchange of shared meaning, encompassing both transmission and ritualistic elements within all communicative acts (Rimal and Lapinski, 2009). This aligns with the Oxford English dictionary's definition, which defines communication as "The imparting or exchanging of information by speaking, writing, or using some other medium" and as "The successful conveying or sharing of ideas and feelings (Oxford)." Both definitions highlight the exchange of information and the shared understanding of ideas and emotions as central components of communication.

Healthy People 2010 offers a definition of health communication as "the art and technique of informing, influencing, and motivating individual, institutional, and public audiences about important health issues." Simultaneously, the Institute of Medicine (IOM) defines public health as "what we, as a society, do collectively to assure the conditions in which people can be healthy." By combining these two perspectives, a new definition emerges: Public Health communication embodies the scientific advancement, strategic distribution, and meticulous evaluation of pertinent, precise, easily accessible, and comprehensible health information conveyed to and from intended audiences, all with the ultimate aim of promoting public health. Public health communication is an indispensable tool in safeguarding the health of individuals and communities. It serves several critical purposes, including disease prevention, health promotion, emergency preparedness, and vaccine advocacy (Bernhardt, 2004). During disease outbreaks, it provides vital information on preventive measures and vaccination campaigns. In everyday life, it encourages healthy behaviors and discourages risky ones, reducing the burden of chronic diseases (Bernhardt, 2004).

Public health communication is also essential in emergency situations, disseminating evacuation instructions and updates during natural disasters and crises. It supports policy development by conveying scientific evidence to policymakers and the public, influencing the adoption of health-promoting policies (Bioterror, 2013). Additionally, it addresses health disparities by targeting vulnerable populations and engaging communities in tailored interventions (Horowitz and Lawlor 2008). Moreover, public health communication empowers individuals to make informed decisions about their health, fostering behaviour change and reducing misinformation. It plays a pivotal role in managing public panic during crises by providing accurate information (Porat et al., 2020) Continuous research and evaluation refine communication strategies, ensuring they are evidence-based and effective. In today's information-rich environment, public health communication bridges the gap between healthcare providers, policymakers, and the public (Hartley, 2004). Its success lies in its ability to inform, educate, and motivate individuals to prioritize health, ultimately contributing to the well-being of society.

HEALTH STATUS OF THE TRIBAL POPULATION

In context to minority population, there is no universally accepted definition for indigenous peoples or ethnic minorities. Typically, they share identity, language, religion, or distinct characteristics and may not be in a dominant position within a nation. This can result from numerical differences, cultural uniqueness, or a desire to preserve their traits, whether due to migration or colonization (World Bank, 2023) . Estimating the global indigenous population varies but ranges from 300 million to 400 million. Counting ethnic minorities is complex due to differing definitions and data collection methods. For instance, in China, 113 million people identified as ethnic minorities in 2010, while India had 104 million Scheduled Tribes and 201 million Scheduled Castes in 2011. Latin America estimated 130 million people of African descent in 2015, and in the United States, over a third identified as diverse racial and ethnic groups in 2016 (UN,2018).

Tribe and Tribal in context to this chapter refers to Tribe is a social group, usually with a definite are, dialect, cultural homogeneity, and unifying social organization. It may include several subs - groups, such as sibs or villages. It may and may have common ancestor as well as presiding deities. The families or small communities making up a tribe, are linked through economic, social, religious, or blood ties i.e. kingship bondage (Sneath, 2016). The "Katkari" is a scheduled tribe in India (The Scheduled Castes and Scheduled Tribes are officially designated groups of people and among the most disadvantaged socio-economic groups in India. The terms are recognized in the Constitution of India and the groups are designated in one or other of the categories) (NCST,2023). The tribal community is considered indigenous because they are the original inhabitants of a particular region, often predating the establishment of modern nation-states. They have a unique cultural, historical, and social identity tied to their ancestral lands. Additionally, tribal communities are often characterized by distinct languages, customs, and traditional knowledge that set them apart. Tribal communities are considered minority communities due to their relatively smaller population compared to the majority population in a given country (Golbéry, 2000). Hence "Katkari" the target population of this research study are termed as tribal in this chapter.

About the health status of the tribal populations- Globally, they experience pronounced health disparities. Approximately 15% of the world's extreme poor are tribal people, and they have limited healthcare access. They face higher rates of infectious diseases, with tuberculosis incidence up to 20 times the global average. Malnutrition and inadequate sanitation are common issues, necessitating targeted interventions and policies to address their marginalized health status (Hall and Gandolfo, 2016).

Equally, in India, with 8.6% of its population belonging to tribal communities, it faces a formidable challenge in narrowing the healthcare disparity between tribal and non-tribal populations. The tribal populace bears a complex burden almost quadruple of diseases, encompassing communicable illnesses, non-communicable conditions, malnutrition, mental health issues, and substance addiction, all exacerbated by suboptimal healthcare-seeking behaviour (Kumar et al., 2020).

Public Health Communication becomes crucial for tribal, as it can empower them with vital information and resources to address the high prevalence of diseases, lower life expectancies, thus reducing health disparities. By effectively delivering health information, it can promote better access to healthcare services and improve overall health outcomes within these communities. Nonetheless, there is a pressing requirement for culturally sensitive communication. Such communication serves as a vital tool in fostering trust, surmounting access barriers, streamlining health information, empowering individuals, involving communities, facilitating precise interventions, advocating for policy changes, and assisting in crisis response (Ramalinareddy,2016).

Given its focus on people, anthropology is another field that can make a significant contribution to public health communication. It is defined as the scientific study of humanity, concerned with human behaviour, human biology, cultures, societies, and linguistics, in both the present and past, including past human species. Particularly "Communication Anthropology," can be seamlessly integrated into public health communication. It goes beyond conventional media-centric approaches, recognizing communication's intricate web, including natural communication forms, cultural metaphors in media, and social and cultural dynamics among message sources, mediums, and receivers. Communication's impact is thoroughly analyzed, considering aspects like value, message content, practices, accessibility, reach, understanding, credibility, response, and the factors influencing message acceptance or rejection (Sinha, 2021).

Citing an example of the Ebola epidemic-anthropology employed the ethnographic method to gain insights into cultures through interviews and observation. For health communication practitioners situated outside the target communities, anthropology's key contribution lay in its ability to act as a bridge, facilitating a "translation" of sorts between these communities. It helped outsiders comprehend the intricacies of a society, as well as the significance it held for its inhabitants. The Ebola crisis demonstrated that the medical, crisis response, and governmental sectors didn't always fully grasp the concerns and perspectives of affected communities or appreciate how profoundly these worldviews could impact the efforts of health workers in containing the disease. That is the reason health communication professionals employed ethnography to comprehend and engage with diverse cultures. They gain insights into the structure of societies and people's self-perceptions. This knowledge helped in promoting health ideas and behaviours to prevent illness within these communities (Cobb, 2015).

An article from US highlights significance of anthropological research in the field of health literacy on the influence of culture and life experiences on health-related communication that enrich the extensive literature on communication and specifically on science communication (Rikard et.al., 2016). In the UK during the COVID-19 pandemic, health communication played a crucial role, especially for ethnic minorities who were disproportionately affected. This study investigates how health information was communicated within ethnic communities during the pandemic, focusing on their experiences with primary healthcare services. Qualitative methods, including focus groups and interviews, were used with community members and leaders from three ethnic minority groups. However, communication and information available to them were reported to be insufficient (Ekezie,2022). These are some of examples of integration of anthropology in the health communication to deal with the public health issues at the global front. However, there is complete scarcity of literature in this particular area in India.

To fill the research void, qualitative research was planned on a specific tribe in western Maharashtra, applying the framework of 'Communication Anthropology' to comprehend cultural sensitivity, contextual understanding, barrier identification, and policy guidance, to strategize culturally tailored healthcare communication and outcomes.

The list of objectives:

1. To study the sources of health communication of the tribals (Katkaris) residing in western Maharashtra.
2. To study the communication process in detail using perspective of "Communication Anthropology" of the tribals (Katkaris) residing in western Maharashtra.

METHODS

The university initiated the Symbiosis Community Outreach Programme and Extension (SCOPE) as part of its health-promotion initiatives in the month of July 2012. The program aims to improve the well-being of the local community surrounding the university by empowering them to identify and advance their health initiatives. SCOPE focuses on proactive, community-driven, sustainable socio-economic, and environmental efforts. The SCOPE team commenced its work in 35 designated villages which comprises 27% of the total Mulshi block population within the western region of the state of Maharashtra, India, operating through two permanent Mobile Medical Units (MMU). MMUs provide weekly primary health check-ups in selected villages with a team including a Medical Officer, Nurse, Medical Social Worker, and a driver. The station sites are selected in coordination with the local village representative and as per the feasibility of MMU movement. Referrals are made for specialist care when needed or Symbiosis University Hospital and Research Centre (SUHRC).

Apart from the MMU the health initiative involves general check-up camps at various locations, including schools, labor camps, and migrant worker areas. Mega camps, of Health Check-up, are organized with the help from inter-institute, inter organizations collaboration. Health awareness sessions are conducted in alignment with government health days, with support for events like the Pulse Polio Immunization drive and National Nutritional Week.

In SCOPE, out of the 35 villages surveyed, 10 contain tribal hamlets. Within these villages, 1005 individuals, comprising 2% of the total population of 48242, have identified themselves as tribal. The Katkari, classified as one of India's 75 Particularly Vulnerable Tribal Groups by the Ministry of Home Affairs, primarily inhabit Maharashtra (Pune, Raigad, and Thane districts) and parts of Gujarat. Often referred to as Kathodis, their name stems from their traditional occupation of crafting Katha (Catechu) from the sap of the Khair tree. The Katkari community is engaged in various activities, including agricultural labor, firewood and jungle fruit sales, fishing, coal production, and brick manufacturing. Unfortunately, they contend with challenges such as low literacy rates, subpar health conditions, and limited livelihood opportunities, highlighting the need for targeted support. The Katkari community has a rich history of rice cultivation, which continues if they possess small plots of land or leased parcels. After the agricultural season, starting soon after Diwali, able-bodied Katkaris traditionally migrate to work as daily wage laborers in brick kilns or construction sites, returning home around Holi (March). Their financial literacy remains poor, lacking a culture of savings, and relying on daily wages. This lifestyle, coupled with a lack of education, contributes to their limited employment opportunities in local industries. Furthermore, their lack of financial knowledge makes them vulnerable to exploitation by traders, especially when selling forest-based products. Girls often drop out of school after marrying in their teenage years, compounding the issue (Dwivedi,2016).

The interview guide encompassed questions regarding health communication sources, techniques, and protocols, alongside the integration of cultural nuances into health communication strategies, individual experiences, and needs regarding health communication. Interviews with Medical Officer, Primary Health Centre, ASHA working in the tribal regions, local stakeholders such as Sarpanch, Grampanchayat, Member of Grampanchayat, Principal of School and with tribal people were conducted. The detailed profile of the respondents is given in the results section. Before the data collection the interview tool underwent pilot testing to confirm its effectiveness, clarity, and cultural appropriateness. This testing phase involved a small sample, during which researchers identified and addressed potential issues, evaluated the interview's flow and timing, and provided training to the two interviewers in qualitative data collection. A total of

20 in-depth interviews are executed by two Medical Social Workers (MSW) of the outreach team of SCOPE. The MSWs, who had been closely connected to the community for over a decade, approached the interviewees and conducted the interviews. The interviewers were proficient in the local Marathi language and conducted the interviews in this native language. The principal investigator provided them with training in qualitative interview techniques. The interviews were audio recorded, transcribed and translated to English. The qualitative data was entered in the MAXQDA (version 11) software for analysis. The data were analysed using inductive approach with thematic framework. Thematic qualitative analysis systematically identifies recurring patterns, themes, and concepts in collected data, providing a deeper understanding of participants' experiences and perspectives. The process involved data familiarization, coding meaningful units, and organizing them into broader themes, yielding a comprehensive narrative and valuable insights. Thematic analysis offered flexibility and rigor, enabling rich interpretations from qualitative data. Participants who could read and write provided written informed consent, while those unable to read and write provided thumb impressions. Prior to this, all participants were thoroughly briefed on the study and the consent procedure.

RESULTS

The sample comprised two Medical Officers from the Primary Health Centers (PHCs), six ASHAs, seven-gram panchayat members, including one village head (Sarpanch), and five tribal individuals from various villages. Both Medical Officers held Bachelor of Ayurvedic Medicine and Surgery (BAMS) degrees. It was observed that ASHAs were qualified up to higher secondary level, while some gram panchayat members were illiterate, and others had studied up to the secondary level. Among the five tribal individuals, three were illiterate, and two had completed education up to the secondary level. Apart from the Medical Officers and ASHAs, most respondents were engaged in farming, daily wage labour, and various small-scale businesses such as fishing and self-help group activities. Furthermore, each Medical Officer had accumulated six to eight years of experience working with tribal communities. Additionally, the current gram panchayat had been operational for the past 2.5 years.

Abbreviations:
SSC: Secondary School Certificate (10th standard)
HSC: Higher Secondary Certificate (12th standard)
ASHA: Accredited Social Health Activist (ASHA)
Definitions:

Gram Panchayat: Gram Panchayat is a basic village institute of a formal and democratic structure at the grassroots level in India. It acts as a cabinet of the village. It is a political institute.

Sarpanch: It is a designation and he/she is the elected head of a village and serves his/her duty in the village level statutory institution called "Gram Panchayat".

Secretary of Gram Panchayat (Vice-Sarpanch): The Secretary of the Panchayat is a non-elected representative, appointed by the state government, to oversees the activities.

Members of Gram Panchayat: The Gram Panchayat is divided into wards and a Ward Member or Commissioner represents each ward, also referred to as a Panch or Panchayat Member, whom the villagers directly elect. The number of members usually ranges from 7 to 31; occasionally, groups

Table 1. Profile of the participants

Sr. No	Code	Type of stakeholder	Sex	Age	Education	Occupation	No. of Years of experience working with Katkari (Tribal)
1	RIHM1	Medical Officer	M	43	BAMS	Medical Officer	6
2	NANM1	Medical Officer	M	48	BAMS	Medical Officer	8
3	AND1	ASHA	F	53	9	ASHA	13
4	NAN1	ASHA	F	43	10	ASHA	9
5	NAN2	ASHA	F	43	10	ASHA	15
6	NAN3	ASHA	F	35	10	ASHA	15
7	RIH4	ASHA	F	30	10	ASHA	10
8	NAN6	ASHA	F	25	10	ASHA	3
9	AND2	Sarpanch	M	32	12	Buisness	2.5
10	AND3	GP member	M	24	7	Daily wages	NA
11	RIH1	GP member	F	35	Not literate	Daily wages	NA
12	ANDS1	GP member	F	42	Not literate	Farming	NA
13	BHD1	GP member	F	55	Not literate	Farming, fishing	NA
14	RIH2	GP member	M	30	10	Daily wages	NA
15	RIH3	GP member	F	45	9	Farming	NA
16	ANDS2	GP member	M	45	12	Buisness	NA
17	ANDS2	Secretary-GP	M	50	12	Farming	NA
18	NAN4	Community	F	53	Not literate	Farming	NA
19	NAN5	Community	M	45	9	Farming	NA
20	BHD2	Community	F	28	8	Farming, Self Help Group Activities	NA
21	BHD3	Community	F	40	Not literate	Daily wages	NA
22	AND3	Community	F	55	Not literate	Farming	NA

are larger, but they never have fewer than seven members. One-third of seats of the Panchayat are reserved for women. Seats are also reserved for Scheduled Castes/ Tribes.

The Panchayat Samiti: It is a body that supervises and coordinates the working of Gram Panchayats. It acts as a link between the Gram Panchayat and Zila Parishad.

Medical Officer of PHC: He is the head of the health team at the Primary Health Centre.

Please find below the themes-the qualitative findings.

UNCOVERING THE SOURCES OF HEALTH COMMUNICATION DYNAMICS IN A TRIBAL COMMUNITY

The source of health communication in this context primarily involves the Ministry of Health and Family Welfare, which channels information through a series of intermediaries to reach the target beneficiaries, particularly the tribal communities. Health information flows from the Ministry of Health and Family Welfare to the Primary Health Centres (PHCs) and then to Accredited Social Health Activists (ASHAs), who are responsible for delivering health messages to the community. The communication flow is predominantly vertical, originating from the Ministry and extending through the health system to the population. Occasionally, special messages are conveyed directly to the Sarpanch (village head), Attendants, and the population. Besides PHCs and ASHAs, voluntary Non-Government Organizations (NGOs) are also active in disseminating health messages related to their projects within the community. The tribal population has limited access to digital gadgets and smartphones, so digital communication methods are not widely used among them. During emergencies, mobile health vehicles are employed to disseminate health messages across villages. WhatsApp groups exist village-wise, but only a few tribal members access these messages. They prefer attending regular community meetings and accessing government benefits through Aadhaar cards and the Ayushman Bharat scheme. Many tribal households have televisions, and health messages aired on TV are sometimes watched and followed. For tribal residing in brick kiln, the brick kiln owners.

ASHA'S CRUCIAL ROLE

ASHAs are instrumental in conveying various health messages related to antenatal care (ANC), postnatal care (PNC), pregnancy care, sanitation, hygiene, children's vaccination, adolescent health, including topics like menstruation, anemia, diet, and nutrition. ASHAs communicate in Marathi, which the tribal population understands, even though their native language is different.ASHA workers are considered the direct source of health information, but they are also in contact with other intermediaries like Multipurpose Workers (MPWs), Auxiliary Nurse Midwives (ANMs), and Anganwadi Workers, as well as members of the gram panchayat (village council). The tribal population trusts government hospitals and health professionals, such as ASHAs, MOs (Medical Officers), and ANMs. They attend health check-up camps organized by these entities.

ASHA mentioned that the tribal community has now become more receptive to me. They no longer evade me as they did before, but I still face significant challenges in imparting knowledge and lessons to them.

The quote is of ....an ASHA

ACCESS TO MOBILE PHONES AND TELEVISION

Most community members have mobile phones, but they are not smartphones, so they can make calls but have limited access to digital resources. Television serves a vital role in the community, providing access to daily news, weather updates, and information about government schemes that assist with housing, electricity, personal cleanliness, and hygiene. Notably, there are only two TV sets available in the entire village.

PREFERENCE FOR PHYSICAL INTERACTION

Despite the availability of digital resources, the community prefers physical interaction to receive health messages and trusts health professionals like ASHAs for health-related information.

In summary, health communication in this context relies heavily on ASHA workers and government health professionals, supplemented by occasional TV broadcasts. Digital communication is limited due to the community's lack of access to smartphones and a preference for in-person interactions.

IMPACT OF MEDIA AND TECHNOLOGY ON TRIBAL COMMUNITY HEALTH AND LIFESTYLE

This qualitative analysis highlights the evolving influence of media and technology on the health and lifestyle of a tribal community. Several key observations emerge from the provided information.

The tribal have limited access to smartphones. Only a small fraction of the tribal population around 10 to 12 individuals out of the 112 people from a single village owns smartphones, which are not widely accessible in the community. Men have smart phones than women. Those with smartphones tend to spend their time on entertainment videos and social media, rather than health-related content. Television also plays a significant role in the community, providing information on various topics, including health, government schemes, and lifestyle changes. Media, particularly smartphone content and television, has led to positive lifestyle changes. These include improved personal hygiene, dietary choices (such as consuming sprouts and leafy vegetables), and awareness of health risks (e.g., chewing tobacco). Younger community members actively engage with social media, experimenting with recipes and adopting new habits from online sources. While social media is used for entertainment and social interaction, it is not a primary source of health information for this community. They tend to trust traditional healthcare providers, like the Primary Health Centre (PHC), over social media for health-related issues. Access to media and technology has contributed to improved socioeconomic conditions, including better housing, transportation (two-wheelers), and job opportunities in private and semi-private sectors.Media, especially television, has a significant influence on children's behavior, as they are influenced by advertisements and often request snacks and products they see on TV.

A few positive impacts as reported by the ASHA

They paid heed to our messages about dengue, taking actions such as adding diesel to stagnant water and maintaining the cleanliness of water storage containers on a regular basis.

The stakeholder observed a change in the health behavior of adolescent girls, specifically a transition from using cloth to sanitary pads due to their exposure to television and media. However, it's important to note that this shift is only accessible to those who can afford sanitary pads.

In summary, the impact of media and technology in this tribal community is multifaceted, affecting lifestyle choices, health awareness, and socioeconomic conditions. While smartphones and television have brought about positive changes, traditional healthcare providers remain a trusted source for health information. The younger generation is more adaptable to new practices and technologies, while children are particularly influenced by media content.

CULTURAL INFLUENCES ON TRIBAL HEALTH BEHAVIOR

The influence of culture on the tribal community's health behavior is profound and pervasive. The tribal feels "Cultural Disconnect". The tribal culture is distinct from the mainstream culture, and this cultural gap results in the community's reluctance to accept health messages and abandon their rituals and traditions. They reflect "Cultural Resilience" they strongly adhere to their cultural practices even when exposed to modern scientific information. They prioritize their cultural traditions over spending money on health or quitting addictions.

It was found that the tribal community maintains a sceptical attitude toward government healthcare services, often preferring to sticking to their cultural practices, including home deliveries. Despite health warnings and tragic incidents, such as a case of oral cancer due to tobacco chewing, the tribal community remains steadfast in their addiction habits, particularly tobacco use and drinking. The negative attitude was also observed during the COVID-19 pandemic, the community exhibited a lack of positive response to health initiatives, such as screening, testing, and vaccination. Their engagement often hinges on expecting monetary benefits from the government.

In context to spreading of the health messages they are very selective tends to share information primarily with those in close proximity, maintaining a sense of isolation. They trust the brick kiln owners, agriculture farm landlords. However, leadership figures like the Sarpanch or any other educated member from their community can influence the community's behavior to some extent, particularly when they perceive the leader as someone who has helped them in the past. There were obvious challenges in the communication especially as they health messages would not translate into any positive behaviour the change would take time. They believe the knowledge gained from their ancestors which has come to them from the previous generation. ASHA incorporates cultural understanding into her approach when delivering health messages within the community.

In summary, the tribal community's culture strongly shapes their health behavior and attitudes. Cultural practices and traditions are deeply ingrained, making it challenging to alter health-related behaviors, even when confronted with health risks. Building trust, delivering culturally tailored messages, and engaging with community leaders are crucial steps in addressing health challenges within this cultural context.

MAINTAINING CONFIDENTIALITY IN THE COMMUNICATION AND UNDERSTANDING HEALTH BEHAVIOUR

Ensuring confidentiality while sharing sensitive information, such as TB and Leprosy positivity or pregnancy status, often relies on non-verbal communication, including sign language and body language within the group. Reinforcing information is a common practice, as the community members understand but don't consistently translate knowledge into behavior change. For instance, while they comprehend

Marathi and Hindi, encouraging practices like proper handwashing before meals may require persistent reminders. Motivation plays a crucial role in their adherence to health instructions. Sometimes, they comply when the message is tied to consequences, like withholding medicine for those who continue drinking. Otherwise, preventive measures tend to be overlooked unless they become serious, chronic, or symptomatic. Group discussions and meetings prove more effective than one-on-one communication. There is optimism that their situation will improve over time, thanks to the efforts of the Sarpanch who has facilitated housing, water supply, toilets, and encouraged tree planting. The community takes pride in their ability to maintain secrecy using their own code language. Approximately 80% of the community members follow instructions, while 20% do not. Interestingly, the influence of TV and smartphones on the community's health has been limited. However, they exhibit a keen interest in messages about vaccination, health check-ups, and government schemes, actively participating in vaccination drives and screening camps. This engagement suggests the potential for positive health outcomes within the tribal community.

ASHA reported

Considering that they are daily wage labourers who are concerned about potential wage losses. In such cases, we coordinate with the owner (brick kiln and agriculture landlord) who then arranges for them to attend the check-up camp. This process has streamlined their access to healthcare, whereas previously, it was challenging for them.

Improving the process of health messages in tribal communities requires a comprehensive approach that takes into account their unique needs and challenges. Here are some key needs to enhance the effectiveness of health messaging in tribal communities:

STRATEGIES TO ENHANCE HEALTH COMMUNICATION FOR TRIBAL COMMUNITIES

Health messages should be culturally sensitive and adapted to the traditions, beliefs, and language of the tribal community. Using local dialects and respecting cultural practices can make the messages more relatable. Involve community members in the design and delivery of health messages. Engage with tribal leaders and respected people from the community.to build trust and credibility within the community. Utilize visual aids, videos, and interactive materials that are easy to understand, especially for those with limited literacy. This can help convey health information effectively. Implement health literacy programs to enhance the community's understanding of health issues, preventive measures, and the importance of healthcare-seeking behavior. Develop behaviour change communication strategies that go beyond information sharing. Encourage active participation and practical demonstrations of health-promoting behaviors. Train and deploy community health workers or ASHA workers who are familiar with the community's culture and language. They can serve as trusted intermediaries in delivering health messages. Explore the use of mobile phones for delivering health messages via text messages, voice recordings, or mobile apps. Ensure that messages are accessible on non-smartphones as well. Strengthen local healthcare facilities, making them accessible, affordable, and culturally sensitive. This can encourage community members to seek medical advice and treatment. Consider providing non-monetary incentives, such as access to clean water, sanitation facilities, or improved housing, to motivate the community to adopt healthier behaviors. Regularly assess the impact of health messaging programs to make necessary adjustments. Gather feedback from the community to understand their perceptions and needs better. Collaborate with tribal leaders, NGOs, and government agencies to create a holistic approach to tribal health. Work together to address not only health but also socio-economic factors contributing to health disparities. Focus on long-term sustainability by involving the community in decision-making and capacity building. Empower community members to take ownership of their health. Develop health for promotions of health messages that align with the tribal community's seasonal or cultural events to maximize engagement and relevance.

By addressing these needs, health messaging in tribal communities can become more effective, leading to improved health outcomes and better overall well-being of community members.

DISCUSSION

The tribal receive health education mostly from the ASHA through the health care system. The finding about her role as health educator is corroborated in different studies. The role of ASHA workers as crucial link workers, facilitating access to antenatal care and hospital deliveries for women. Their responsibilities include conducting regular home visits to identify and enroll pregnant women for antenatal care, improving accessibility to the Pradhan Mantri Matru Vandana Yojana (PMMVY) scheme, providing health education, distributing iron and folic acid tablets, arranging antenatal check-ups at Primary Health Centers (PHC), and accompanying women in labor to government health facilities for safe deliveries. This fulfilling but demanding role demands constant resourcefulness and presence of mind from ASHA workers (Kawade et al., 2021; Gore et al., 2022). Furthermore, ASHA workers established strong community connections as they were recruited from within the same locality, even though they were not tribal themselves but residents of neighbouring villages.

The research findings show that smartphone ownership among tribal communities varies significantly. Mostly men and young adults had smart phones than women. In some areas, particularly among young adult men, smartphones are prevalent, mainly used for entertainment and social media access on platforms like WhatsApp, Instagram, and Facebook. For instance, in Jharkhand, a study found that one-third of the surveyed tribal population had smartphones primarily for communication and entertainment (Singh, 2019). In contrast, central India, specifically Madhya Pradesh (MP), exhibits a higher smartphone penetration, with around 80% of tribal individuals having access to smartphones, primarily for entertainment purposes (Goswami,2017). Additionally, a study conducted in a north eastern state of India concerning mobile phone usage among students highlights a concerning trend of excessive smartphone usage, potentially indicative of addiction. This pervasive mobile phone use has notably negative consequences, impacting the students' overall well-being and academic performance (Chattopadhyay and Mohanty, 2022). It's worth noting that while there is research on various aspects of smartphone usage within tribal communities, there is a notable gap in studies explicitly addressing the use of mobile phones for health education in these populations. This suggests an area for potential future research and intervention to leverage mobile technology for improving health education within tribal communities.

The positive impact of media and technology on the lifestyle of tribal communities is a topic of increasing importance, as these advancements can bring about significant changes in various aspects of their lives, including housing, food, clothing, fashion, and entertainment. While traditional tribal lifestyles have unique cultural value, integrating modern media and technology can enhance the overall quality of life for these communities. However, a study in north eastern state of India reflected a direct connection between the consumption of new media and a growing cultural disconnect among the tribal youth. These young tribals were increasingly transitioning from their traditional cultural heritage towards a more urbanized lifestyle, which markedly differs from the way of life experienced by their ancestors. But whether the shift in the culture was having a positive impact on the tribal health need to be studied further (Chattopadhyay and Mohanty, 2022). In the context of American Indian and Alaska Native (AI/AN) adolescents and young adults, significant disparities exist in behavioral and mental health. Digital and media-based health interventions offer promise by overcoming geographical barriers. A study of 210 self-identified AI/AN students at tribal colleges revealed diverse and widespread technology usage, indicating the potential for technology-driven interventions to provide relevant information and behaviour change tools tailored to AI/AN young adults' unique perspectives and social contexts. (American). Though this study has shown a few of the events where the positive effect of media and technology is observed, but there is scarcity of research in this area (Sabato, 2018).

The study's findings underscore the significant influence of culture on the reception of health messages within tribal communities. While tribal individuals attentively listen to these messages, they remain steadfast in preserving their cultural norms and practices. This cultural adherence often manifests as resistance to abandoning addictive behaviors, getting vaccinated, or seeking medical treatment, resulting in suboptimal health-seeking behaviors.

The short review discusses the factors influencing health-seeking behaviour among tribal communities, emphasizing the interplay of socio-cultural beliefs, accessibility to modern healthcare, and changing dynamics due to globalization. Traditional tribal medicine is deeply rooted, influenced by cultural and supernatural beliefs. However, modern healthcare accessibility and affordability, as well as education, are leading some tribal groups, particularly the younger generation, to adopt modern medical practices. Factors such as the effectiveness of treatment and perceptions of disease causation influence this shift. Nevertheless, the write-up highlights the complex medical pluralism in tribal healthcare systems, with some communities still preferring traditional remedies for both simple and complex diseases. Overall, the transition toward modern healthcare in tribal communities is shaped by a combination of socio-cultural, economic, and healthcare accessibility factors (Islary, 2014). Tribal following gestures and code language to maintain confidentiality in the communication is the naïve finding of this research study. There is no research to confirm or contrast the finding. This mode of communication enables the preservation of confidentiality while disclosing sensitive information.

In the discussion section, we will explore the various strategies employed to improve health communication in diverse regions and among different populations. One of the critical aspects of effective healthcare delivery is the ability to communicate health information clearly and efficiently. In our study, we engaged key stakeholders to gather their insights on how to enhance communication with specific populations. The feedback we received emphasized several essential points. First, cultural sensitivity emerged as a crucial consideration. Tailoring health messages to the cultural norms and beliefs of the target population can significantly improve their reception and impact. Another notable suggestion was the involvement of the community in creating health communication materials. Engaging the community not only ensures that the content is relevant and relatable but also fosters a sense of ownership and trust in the information being shared. Additionally, aligning health campaigns with cultural occasions can be a powerful strategy. This timing can help integrate health messages seamlessly into the community's existing traditions and practices. Moving beyond theoretical discussions, our research also explored practical examples of innovative health communication strategies. In the Indian context, two states, Rajasthan and

Tamil Nadu, demonstrated creative approaches to reach their target populations. In Rajasthan, health messages were effectively disseminated through live performances by local artists, including drummers, dancers, folk musicians, magicians, and puppeteers. This approach leveraged entertainment and cultural expressions to engage tribal communities actively. Moreover, incentives were provided to Accredited Social Health Activists (ASHAs) for successfully executing these activities, creating a motivation for community health promotion (World Bank, 2012).

In Tamil Nadu, a blend of traditional and modern communication methods was employed. In addition to posters and hoardings, radio jingles and videos featuring popular film stars were used to communicate health messages to tribal communities. Personalized letters were also employed for literate family members, ensuring a comprehensive and inclusive approach to health communication (World Bank,2012). Looking beyond India, our discussion extends to a global perspective. In the context of Indigenous Australian adults, a systematic review encompassing six databases revealed various interventions aimed at boosting health literacy. These interventions included workshops, exercise classes, and discounted produce, all aimed at improving nutrition and oral health literacy (Nash and Arora,2021). Furthermore, addressing health communication challenges extends beyond regional borders. To tackle these challenges effectively, healthcare personnel and community leaders must develop the capacity to bridge Western and traditional medicine. This necessitates the use of participatory communication strategies and ethnographic methodologies to make informed decisions. The Pan American Health Organization/World Health Organization (PAHO/WHO) has successfully applied these strategies in various regions, including indigenous communities in Colombia and the Amazon, Nariño, and Magdalena regions. Through a dialogue-based and ethnographic approach, these initiatives aim to provide relevant information and foster voluntary access to life-saving therapeutic options such as vaccines while minimizing physical and psychological harm (Ferrante and Ferrante, 2020).

CONCLUSION

This was a qualitative research implemented to identify the sources, process of health communication, and strategies for improvement in a tribal community located in the western regions of Maharashtra state in India. In depth interviews were conducted with key stakeholders and the community by a trained qualitative researchers. The findings revealed the operation of a vertical health system, where health communication content is conceptualized and validated with resources from the Ministry of Family Welfare and Health. These resources are then disseminated to Primary Health Care Centers, where ASHA workers, supervised by PHC staff, execute the messages and activities at the grassroots level. They impart health education related to Nutrition, Family Planning, Pregnancy ANC and PNC care and Child Health, Adolescent Health, Infectious Diseases, Non-Communicable Diseases and other diseases to the community. In this specific role they are supported by local stakeholders of the villages. The findings also revealed about the effect of "Cultural Disconnect" and "Cultural Resilience" on the acceptance of health messages. Lastly, findings about the importance of confidentiality in imparting sensitive health messages, detail strategies to improve the health communications emerged from the study.

Improving health communication for India's tribal populations will involve culturally tailored strategies. Local communities should engage in crafting health messages to ensure relevance and trust. Traditional art forms and local artists to be leveraged for live performances to make health information engaging and accessible. Multimedia approaches, including radio jingles and videos featuring celebrities, can be used with traditional methods like posters. Incentives to the ASHA to ensure the successful execution of health communication activities would help. Furthermore, emphasis should be placed on language diversity, with special attention given to accommodating low-literacy populations through the use of visual aids and simple language. By integrating these strategies, India can bolster health communication efforts and foster improved health outcomes within its tribal communities in the future.

REFERENCES

Chattopadhyay, K., & Mohanty, S. (2022). New media and cultural disconnect: A study on the lodha tribal community of India. Asian Journal of Social Science, 50(2), 137-146.

Cohen, J. A. (Ed.). (2008). *Challenges and successes in reducing health disparities: Workshop summary*. National Academies Press.

De Golbéry, L., & Chappuis, A. (2000). Underprivileged minorities in India: Dalits and tribals. A cartographic Approach. *Essays on Population and Space in India.* French Institute of Pondicherry.

Desa, U. (2018). Promoting Inclusion through Social Protection: Report on the World Social Situation 2018. New York: United Nations.

Dwivedi, P. (2016). An Introduction To Katkari Tribes Of Maharashtra. Retrieved from https://indiafellow.org/blog/all-posts/an-introduction-to-katkari-tribes-of-maharashtra/

Ekezie, W., Maxwell, A., Byron, M., Czyznikowska, B., Osman, I., Moylan, K., ... Pareek, M. (2022). Health communication and Inequalities in primary care access during the COVID-19 pandemic among ethnic minorities in the United Kingdom: lived experiences and recommendations. International Journal of Environmental Research and Public Health, 19(22), 15166.

Ferrante, L., & Fearnside, P. M. (2020). Protect Indigenous peoples from COVID-19. Science, 368(6488), 251-251.

Gore, M., Kawade, A., Smith, P., Pinnock, H., & Juvekar, S. (2022). Working as frontline health facilitators, service providers, program supporters, and social health activists in Indian hilly terrain areas: A qualitative study of accredited social health activists' experiences before and during the COVID-19 pandemic. *Journal of Global Health, 12*, 12. doi:10.7189/jogh.12.05052 PMID:36579668

Goswami, M. P. (2017). Mobile Phone, Entertainment and Tribal Life. Media Mimansa.

Hall, G., & Gandolfo, A. (2016). Poverty and exclusion among Indigenous Peoples: The global evidence. World Bank Blogs. Retrieved from https://blogs.worldbank.org/voices/poverty-and-exclusion-among-indigenous-peoples-global-evidence

Islary, J. (2014). Health and health seeking behaviour among tribal communities in India: A socio-cultural perspective. Journal of Tribal Intellectual Collective India, 1-16.

Kawade, A., Gore, M., Lele, P., Chavan, U., Pinnock, H., & Smith, P. (2021). Interplaying role of healthcare activist and homemaker: a mixed-methods exploration of the workload of community health workers (Accredited Social Health Activists) in India. Human Resources for Health, 19, 1-12.

Kumar, M. M., Pathak, V. K., & Ruikar, M. (2020). Tribal population in India: A public health challenge and road to future. Journal of family medicine and primary care, 9(2), 508.

Nash, S., & Arora, A. (2021). Interventions to improve health literacy among Aboriginal and Torres Strait Islander Peoples: a systematic review. BMC Public Health, 21(1), 1-15.

National Commission For Scheduled Tribes. (n.d.). https://ncst.nic.in/sites/default/files/documents/NCST.pdf

Porat, T., Nyrup, R., Calvo, R. A., Paudyal, P., & Ford, E. (2020). Public health and risk communication during COVID-19—Enhancing psychological needs to promote sustainable behavior change. *Frontiers in Public Health*, *8*, 637. doi:10.3389/fpubh.2020.573397 PMID:33194973

Ramalingareddy, K. (2016). Improving health services for tribal populations. International Journal of Research in Social Sciences, 6(11), 345-357.

Rikard, R. V., Thompson, M. S., McKinney, J., & Beauchamp, A. (2016). Examining health literacy disparities in the United States: a third look at the National Assessment of Adult Literacy (NAAL). BMC public health, 16, 1-11.

Rimal, R. N., & Lapinski, M. K. (2009). Why health communication is important in public health. Bulletin of the World Health Organization, 87, 247-247a. doi:10.2471/BLT.08.056713

Sabato, T. M. (2018). Utilization of media-driven technology for health promotion and risk reduction among American Indian and Alaska Native young adults: An exploratory study. Journal of Health Disparities Research and Practice, 12(1), 4.

Singh, P., & Kumari, R. (2019). Usage pattern of mobile phone among tribals of Jharkhand. Mass Communicator: International Journal of Communication Studies, 13(1), 27-31.

Sinha, A. (n.d.). Communication Anthropology: A realization. World Anthropology Congress. Retrieved from https://wac.kiss.ac.in/blog/communication-anthropology-a-realization/

Sneath, D. (2016). Tribe. Cambridge Encyclopedia of Anthropology. doi:10.29164/16tribe

World Bank. (2023). Indigenous Peoples. Retrieved from https://www.worldbank.org/en/topic/indigenouspeoples

Chapter 7
President's Speech and Terminology Used During the COVID-19 Pandemic:
The Interpretation of Linguistic Meaning in Context and Situational Context

Kgomotso Theledi
University of the Witwatersrand, South Africa

Violet M. S Pule
Sol Plaatje University, South Africa

ABSTRACT

This chapter investigates the interpretation of the South African President's terminologies during family meetings in a linguistic and situational context. During the COVID-19 pandemic, South African President Cyril Ramaphosa addressed the nation to communicate important information and updates about the virus and the measures taken by the government to curb the spread of the virus. The authors argue that most South African people do not know how to write and speak English; however, the information was delivered through the medium of English, excluding those who do not know the English language, with special reference to Setswana speakers. Hence, the chapter focuses on the South African President's speeches during the COVID-19 pandemic era. A theory of Afrocentricity will be employed in a qualitative approach to address the research questions and objectives of this chapter. At the end of this chapter, communication strategies are addressed in line with language use and cultural appropriateness.

DOI: 10.4018/979-8-3693-0624-6.ch007

1. INTRODUCTION

1.1 The Significance of the Chapter

In this chapter, the aim is to reveal the importance of considering the linguistic and situational context when forming new terms for the community. The chapter highlighted the impact of new terms or instructions on cultural beliefs, Christianity, and spirituality. The outcome of this chapter can serve as a guide in forming new terms, considering the linguistic and situational context. The chapter's target is to assist organisations, universities, and government departments that deal with language translation or terminology, to create terms considering the linguistic and situational context of the community for the information to be well received and understood. This chapter focused on the dissemination of information during COVID-19, the language, culture, and identity of Batswana, the interpretation of terminology and its impact on society, and finally the marginalisation of society.

The primary purpose of this chapter is to explore the president's speech and terminology used during the COVID-19 pandemic with special reference to the interpretation of linguistic meaning in context and situational context in the case of the Setswana language. A qualitative desktop research methodology was employed in this research. Secondary research or desk research is a research method that involves using already existing data. Existing data was collected from reliable sources such as television broadcasts, newspapers, and governments' regulations and guidelines regarding COVID-19.

A theory of Afrocentricity was employed in a qualitative approach. Afrocentricity theory provides a lens through which to analyse and address the unique challenges faced by African and African diasporic communities during the COVID-19 pandemic. This theory places the experiences, perspectives, and cultural values of people of African descent at the center of analysis, emphasising the need for self-determination, cultural affirmation, and collective action. By applying the theory of Afrocentricity to the pandemic context, it becomes possible to understand the specific impact on these communities and develop strategies for resilience and empowerment. This theory helps to highlight the importance of acknowledging historical and structural factors that contribute to these disparities. To encourage the examination of how systemic racism, economic inequality, healthcare access, and other social determinants of health impact the well-being of these communities during the pandemic

1.2 Background

There were misunderstandings and misinterpretations based on terms used that led to some regulations not being followed by all old and young South Africans. While many South Africans appreciated President Ramaphosa's efforts, there were also critiques and concerns voiced by some segments of the population. These included concerns about the impact of restrictions on livelihoods, disparities in the distribution of relief measures, and the effectiveness of certain strategies. However, the overall sentiment was that the family meetings served as a vital platform for open communication and dialogue on how terminology and messages were interpreted and received by South Africans. Indigenous communities often rely on traditional communication channels within their own networks, such as word of mouth, community gatherings, and local leaders. Trusted community members and leaders play a crucial role in disseminating information and interpreting it in a culturally appropriate manner.

When addressing the nation on the issue of the COVID-19 pandemic, the president used English as the language of communication. Language of communication is a choice, but it can disadvantage cultural communities if it benefits only the speaker or the people who know and understand that language. Since language embodies and expresses cultural relativity the president's speech disadvantaged cultural communities who are in the majority and cannot speak a foreign language. Language is used for human social interactions and so its origins and capacities are dependent on its role in our social life. Linguistically, language is categorised as spoken and written language. There are no grammatical rules in spoken language but in written language, there are standard forms and grammatical rules.

South Africa is a plurilingual country accommodating different cultural groups. The majority of these groups do not know how to write, speak, and interpret the English words. English is one of the official languages in South Africa. In Rudwick et al. (2021) English in South Africa is the home language of just over 8% of the entire population (cited in Statistics South Africa 2019). Therefore, monolingualism in South African languages is still rather prevalent in rural society. Language limitations may keep certain groups out of the picture. It is therefore evident that the use of terminology to address a crucial issue such as the COVID-19 pandemic was an exclusion of the majority of people in South Africa. However, in this chapter, the focus is on the Setswana mother tongue speakers whom we believe were marginalised using the English language during the COVID-19 pandemic.

Batswana, like other social groups, have their own language that they can interpret and understand better. Their language and culture are intertwined towards decolonising their cultural identity. However, the presidential speeches during the COVID-19 pandemic seem to have not addressed the issue. On the other side, in the Batswana culture, when there are gatherings such as funerals and weddings, people gather in big numbers to give their last respects or to celebrate the life of the deceased. However, during COVID-19 there were restrictions and regulations that were imposed by the government to be followed by groups of people. People were not allowed to gather in numbers, e.g., less than 50 people were allowed to attend the funerals, which was a taboo in Setswana.

The use of the English language in addressing non-English speakers is a linguistic barrier. In this chapter, a linguistic barrier is a recognised source of health inequities for ethnic minority communities whose health communication needs cannot be adequately met. This multilingual communication crisis has emerged as a global challenge during the COVID-19 pandemic. Rudwick et al. (2021) mentioned that Ngcobo (2009, 118) long argued that communication in English by government officials violates the concept of equity which relates to the perception of fairness as enshrined in the South African Constitution. The indication is that public health communication is characterised by the large-scale exclusion of linguistic minorities from this most important information. Our understanding is that linguistic context can help clarify the meaning of a particular word or phrase and can also help to convey additional meaning beyond the literal definition of the words.

The severe limitations of multilingual crisis communication that the COVID-19 crisis has laid bare result from the dominance of English-centric global mass communication; the longstanding devaluation of minoritised languages; and the failure to consider the importance of multilingualism for building trust and resilient communities. Our government could have organised different interpreters of all African languages, even after the president agreed to explain the speech in their spoken language or could have made means on how to address people in their own languages. To give an example, in isiZulu Blade Nzimande, South African Minister of Higher Education starts speaking in isiZulu to explain the issue effectively to a broader audience such as tertiary students, parents, and academics in the country, about the delay in the distribution of laptops to students. For example, in saying 'Ningixolele ngane zakwethu ningamane nithi ukulibala kancane' ('Please forgive me here, children of my home/my siblings, you will rather have delays'). Whereas the South African president has started by saying, "Fellow South Africans …" in English and not in any of the African languages.

Batswana also requires information in a language and manner that they can comprehend. It must also be presented in a style that is relevant to them and accessible through a channel they can access and trust. Culturally, Batswana like other African cultures would prefer the language that they use and understand better because most of them do not rely on Western medicines. While the president's advice was mainly based on foreign medicine, it is vital to note that the Batswana, also believe in traditional doctors and medicines. For some, it was not an easy task to convince them to visit foreign doctors and take vaccines for instance.

Culturally the Batswana would use traditional medicine such as *'lengana'* (Wormwood) or *'mologa'* (Acacia ataxacantha) to heal colds and influenza. That is why most of the people during COVID-19 prefered their concoctions including '*lengana*', garlic, and lemon to drink. *Lengana* is a popular medicinal plant used by Batswana to treat coughs, colds, diabetes, bladder, malaria, and other diseases. This medicine is also good for children, e.g., when children have fever or constipation, they use an enema to stimulate the empty their bowels. Therefore, some of the English terms used by the president during his speech might not be effective regarding the cultural background of the Batswana.

Another example is traditionally, Batswana people use *'boloko'* cow-dung as a disinfectant, when a child is born, they will smear and decorate the hut with the cow-dung to protect the young child and mother from any infections. Sanitiser was something new for them. Madagascan President Andry Rajoelina had officially launched a medicine he believes can prevent and cure patients suffering from COVID-19 (Abdur Rahman Alfa Shaban with AGENCIES 22/04/2020). This shows how the indigenous communities view the world, and their role can greatly influence how they approach problems and resolve issues.

It is evident that language (terminology), culture, self-identity, and social contact patterns have been shown to be crucial factors behind the risk of exposure to diseases. Furthermore, the language spoken, which is an important component of any cultural heritage, can have an additional impact on exposure to disease. This is especially true in the case when a virus can spread via airborne transmission and therefore when the interaction with affected individuals or communities facilitated using a common language becomes a critical factor.

2. DISSEMINATION OF INFORMATION DURING LOCKDOWN IN SOUTH AFRICA

2.1. How the Information Disseminated

The COVID-19 virus emerged in March 2020, causing a disaster in the entire world. It was a new sickness that threatened the lives of everyone. As a result, significant information sharing, and illness education were required in all languages. When disseminating information about COVID-19, several organisations and government departments employed new terminology that had to be translated into different languages for everyone to understand. Global response plans for COVID-19 identify risk communication and community engagement as a priority. That requires all responders to communicate effectively with communities, counter misinformation, and make sure people can hold them accountable. This brief outlines findings and recommendations on four key aspects to achieve these aims: language, format, relevant content, and channel.

The very first death due to the illness was recorded on March 23, and a nationwide lockdown was announced to begin on March 27, 2020, via a news broadcast and the government website. To mitigate the spread of coronavirus and reduce its impact in the country, a national command council for the coronaviruse was established, which intended to guide the country's strategy. In the wake of the COVID-19 virus spreading across South Africa, the president of South Africa Cyril Ramaphosa held 14 family meetings in which he briefed the nation on its situation and response from the government. These addresses have all been aired on the South African state television channels and uploaded to YouTube, as well as the social media page of Cyril Ramaphosa which is managed by the government in South Africa.

Moreover, the content of all speeches was made available on the government's website. The speeches were scripted monologues, with no questions and answer sessions attached, and no press presence, apart from the first one. A sign interpreter was shot separately, but at the same time as this recording was displayed to the right of the screen. The speeches were typically delivered in ceremonial settings such as the president's office, with President Ramaphosa sitting in a high-backed chair or standing at a podium, flags displayed to his right and either wood-paneling or wallpaper with national symbols were visible behind him. Although the speeches' content was mainly in English, Ramaphosa occasionally included phrases or words in one of the other official languages, especially by beginning or finishing a speech by welcoming the addressees in multiple languages. He kept his eyes focused on the camera or just below it for most of the time, and his facial expression was serious.

During the COVID-19 pandemic, South African President Cyril Ramaphosa addressed the nation through a series of family meetings to communicate important information and updates about the virus and the measures taken by the government. Many South Africans viewed President Ramaphosa's family meetings as an important source of information and guidance. His calm and measured approach, combined with his reputation as a respected leader, helped instill a sense of trust and confidence in the messages he delivered. The president used the term 'family meeting' which in Setswana, a family meeting is held when there is an urgent or important thing that affects the whole family. The word 'family meeting' was used intelligibly to attract listenership. President Ramaphosa's family meetings played a crucial role in emphasising the seriousness of the pandemic and the need for compliance with regulations and restrictions. His messages about social distancing, wearing masks, practicing good hygiene, and adhering to lockdown measures were not generally well-received.

Communicating in an international lingua franca or a national language increases the vulnerability of marginalised individuals. For example, English is an official language in 35 nations. Nonetheless, only a minority of people in those countries learnt English as their first language. Women, the elderly, and individuals with disabilities, in particular, are typically denied educational opportunities and are less likely to speak or read a second language. People also tend to communicate in their mother tongue as they get older. Language limitations may keep certain groups out of the picture. During the 2014-16 Ebola outbreak in West Africa, language was a barrier to curbing the disease's transmission. A lack of informative material for local language speakers and non-literate audiences at the outset put segments of the people in danger.

During these epidemics, millions of marginalised individuals lacked fundamental knowledge on how to keep themselves and their communities safe and healthy. This includes those who do not speak the dominant language in their area, people with no or low literacy, and people who do not have access to alternative ways of communication. As a result, individuals may be unable to make informed decisions about how to act, which will not slow the spread of disease. Marginalised people, like everyone else, have the right to clear, accurate, and easily accessible information about the disease and response actions. They require information in a language and manner that they can comprehend. It must also be presented in a style that is relevant to them and accessible through a channel they can access and trust.

2.2. The Family Meetings and the Use of Colonial Language

This chapter outlined how the information reached the South African people by using government briefings, family meetings by the South African president, media like television, radio, and other social media platforms such as Twitter, WhatsApp, YouTube and so forth during the COVID–19 pandemic. The concept of best practices is a popular approach to improving organisational and professional practice in a wide array of venues, including many communication contexts (Seeger, 2006). The South African president used a family meeting to reach out all diverse South African people.

The family meeting was held at night where everyone had a chance to listen to the updates on the COVID-19 pandemic. Culturally, in Setswana the family meeting is led by the head of the house (fathers, uncles, or the elderly), and in other circumstances children are not invited to family meeting. Therefore, this chapter concludes that the expectation of holding these meetings at night was that children were sleeping. Family meetings were used as a communicational tool. Traditionally, it is the most common way to communicate family matters or solve family disputes. Hence, many individuals responded positively to these briefings.

During the COVID-19 pandemic, South Africa implemented several lockdown measures to curb the spread of the virus. Mirbabaie, et al. (2020) indicates that in recent times societal crises such as the coronavirus disease 2019 outbreak have given rise to tension between formal 'command and control' and informal social media activated self-organising information and communication systems that are utilised for crisis management decision-making. It's important to recognise that effective dissemination of information is vital in combating misinformation and ensuring that citizens have access to accurate and reliable information to make informed decisions about their health and well-being. However, challenges such as limited access to technology in some areas and language barriers may have impacted the reach and effectiveness of information dissemination in other parts of South Africa during the COVID-19 pandemic.

The dissemination of information during these lockdowns played a crucial role in keeping the public informed about government regulations, health guidelines, and updates on the pandemic. There were multiple channels employed to reach the population effectively but one of the challenges of the strategies to disseminate messages was the use of a foreign language such as English. People who use English sometimes forget that not all people know or understand it. This shows that language excludes or includes people in conversations or in the decision-making process. South Africa is a plurilingual country accommodating different cultural groups. Most of these groups do not know how to write, speak, and interpret the English words. It is therefore evident that the use of scientific western terminologies to address a crucial issue such as the COVID-19 pandemic results in the exclusion of most people in South Africa.

We therefore argue that the use of the English language in addressing non-English speakers is a linguistic barrier. In this chapter, a linguistic barrier is a recognised source of health inequities for ethnic minority communities whose health communication needs cannot be adequately met. This multilingual crisis in communication emerged as a global challenge during the COVID-19 pandemic. This public health communication is characterised by the large-scale exclusion of linguistic minorities from this most important information. The severe limitations of multilingual crisis communication that the COVID-19 crisis has laid bare results from the dominance of English-centric global mass communication;

the longstanding devaluation of minoritised languages; and the failure to consider the importance of multilingualism for building trusting and resilient communities.

This chapter argues that the government could have employed other strategies to reach all the people such as makgotla (Lekgotla is a meeting place of village leaders) where chiefs or community leaders could have fairly and effectively disseminated information during the COVID-19 pandemic. Misinformation and rumors related to COVID-19 may have spread in local languages without proper fact-checking and verification, leading to further confusion and fear within linguistic minority communities. Social distancing measures and lockdowns may have impacted traditional cultural practices and gatherings, affecting the transmission and preservation of languages and cultural knowledge. Again, the government could have used professional interpreters to avoid stigmatisation or discrimination due to the perception that the pandemic originated from certain regions or linguistic communities. Language barriers can lead to misunderstandings and hinder effective communication.

During the COVID-19 pandemic, the South African indigenous languages were marginalised in various ways, particularly concerning information dissemination, access to resources, and support services. The marginalisation of languages can impact certain linguistic communities, especially those with minority or indigenous languages. In many regions, official information related to COVID-19, such as government guidelines, health advisories, and safety measures, were primarily provided in dominant or official languages. This resulted in limited access to crucial information for speakers of minority languages who were not proficient in the dominant language (English). We must be cautious about the naturalising of monolingualism (in this instance English being the language of choice) through a system of educational qualifications which reinforce the standardised values of normative language and legitimises itself on the grounds that we have a labour market in which employment depends upon such qualifications (Gaganakis, 2006).

Research and studies related to COVID-19, including vaccine trials and public health surveys, may have been conducted primarily in dominant languages, potentially excluding linguistic minority groups from participation or representation. The demand for accurate translation and interpretation services during the pandemic increased significantly. However, not all languages had adequate resources for timely and accurate translation, leaving some communities without access to translated information.

Drawing attention to address language marginalisation during a crisis like COVID-19 required proactive measures, such as:

- Providing multilingual information and resources to ensure equitable access to critical information.
- Strengthening language support services in healthcare settings to improve communication with diverse linguistic communities.
- Encouraging research and studies in various languages to ensure inclusive participation.
- Supporting translation efforts for vital information and debunking misinformation in local languages.
- Promoting and preserving linguistic diversity and cultural practices during and after the pandemic.
- By recognising and addressing language marginalisation, policymakers, and organisations can better serve linguistic minority communities during public health emergencies and create a more inclusive and resilient response to crises.

2.3 Information Through Social Media

The South African government regularly held press briefings to provide updates on the lockdown restrictions, COVID-19 statistics, and measures put in place to combat the virus. Key figures, such as the president and health minister, addressed the nation through televised broadcasts and social media platforms. Broadcast media, including radio and television, played a vital role in reaching populations without internet access or limited digital literacy. Regular public service announcements and educational programs were aired to communicate critical information during the lockdown.

It's important to recognise that information dissemination during the lockdown aimed to combat misinformation and ensure that citizens had access to accurate and reliable information to make informed decisions about their health and well-being was made available. Nevertheless, lockdowns, business closures, and job losses during the pandemic have disproportionately affected low-income individuals and marginalised communities. People working in informal sectors, daily wage laborers, and vulnerable populations have faced financial hardships and struggled to meet their basic needs. Mostly it was thewomen who were affected, as they often bear the brunt of caregiving responsibilities and may face increased risks of domestic violence and economic hardships. Hence, this chapter showed how the South African people reacted to information spread using social media.

According to Stieglitz, et al. (2017) social media is becoming increasingly important during crisis situations. Hence, affected people are now enabled to provide helpful on-site information, and emergency service organisations can use social media to inform people and communicate with them. The COVID-19 outbreak highlighted the necessity for the development of a comprehensive social media communication strategy to enhance and support crisis response. Social media has become the most used and active way of communication (Apuke and Tunca, 2018). Social media platforms were extensively used to disseminate information to the public, but this begs the question as to the exclusion ofelderly people who do not know how to use social media platforms?

Government agencies and health departments actively posted updates, guidelines, and educational content about COVID-19. Citizens could follow official accounts to stay informed about the latest developments. The nature of social media was to transform the communication crisis to allow more interaction. This chapter maintained that although social media dissemination of information during COVID-19 was effective in other parts of the world, not all people were reached in South Africa, particularly the so-called poor people or disadvantaged communities. Therefore, the message and information from the government during the COVID–19 pandemic did not reach them all.

Most people in South Africa are unemployed and there is inequality among the urban and rural people. Some of the rural people unlike urban people do not have access to electricity and other resources such as televisions, radios, or money to buy newspapers. This shows that the COVID-19 pandemic has exposed inequality among the people of South Africa. Mirbabaie, et al. (2020) points out that social media distrust affects the dissemination of disaster information as it entails shifts in media perception and participation but also changes in the way individuals and organisations make sense of information in critical situations.

It was not only Batswana who experienced problems with the use of social media. There were some individuals from other countries who resisted following health guidelines or adhering to lockdown measures for various reasons, such as economic concerns, perceived infringements on personal freedoms, or disbelief in the severity of the virus. It's important to recognise that people's reactions were diverse and influenced by various factors. Governments and health authorities faced challenges in effectively

Figure 1. Virus shut out
(United States Environmental Protection Agency)

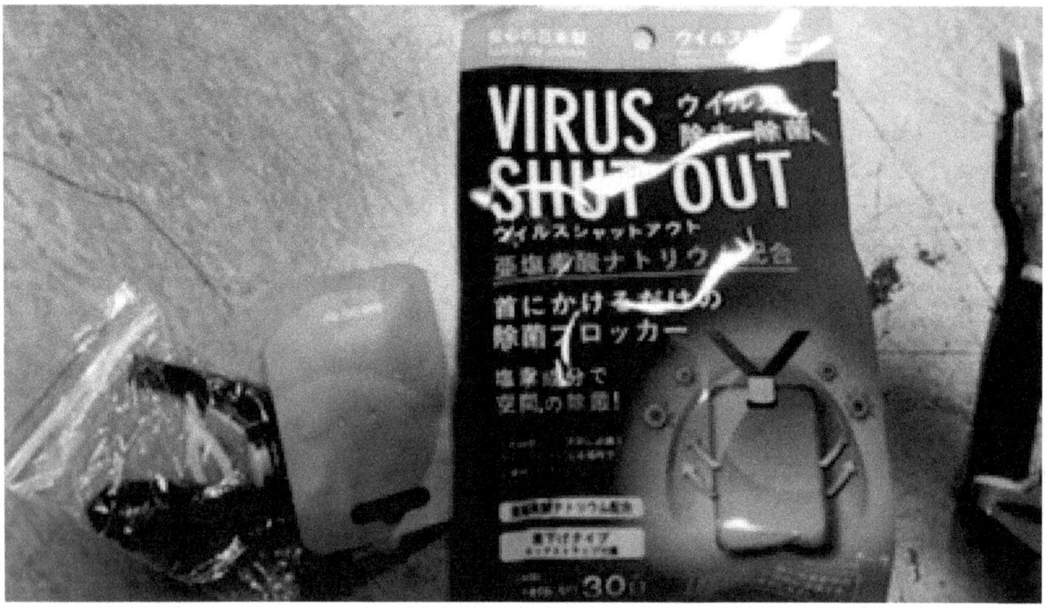

communicating with the public and addressing the concerns and behaviors that emerged during the pandemic. Providing accurate and consistent information, combating misinformation, and understanding the needs and concerns of different communities were essential in fostering a united response to the COVID-19 pandemic. This chapter shows how people reacted to the COVID-19 information worldwide and locally in South Africa. For example:

- FDA (2023) reported that the U.S. Food and Drug Administration was issuing warning letters to firms for selling fraudulent products with claims to prevent, treat, mitigate, diagnose, or cure the coronavirus disease 2019 (COVID-19).
- According to BOSTON (CBS) (2020) a Quincy man has pleaded guilty to charges that he was selling a lanyard that falsely claimed to protect people from viruses.

Gualtieri in CBS News May 13, 2021/5:17 pm states that New York Mayor Bill de Blasio downed some Shake Shack fries during a virtual press conference one Thursday, touting a new partnership to encourage New Yorkers to get vaccinated. "I want you to look at this and think about — again, some people love hamburgers, some don't, and we want to respect all ways of life — but if this is appealing to you, just think of this when you think of vaccinations," he said. "Mmm, vaccinations. Mmm. I'm getting a very good feeling about vaccinations right at this moment."

Fake news in SA:
Fake news 1 and 2 from the government website.
Fake news 1:

Figure 2. Fake news 1

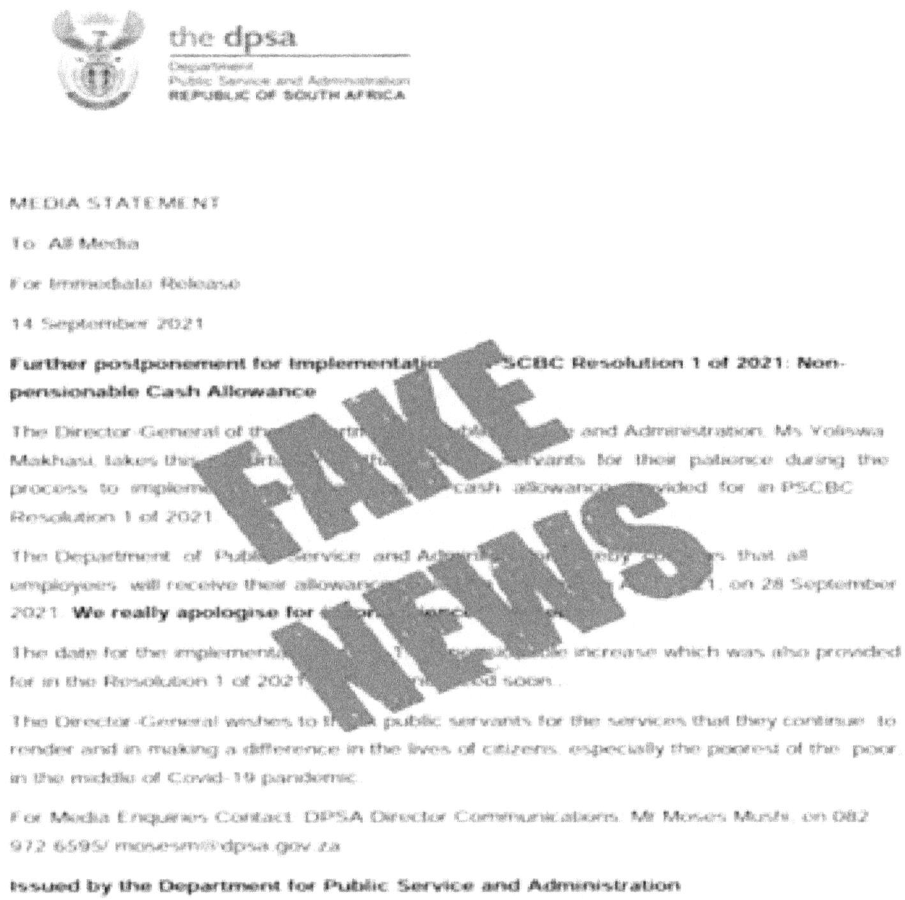
the dpsa
Department:
Public Service and Administration
REPUBLIC OF SOUTH AFRICA

MEDIA STATEMENT

To: All Media

For Immediate Release

14 September 2021

Further postponement for Implementation [illegible] PSCBC Resolution 1 of 2021: Non-pensionable Cash Allowance

The Director-General of th[illegible] and Administration, Ms Yoliswa Makhasi, takes thi[illegible] servants for their patience during the process to impleme[illegible] cash allowanc[illegible] vided for in PSCBC Resolution 1 of 2021.

The Department of Publ[illegible] ervice and Ad[illegible] s that all employees will receive their allowanc[illegible] 1, on 28 September 2021. **We really apologise for [illegible]**

The date for the implement[illegible] increase which was also provided for in the Resolution 1 of 202[illegible] soon.

The Director-General wishes to th[illegible] public servants for the services that they continue to render and in making a difference in the lives of citizens, especially the poorest of the poor in the middle of Covid-19 pandemic.

For Media Enquiries Contact: DPSA Director Communications, Mr Moses Mushi, on 082 972 6595/ mosesm@dpsa.gov.za

Issued by the Department for Public Service and Administration

Fake news 2:

The period also saw a sharp rise in reliance on social media platforms and websites for interaction due to physical restrictions by the South African government. These served as both a source of entertainment as well as a source of education for many. Government and news platforms thus also started to focus greater efforts on using such platforms for dissemination and engagements. This newly adopted focus also led to the more privileged schools choosing to engage students through such, and thereby polarising the education system within the 'haves' and 'have-nots'. According to South African Stats (2022), while remote learning programmes were designed, this did not guarantee that the children participated in the instruction. According to a new report, "COVID-19 and barriers to participation in education in South Africa, 2020" released by Statistics South Africa, only 11,7% of schools offered remote learning options nationally. Most schools offered rotational options instead of remote learning and the urban-rural divide was prominent, as twice as many individuals were given the option of remote learning in urban areas compared to rural areas.

Figure 3. Fake news 2

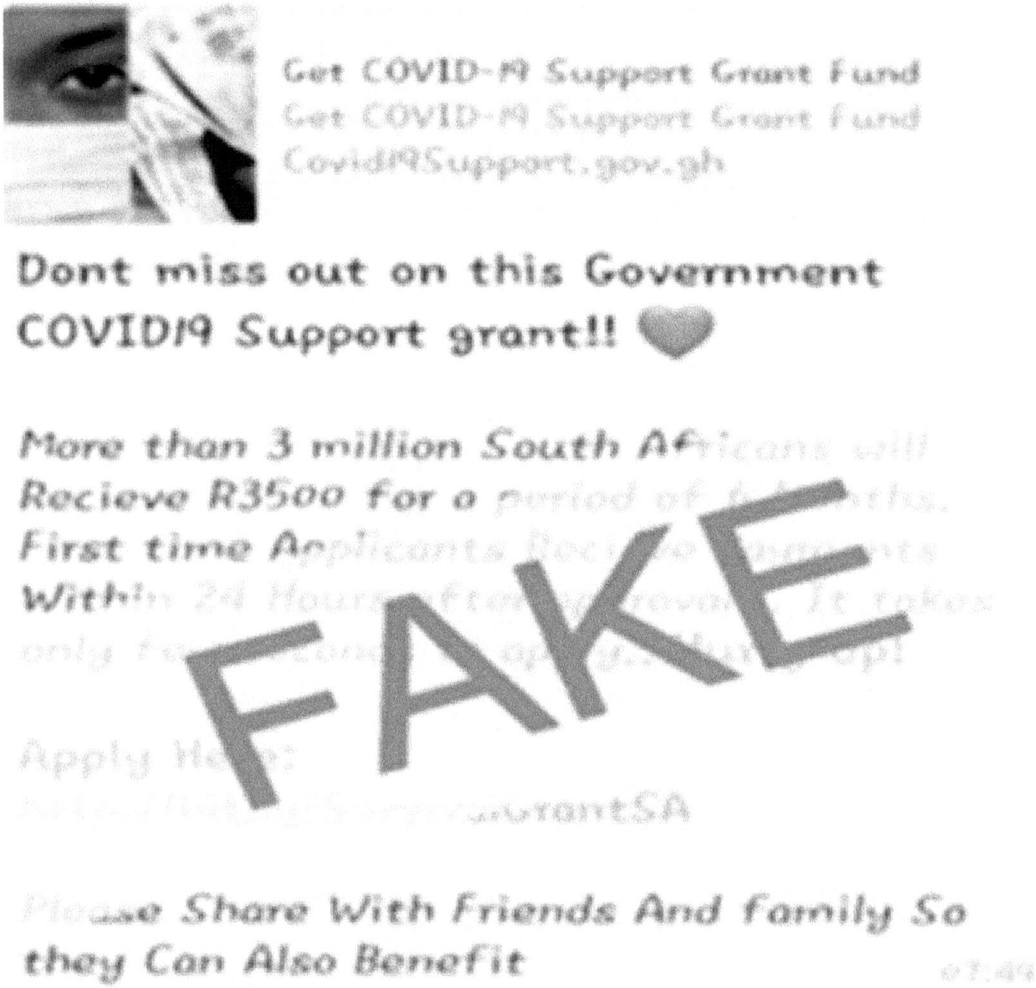
Get COVID-19 Support Grant Fund
Get COVID-19 Support Grant Fund
Covid19Support.gov.gh
Dont miss out on this Government COVID19 Support grant!!
More than 3 million South
Recieve R3500 for a
First time
FAKE
Share With Friends And Family So they Can Also Benefit

These interventions were not without their perils and a rise in fraud and scam incidents due to a lack of prior protocols having existed beforehand.

3. LANGUAGE, CULTURE, AND IDENTITY

Setswana is an indigenous language spoken by an estimated four million people in South Africa. It is one of the South African official languages. Setswana is also spoken in Botswana and Namibia. The culture of the Batswana is communicated through Setswana language and traditional music. Culture is also based on local food, dance, traditional attire, rituals and other ceremonies like wedding celebrations.

Approximately 25 different languages are spoken in South Africa, of which 11 have been granted official status in terms of section 6 of the Constitution (Act No. 108 of 1996), on the grounds that their usage includes about 98% of the total population. The 11 official languages are isiNdebele, isiXhosa,

Figure 4. Remote vs. nonremote schooling

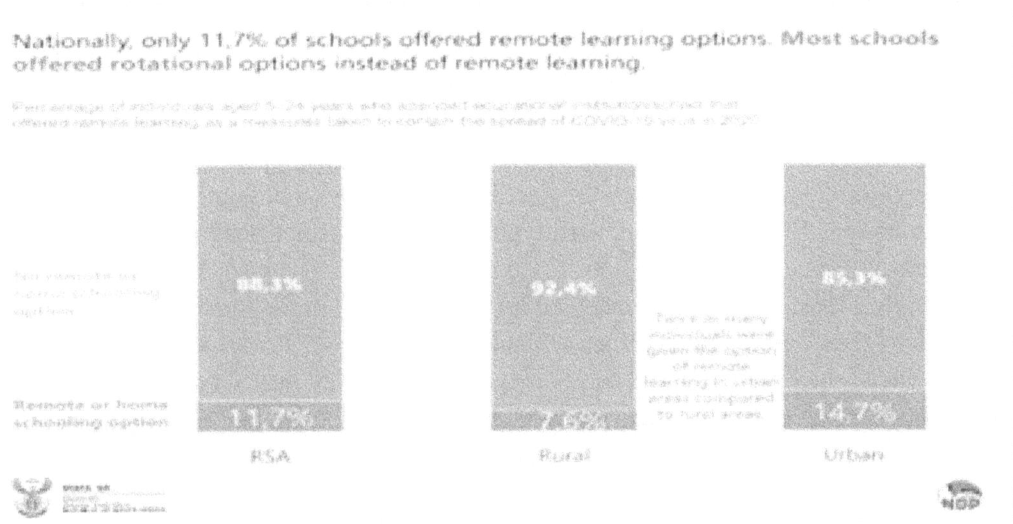

isiZulu and siSwati (referred to as the Nguni language group); Sesotho, Sepedi and Setswana (referred to as the Sotho language group); Tshivenda, Xitsonga, English and Afrikaans.

Culture is a customary belief and values that ethnic, religious, and social groups transmit unchanged from generation to generation. In this chapter we regard the Setswana language as a vehicle for cultural practices and self-identity. As such, cultural origins can expose certain groups/communities to epidemics more than others and influence the way in which these groups/communities react to public policy.

Traditionally the Batswana have different types of ceremonies including bride-wealth payment (lobola), marriage, and death. Religious rites include bogwera and bojale (male and female initiation ceremonies) and fetlha pula or rain-making rites. Unlike in western culture, the Batswana are the people who come together to support each other during these ceremonies. In a nutshell, it can be said that Batswana people do not work in silos but in a communal way. It is therefore difficult to convince the Batswana people to keep the required social distancing from each other, even under difficult circumstances.

Regarding marriage the Batswana wedding celebrations would start at the bride's home where all the guests would sing wedding songs, ululate, and eat their fill. By singing together at wedding celebrations, the Batswana gather together as a unit. Setswana music, which is also part of folk songs is mostly vocal and performed without instruments. When people sing, they come close to one another and exchange voices. This type of singing also brings unity among the people. Folk songs are also performed in initiation ceremonies such as bogwera and bojale (male and female initiation ceremonies) whereby youth are prepared for adulthood.

In the case of bereavement, the Batswana can also not be separated. They need to be a unit. The wake, also known as night vigil, is held at the deceased's home or a family member's home. Mourners pay their respects by praying, singing, and giving speeches in honor of the deceased. The deceased's family also may provide snacks and tea for everyone while mourning continues until the morning. A Batswana funeral is a sad occasion rather than a celebration. It's a large event whereby many people attend from family and friends to neighbors and community members. Funerals are typically on Saturdays starting in the early morning and lasting the entire day. This implies that all preparations are done during the whole week whereby community members visit the bereaved family to assist in arrangements.

Where Christianity is the religion of Batswana, a Batswana funeral typically follows these traditions. Traditionally, families buried the deceased in their home village and wrapped the body in black cattle skin. They place the body in the fetal position and buried them facing west - which they believe is the direction of the ancestral world. Today, they're buried in cemeteries typically outside of their village. Those who live in rural areas tend to bury the deceased as quickly as possible. At the burial, everyone sings Christian hymns. However, this modern type of burial does not deny the Batswana from their communal duties.

There's usually a meal to honor the deceased after the burial, but like the funeral, it isn't a celebration. Traditionally, they serve simple dishes without salt. The food is prepared by a group of women and men who gather together for the preparation event. Today, they may serve beef dishes and a non-alcoholic beverage called gemere (ginger) made of ground ginger, cream of tartar, sugar, and a few other ingredients. The Batswana have a strong belief in the supernatural, and they use traditional healers to treat illness and injury.

The Batswana culture also embraces what is known as letsema (working as a group). For instance, in this case, the Batswana will work a particular field owned by one of the community members to harvest the crops. This will be done to all the fields in the community. Those who did not get harvested will be provided with some food. During letsema the Batswana would sing folk songs to bring them strength and unity. It is therefore evident that it is not an easy task to convince the Batswana to keep a long distance from one another.

For people living in rural areas and informal settlements, social distance was enforced as a major prevention mechanism. This was impossible for certain sectors of the population, for example, the people living in an informal settlement who use a communal bathroom and a water tap with no access to warm water or electricity and who cannot keep the social distance regulations and keep up with the hygiene standard expected during the pandemic. It was evidence that poor people were at high risk.

Researchers who conducted interviews in different informal areas over the first 21 days of the national lockdown, provided insight into how the national lockdown has impacted some of South Africa's poorest and most vulnerable communities in informal areas (Business Tech 2020). In most media reports, it became apparent that in most informal areas, lockdown was more of a soft lockdown, not because of ill-discipline or out of a sense of defiance, but rather because of limited options and necessity.

There are reasons for the lack of adherence to lockdown rules, especially in informal areas such as the understanding of the spread of virus, living in lockdown was not possible for those who lived on the streets (selling on the streets) and believed that COVID-19 was no more hazardous than their daily realities. It was clear that social distancing, one restriction that was encouraged, was indeed unachievable in those areas.

4. COVID-19 TERMINOLOGIES IN THE RAMAPHOSA SPEECHES

4.1 Use of Terminologies

It is evident that language (terminology), culture, self-identity, and social contact patterns have been shown to be crucial factors behind the risk of exposure to diseases. Furthermore, the language spoken,

Table 1. Setswana terms were extracted from COVID-19 multilingual terminology 2021

English Term	Setswana Term
1. Family meetings	Kopano ya lelapa
2. Lockdown	taolelometsamao
3. Close contact	Moatamelwa
4. Cloth face mask	Thibedi ya lesela
5. Community spread	moanamisabolwetse
6. Isolation	Tlhaolo
7. self-isolation	itlhaolo
8. self-quarantine	itebelo
9. social distancing	mokatologano
10. Regulation	Melawana

which is an important component of any cultural heritage, can have an additional impact on exposure to disease. This is especially true in the case when a virus can spread via airborne transmission and therefore when the interaction with affected individuals or communities facilitated using a common language becomes a critical factor. Below we highlight the most common English terminology that was used in the president's speeches and the Setswana term as stated in the COVID-19 Multilingual Terminology 2021 booklet. See the table below:

4.2 Interpretation of terminology and Its Impact on Society

Below Table 2 shows how the terms were interpreted in English and how this was related in Setswana based on their daily lives. We also give the Setswana terminology and its impact on the understanding of the president's speeches in general taking into account of the language, culture, and identity of the majority of people in South Africa. See the table below:

Linguistic understanding influenced participation during COVID-19. This misinterpretation of scientific terminology could have been avoided if it was used in their own languages. For example, Table 2 shows that Setswana does have terminologies that could have been used during COVID-19.

5. CONCLUSION

This chapter is based on its own originality in exposing how the interpretation of the linguistic meaning in the context of the COVID-19 pandemic has a multifaceted process influenced by situational and broader contexts. The finding is that the impact of situational context can navigate the linguistic challenges posed to individuals.

The chapter recommends the design of one South African language that can serve speakers in several related discerned languages for formal domains. Something similar to Germany where there are 15 discerned spoken languages: Alemannic, Bavaria, Saxon, Swabian, German, Limurashaish, Westphalian, Ripuarian, Franconian, Plautdietsch, Luxembourgish, Yiddish, and others use standard high German as

Table 2. English vs Setswana colloquial terms

English Definition	Setswana Culture/Beliefs
Family meeting The president meets with the nation to address the important thing that is affecting the country.	**Kopano ya lelapa** Batswana also has a family meeting to address family issues or deliver a message to the entire family (close relatives or extended relatives). The meeting is chaired by the head of the house. It can be the father/uncle /any elderly person in the family. That is why the South Africans respected the family meetings conveyed by the president.
Lockdown The restriction of movement of persons during the period for which this regulation is enforced and effect namely, an emergency measure where the control of exposure to or transmission of the disease.	**Taolelometsamao** In Setswana, the word lockdown is a taboo to be referred to by people because in Setswana you cannot keep a person locked up. They associated lockdown with prison which traditionally was not used. In the past Batswana did not have prisons because they used lekgotla to solve their problems and to punish the offenders who committed crimes.
Close contact A person who may be at risk of getting a contagious disease due to proximity or exposure to a known case.	**Moatamelwa** Batswana have different types of ceremonies which include lobola, weddings, welcoming chiefs, funerals, and so on and the attendance is always in numbers. Their belief is to hug one another to bring comfort, when meeting or after seeing one another long time, greet by hand and sit closer to one another. Therefore, it was difficult to convince Batswana to keep a long distance from each other, even under difficult circumstances.
Cloth face mask A face covering that provides enhanced protection against the transmission of viral and bacterial disease.	**Thibedi ya lesela** In Setswana, culturally, the bride is covered in the face when she gets married. Animals like donkeys are covered to only look straight on the road.
Community spread When a person in a community is infected with a virus without having had any known contact with a sick person.	**Moanamisabolwetse** In Setswana, a widow is not allowed to visit people's homes because it is believed that she will spread bad luck.
Isolation The act of separating people with a contagious disease from those who are not sick.	**Tlhaolelo** In Setswana a woman is kept indoors for three months after she has delivered a baby under the care of an elder person.
Self - isolation The act of putting oneself in isolation in order to prevent others from being infected with a contagious disease.	**Itlhaolo** In Setswana there are sicknesses such as mmoko (measles). The person needs to be put in her or his own place for days. Mainly because he/she might spread it or for a speedy recovery.

a common designed language. It is possible to adopt this method of designing a language but not closing doors for other South African indigenous languages.

REFERENCES

Apuke, O.D. & Tunca, A. (2018). Social Media and Crisis Management: A review and Analysis of Existing Studies. Laü Sosyal Bilimler Dergisi (IX – II: 199 – 215).

Department of Public Service and Administration. (2021). Postponement of Cash allowances. Available at: www.gov.za/covid-19/resources/fake-news-coronavirus-covid-19

Fraudulent Coronavirus Disease. (2019). (COVID-19) Products. Available at: 11: 41 pm on 25/08/2023 https://www.fda.gov/consumers/health-fraud-scams/fraudulent-coronavirus-disease-2019-covid-19-products

Gaganakis, M. (2006). Language and ethnic group relations in de-segrated South African Schools. . doi:10.1080/0159630940150103

Gualtieri, A. E. (2021). New York Mayor Bill de Blasio tempts New Yorkers with free fries: "Mmm, vaccinations. Available at: https://www.cbsnews.com/news/covid-vaccine-new-york-shake-shack-fries/

Mirbabaie, M., Bunker, D., Stieglitz, S., Marx, J., & Ehnis, C. (2020). Social media in times of crisis: Learning from Hurricane Harvey for the coronavirus disease 2019 pandemic response. *Journal of Information Technology*, *35*(3), 195–213. doi:10.1177/0268396220929258

Rudwick, S., Sijadu, Z., & Turner, I. (2021). Politics of language in COVID-19: Multilingual perspectives from South Africa. *Politikon: South African Journal of Political Studies*, *48*(2), 242–259. doi:10.1080/02589346.2021.1917206

Seeger, M. W. (2006, August). Best Practices in Crisis Communication: An Expert Panel Process. *Journal of Applied Communication Research*, *34*(3), 232–244. doi:10.1080/00909880600769944

Stieglitz, S., Mirbabaie, M., Schwenner, L., Marx, J., Lehr, J., & Brΰnker, F. (2017). Sensemaking and Communication roles in Social Media Crisis Communication. Academic Press.

KEY TERMS AND DEFINITIONS

COVID-19 Pandemic: Is known as the coronavirus pandemic. It is caused by severe acute respiratory syndrome coronavirus 2 (SARS- Cov-2). It is infectious and can led to widespread illness, hospitalisation and deaths in many countries around the world.

Interpretation: A process of making sense of or assigning meaning to something or any other form of communication. It involves examining and understanding the context, content, or elements to derive a meaningful understanding or explanation.

Linguistic Context: Helps to clarify the meaning of a particular word or phrase and can also help to convey additional meaning beyond the literal definition of the words. In understanding the linguistic context, one requires an understanding of the grammatical structure of the sentence and the meaning of the individual words.

President's Speeches: Speeches are crafted carefully to communicate specific messages to diverse audiences or communicate directly with the public.

Setswana: Setswana, is an indigenous language spoken in South Africa, Botswana, and Namibia. It is one of the South African official languages.

Situational Context: Situational contexts explain how speakers use language to achieve their goals, how listeners interpret language considering their knowledge and expectations, and how meaning is negotiated through interaction between speakers and listeners.

Terminology: A term, word or expression used within a particular field, subject, profession, or domain to convey specific meaning. It is important for communication.

Chapter 8
Public Health Communication and the Exclusion of Minority Languages in Zimbabwe:
Analysis of Community Radio Awareness Campaigns in Facebook Posts

Limukani Mathe
https://orcid.org/0000-0002-6776-0683
North-West University, South Africa

Gilbert Motsaathebe
North-West University, South Africa

ABSTRACT

Public health communication is imperative to every livelihood including minorities. Language, however, remains one of the fundamentals of communication that can make the message reach the people. This chapter focuses on health awareness campaigns on Facebook community radio to analyse public health communication in Zimbabwe's minority languages. The authors used community radio platforms on the assumption that local languages such as minority languages can at least find space on community radio. However, a qualitative content analysis on radio content on Facebook reveals the dominance of Shona (major indigenous language) and English in public health communication by health authorities and representatives of the ruling party. There were a few exceptions of minority languages used in code-switch with English. Theorising effective communication to minorities, this chapter notes that governments should prioritise public health communication in minority languages through open collaborative networks by making use of language translation and community leadership in health awareness campaigns.

DOI: 10.4018/979-8-3693-0624-6.ch008

INTRODUCTION

The internet and digital forums have become platforms for local cultures and interactions in indigenous languages (Mathe, 2023; Lister et al., 2003). Although largely dominated by the English language in former British colonies, local people can localise digital platforms to reflect their own culture on matters of local interest (Mpofu & Salawu, 2020; Arora, 2019; Mignolo, 2007; Waisbord & Mellado, 2014; Willems & Mano, 2016). Literature reflects language mix and switching in contemporary media space and in indigenous language media such as *Kwayedza* and *Mthunywa* newspapers and radio public sphere in Zimbabwe with Shona and Ndebele as dominant languages (Mathe & Motsaathebe, 2023a; Mathe & Motsaathebe, 2023b; Mpofu, 2023). In a critical analysis of minority language representation on talk radio programmes in Zimbabwe, Mathe and Motsaathebe (2023a) report language hybridisation with evident code-switching to major indigenous languages at the disadvantage of minorities. This chapter focuses on public health communication to minorities in minority languages on community radio platforms. Given the dominance of Shona and Ndebele in Zimbabwe's indigenous language media, the chapter specifically focuses specifically on community radio that broadcasts and disseminates local content through audio-visual formats and textual versions on Facebook.

Minority languages had no exclusive media coverage of their own in Zimbabwe until the licensing of community radio stations between 2021 and 2022. There are 14 community radio stations in Zimbabwe and all have digital Facebook communication platforms (Mathe & Motsaathebe, 2023c). The dominant and widely spoken languages in the country are English, Shona and Ndebele and have had dominance in Zimbabwe's media landscape since 1980. In 2013, the Constitution of Zimbabwe officialised 16 languages namely English, Shona, Ndebele, Kalanga, Nambya, Venda, Shangani, Tonga, Xhosa, Sotho, Tshwawo, Tswana, Barwe, Doma, Chikunda, Chewa, and Sena. This chapter defines non-dominant indigenous languages such as Kalanga, Nambya, Venda, Shangani, Tonga, Xhosa, Sotho, Tshwawo, Tswana, Barwe, Doma, Chikunda, Chewa, and Sena as minority languages. We thus apply a qualitative content analysis on health awareness campaigns to answer questions: did community radio platforms communicate public health in minority languages, what were the health awareness campaigns in minority languages and how was the audience reception to health awareness campaigns in local languages?

Public heath communication has no fixed definition. It might mean the dissemination and evaluation of accurate information on heath for the protection of the public (WRHA Professionals, 2023). Healthy People (2010) defines health communication as "the art and technique of informing, influencing, and motivating individual, institutional, and public audiences about important health issues". Public heath communication normally intervenes by seeking to promote public health (Healthy People 2010). The agreement among scholars is that public health communication should be relevant or accurate, accessible and understandable in various languages (Eberhard, Simons & Fennig, 2020; Citron, Michaelis & Goldberg, 2020; Piller, Zhang & Li, 2020). This chapter, therefore, analyses public heath communication in various minority languages in Zimbabwe.

MINORITY LANGUAGES AND THE MEDIA IN ZIMBABWE

In 2021 and 2022, the Broadcasting Authority of Zimbabwe (BAZ) licensed 14 community radio stations. These community radio stations broadcast in indigenous languages as shown in table 1 below. The recognition of the minority languages in the 2013 Constitution of Zimbabwe paved ways for their

Table 1. Minority indigenous language per community radio station in Zimbabwe

Name of Community Radio	Area	Minoritised Indigenous languages
Ntepe-Manama CRT	Manama Gwanda	Sotho and Ndebele
Lyeja FM	Hwange	Nambya & Dombe
Ingqanga FM	Mbembesi	Xhosa
Radio Bukalanga	Plumtree	Kalanga
Bayethe FM	Matobo	Ndebele and Kalanga
Beitbridge- Shashe CRT	Beitbridge	Venda, Shangani, Sotho & Pfumbi
Twasumpuka FM	Binga	Tonga
Nyangani FM	Nyanga	Manyika, Hwesa, Buja (classified as Shona)
Avuxeni FM	Chiredzi	Shangani, Shona, Ndau, Ndebele
Chimanimani CRT	Chimanimani	Ndau/Shona
Vemuganga CRT	Chipinge	Ndau
Ndau CRT	Mahenye (Garahwa)	Ndau/Shona
Kasambabezi FM	Kariba	Tonga/Shona
Madziwa FM	Shamva	Shona

Source: Authors

recognition in the formal educational system. The Constitutional recognition of indigenous languages also opened up opportunities for local communities to run own local media in their own indigenous languages. Literature shows that there has not been media diversity in Zimbabwe (Chiumbu 2009; Mathe 2020) due to state control. Zimbabwe has a modicum of print media, (state-controlled by Zimpapers and privately owned media) and public broadcasting radio stations and television (ZTV) controlled by Zimbabwe Broadcasting Corporation (ZBC). Public radio stations run by Zimbabwe Broadcasting Cooperation are National FM, Khulumani FM, Power FM, Radio Zimbabwe and Classic 263. However, minority indigenous languages have had limited airtime on the National FM (formally known as radio 4) and Radio Zimbabwe (formerly known as Radio 2) dominated by Shona and Ndebele languages (Dube & Wozniak, 2021).

Embracing the three-tier system, the Broadcasting Authority of Zimbabwe (BAZ) licensed commercial radio stations between 2015 and 2018 and community radio in 2021-2022. However, minority indigenous languages still find limited airtime in commercialised radio broadcasting. As usual, community indigenous languages found more cultural independence in community radio broadcasting. Community radio licensing since 2021 opened up hopes for more radio airtime for indigenous minority local languages (Tshuma, 2021). As put by De Beer (1998) community radio aims to open up opportunities for local participation through the redistribution of power communication for socio-politically marginalised groups, in this case, minority indigenous language groups

Community radio broadcasting defies communication barriers, illiteracy and lingual diversity by reaching people in their local languages. Community radio also promotes socio-cultural and community development of local people (Mano, 2012; Mathe & Motsaathebe, 2023a; Mathe & Motsaathebe, 2023b). Mainly community radio broadcasting is not meant for profit making. We, therefore, followed the Facebook pages of every community radio as shown in Table 1 to analyse the online visibility of the minority indigenous language in public health communication. Table 1 below shows the representation of minority indigenous language per community radio in Zimbabwe. Thus, this chapter evaluates health awareness campaigns in the minority languages per the indigenous languages on community radio Facebook platforms.

Digital technologies and social media have enabled a broader network of community networking and access to information. Communities have now become abstract and unlimited by geographical boundaries (Mathe & Motsaathebe, 2023c) what Moyo (2012) describes as symbolically connected netizens. Beforehand, radio audiences used to engage the presenter through phone calls but now they engage the media through social media such as WhatsApp and Facebook. This means even local people beyond the geographical reach of the traditional radio waves can now access radio through the internet and social media platforms. The public sphere is no longer restricted through analogy radio but has become interactive through new media technologies and radio convergence (Wasserman, 2005). Now audiences can text on commentary platforms attached to Facebook Posts as they share links of radio content even on WhatsApp (Croteau & Hoynes, 2000). The dissemination of radio content and the storytelling have also changed into new techniques (Pavlik, 2001) through navigable ways in audio-visual, posters, captions and other textual version (Bosch, 2013).

Although what is known as radio has not changed- its aural culture in audible voices, social media artefacts such as text and other affordances are described as the implants to the body of radio (Bonini 2012; Berry, 2016). Thus, the convergence of radio on social media has now become communication from one to many or many to many through opportunities of interaction between producer and consumer (Benkler, 2006; Bonini, 2012). Dissemination of radio content on social media is somehow likened to citizen journalism due to its participatory nature, even community radio as more participatory at grassroot level in local languages than any other media (Bosch, 2014). However, some studies question the accessibility of radio on the internet and social media due to digital divide and many localities having no access to the digital technologies(Bosch, 2014; Tkach & Williams, 2018). Mathe and Motsaathebe (2023c) questions the opportunities for indigenous languages in Facebook posts of radio content which are inaudible. The relevance of Facebook posts in video and print posts as radio content remains debatable. This chapter takes the print posts and cut videos on radio platforms as implants to the body of radio or the output of radio (Bonini, 2012; Berry, 2016; 2014). We make use of print posts, captions, live recorded videos of radio studio sessions to analyse public health communication in minority languages.

THEORISING EFFECTIVE COMMUNICATION IN HEALTH CRISES

Effective communication studies show that the success of health awareness campaigns is usually determined by the languages relevant to the audiences (Eberhard, Simons & Fennig, 2020; Puntoni, De Langhe & Osselaer, 2009; Citron, Michaelis & Goldberg, 2020; Piller, Zhang & Li, 2020). A study by the crisis and emergency risk communication also reflect this perspective that communication campaigns should reflect the diversity of the people intended by the message (Crisis & Emergency Risk Communication, 2014). Diversity in this case refers to lingual diversity of the audience. Diversity involves customising communication and translating into different local languages of the miscellaneous audiences. The problem now and then is that public health communication is often disseminated in majority languages, for instance, the world entered in the COVID-19 pandemic with English as the most spoken language (Piller, Zhang & Li 2020). This means public health communication in the COVID-19 pandemic was largely in English. The linguistic hierarchy favoured the elite and the World Health Organization (WHO) made information accessible in six languages Arabic, Chinese, English, French, Russian, Spanish of the United Nations with additional languages German, Hindi, Portuguese. English language, however, dominated the press conferences and was the immediate language on record in the new media (Coronavirus disease (COVID-19) pandemic, 2020).

Nonetheless, knowing the need for effective response to the pandemic, WHO tasked United Nations member states to disseminate information in local languages through national health authorities. The national states had key roles to exercise effective communication through local languages even for linguistic minorities. Thus, member states had the mandate to translate COVID-19 information from English to diverse indigenous language including "linguistic minorities within those states whether indigenous or migrant, face significant language barriers" (Piller, Zhang & Li 2020, p. 505). Marketing studies show that messages delivered in person's first language have more impact and tend to provoke emotional reaction than messages delivered in person's second language (Puntoni, De Langhe & Osselaer, 2009; Citron, Michaelis & Goldberg, 2020). Other scholars note that messages in person's first language make the content more memorable and effective in changing behaviour [REMOVED HYPERLINK FIELD] (Mohanty, 2020; Tyng, Amin, Saad & Malik, 2017). There is always an assumption that minority language speakers will understand messages communicated in majority languages (Piller, Zhang & Li, 2020). In many cases awareness campaigns overlook the effect of language choice and the histories of majority language domination and exclusion of minority language speakers (Eberhard, Simons & Fennig, 2020). The marginalisation of minority communities is common around the world (Avineri et al., 2018; Piller, 2016) and often due to time limitations, negative influences on audience trust and effective communication tend to be less valued (Piller, 2016). Global public communication has always disadvantaged the minorities because it privileges the people who speaks majority languages at the expense of grassroot communities. In 2015, Wikipedia entries reflected 291 (5%) languages out of 5000-6000 world's languages as global knowledge repository and English came out as the most used language in the World; 2,5 times more than the second majority spoken languages (Piller, 2016). .

According to a report by Endangered Languages Project (2020); the COVID-19 outbreak saw the translations of preventive measures into 700 languages. Amongst the 700 languages, 630 were majority languages as it was assumed that minority language speakers are proficient in major languages (Eberhard, Simons & Fennig, 2020). Regardless of numerous translations, Eberhard, Simons and Fennig (2020) note that the success achieved was substantial because of misinformation in the infodemic. A report by the Global Preparedness Monitoring Board (2020) notes that building trust during the COVID-19 pandemic was the most crucial aspect in communication. Communication in dominant languages are historically perceived as tools of oppression and stigmatisation by minorities (Piller, Zhang & Li, 2020). Distrust in government authorities and health communicators also contributed to poor audience reception (Mathe & Motsaathebe, 2023d). The COVID-19 preventive measures such sanitising, social distancing and wearing of mask were largely communicated in major languages, of course with sign language (non-verbal language) (Piller, Zhang & Li, 2020). According to the Crisis and Emergency Risk Communication (2014) public health communication in local languages should be accompanied by local styles of delivery to promote audience' trust. Such an approach local styles of delivery includes making use of community leaders in delivering health campaigns in local languages (Eberhard, Simons & Fennig, 2020).

Open collaborative networks between linguists, specialist in the health sector, academics and marginalised communities is one example of co-creation for effective communication in health crisis (Austin, 2016; Henderson, 2015; Eberhard Simons & Fennig, 2020). Open collaborative network as a model enables the prioritisation of message preferences in language and cultural norms (Eberhard Simons Fennig, 2020). Thus, involving local community leaders in the model also builds trust as they deliver the health messages in local languages. Disaster times always demand high quality of information and timely health campaigns in various languages also for decision makers and health practitioners (Xiang et al., 2020). Uekusa (2019) argues that a mismatch of language and linguistic repertoires of the people targeted by the information worsens the effects of the disaster more on linguistic minorities than majority populations. Misinformation during the disaster occurs because there will not be one centre of communication instead of a variety of social actors namely the state, media, political parties, community leaders and grassroot groups. This means even if state actors do not translate messages in minority languages, some of the social actors at grassroot level can (Haimovich & Márquez, 2020; Lising, 2020; Yu, 2020). In other, words avoiding community leaders and social actors in public health communication, worsens the level of misinformation as they will be no responsibility and accountability as shown by Mathe and Motsaathebe's (2023d) article entitled play in the health crises reflecting dissent on Twitter during the COVID-19 pandemic against the ruling government in such a way that pandemic was further used as a counterpoint to highlight corruption, political violence and poor health infrastructure. Thus, many social actors especially in advent of social media contribute to the infodemic with misleading information and simultaneously getting populations misinformed (Zarocostas, 2020; Mathe & Motsaathebe, 2023d)). Above this involves lack of trust, language barriers. misinformation and fake news endangering minority populations as noted by the European Union research (van Liempt & Kox, 2020; Burke, 2020)

Piller, Zhang and Li (2020) reflect the complexity of language in China during the COVID-19 pandemic where linguistic minorities particularly the Mandarin speakers had to learn Putonghua language (which is a majority language) for communication posing language barriers to access health information. China health authorities communicated in Putonghua during the COVID-19 but the country realised in the middle of pandemic that there was a need to be multilingual to ensure universal compliance with public health regulations (Grey, 2017; Li, 2020; Li et al., 2019). COVID-19 studies in China reflect that China discovered later that multilingual approach was effective (Ahmad, 2020; Grey, 2020; Piller, 2020). Thus, the approach for effective in health crisis is the multilingual approach. English, of course has been dominant in former British colonies as a hegemonic culture in the global media (Motsaathebe, 2010). English has been dominant not only as a language during the pandemic but also as a hegemonic culture in the global media. Gazzola and Grin (2013) note that English as a language privileges countries who take it as a national language and do not need to invest resources in making people learn it as a foreign language. English as a language advantages countries where it is taken as the mother language and disadvantaging English non-speakers. Critiquing radio talkshows in multilingualism, Mathe and Motsaathebe (2023a) note that minorities often get dominated by major languages such as English, Shona and Ndebele. The African multilingual public sphere reflects code-switching and mixing into dominant languages at the expense of minorities and the supremacy of the major indigenous reflects their dominance in the African polity (Mathe & Motsaathebe, 2023a).The code-switching and mixing refers to language deviation and hybridisation opposite to the well-known standard writing (Chan, 2018). The code-switching and mixing disadvantages minorities yet multilingualism should occur without advantaging dominant languages (Mathe & Motsaathebe, 2023a). Gazzola and Grin (2013) note that English as a language privileges countries who take it as a national language and do not need to invest resources in making people learn it as a foreign language.

Communicating in different language, however, does not guarantee effective response to health crisis .O'Brien et al. (2018) and O'Brien and Federici (2019) argue that there must availability of information as essential service, accessibility of information in various forms of the media (radio, print and television even digital) in all languages, acceptability meaning the message should be accurate and appropriate for acceptance by the people, and lastly adaptability to shifting requirements for mobile populations and technological demands. This is why this chapter analyses health awareness campaigns in text, video, posters and every textual versions as radio content on Facebook.

METHODOLOGY

Methodologically, we applied a qualitative content analysis on print posts, captions and live recorded videos of radio studio sessions on health awareness campaigns to unveil public health communication in minority languages. To extract content on health awareness campaigns, we focused on all community radio platforms as shown in Table 1. From 20 July to 18 September 2023, we manually browsed community Facebook pages to identify any health issue communicated. It noteworthy that COVID-19, Malaria and campaigns against drug abuse were common health issues. Facebook has a search button below the profile of the community radio page. Thus, having preconceptions of the health issues in Zimbabwe, we entered COVID-19, Malaria and Drug abuse as keywords in the search engine. It is important to note that not every community radio forum unveiled content on health awareness campaigns. Community radio platforms that opened up much content on heath awareness campaigns include Vemuganga FM, Avuxeni, Nyangani, Lyeja FM just to mention a few. The Facebook posts analysed on health awareness campaigns were around 200 dating from September 2021 to July 2023. This timeframe was not determined by our selection but showed as the dates on the Facebook posts extracted.

COVID-19 refers to coronavirus which affected many livelihood in the late 2019 resulting in the pandemic which was controlled through lockdowns, sanitising, distancing and vaccinations Malaria is a life-threatening disease caused by malaria mosquitos and is common in Zimbabwe (WHO, 2023). In recent years, the country has had a many cases of drug abuse especially between 2022 and 2023. We thus analysed content on the above-mentioned health issues. Moreover, we also captured readers comments on selected videos to ascertain audience reception and interactivity on health awareness campaigns in local languages. We made use of comments on Facebook posts which had more readers' comments. Ethically we avoided screen shooting physical identities of presenters in the studio and we also hid the usernames of readers commenting on the Facebook commentary forum. The study uses Facebook post as a unity of analysis.

FINDINGS

A qualitative content analysis on radio platforms reveals three common public health issues communicated to minorities in various languages. The public health communication was based on (a) COVID-19, (b) drug use and abuse (c) malaria. The purpose was to reflect public health communication using different cases of health crises. COVID-19 is of course more emphasised in this chapter in figure, 4, 5, 6. 7 and cases on drug abuse and malaria are added as additional to the argument Given that not all community radio platforms had adequate content for analysis, the study made use of content largely from four community radio platforms namely Vemuganga, Avuxeni, Lyeja FM, Nyangani FM, Ntepe-Manama Community radio platforms. Vemuganga radio forums broadcasts and disseminates content mainly in Ndau. It is mandated by its licence to broadcast in broadcasting and publishing in Ndau language against drug use and abuse. Vemuganga broadcasting mandate is 85% Ndau, 10% English, 2% Shangani and 3% Ndebele. Ntepe-Manama is mandated to broadcast 5% English while the 95% goes to Sotho, Ndebele and Venda.

HEALTH AUTHORITIES COMMUNICATING IN MAJOR INDIGENOUS LANGUAGES

The qualitative content reveals bias of language in public health communication. Community radio stations reflected health awareness campaigns communicated by health authorities. This means mass communication on public health was centralised or was disseminated through radio stations but by health authorities. Public health communication was mainly communicated in Shona by health authorities, undermining the very minority languages on community radio stations. The Facebook community radio platforms did not reflect much of public health communication in minorities. Most speakers on community radio were health authorities. Figure 1 below gives an example of health awareness campaign on Vemuganga radio by government and the Vice President Chiwenga being the speaker against drug use and abuse. Vice-President Chiwenga assumed the role of Minister of Health during the COVID-19 pandemic. The video in the post reflects the speaker communicating in Shona against drug abuse in the area. Shona acted as a dominant hegemonic language negatively received by minorities (as shown in Figure 2 and 3). Public health communication by ZANU-PF government officials worsened the negative political reception of the public health messages. As shown by Eberhard et al. (2020); awareness campaigns tend to overlook the effect of language choice and the histories of majority language domination and exclusion of minority language speakers. The comments attached to the video reflects politicisation of health awareness event and rejection of the message by minorities. Figure 1 caption is written in Ndau and reads "the words of Minister of Health who is also the Vice President Dr C.D.N Chiwenga against those abusing drugs".

Readers messages attached to the commentary section of the video rejected the speakers as political. Audience reception reflected political sentiments instead of a positive reception towards drug abuse.

Thus, public health communication by politicians in their dominant indigenous languages negatively influenced audience reception. We argue that politicians become the symbol of histories of oppression and dominance, misgovernment, corruption and political violence, hence it becomes ironical for them to be delegates of health awareness campaigns when the health infrastructure collapsed under their rule. Mathe and Motsaathebe (2023d) show dissent on Twitter during the COVID-19 pandemic against the ruling government in such a way that pandemic was further used as a counterpoint to highlight corruption, political violence and poor health infrastructure. Readers comments in Figure 2 illustrate negative audience reception as a response to the awareness campaigns against drug abuse in Figure 1.

(a) "Iwe ukunakirwa nayo here mari"- yourself are you enjoying the money (when the Vice President said how do you enjoy money earned from selling drugs)
(b) "Ko vaarikuba gold"- What about those stealing gold (meaning politicians are doing the same crime done by drug dealers)
(c) "Mabwidi evanhu" - stupid people

Another comment reflects a minority language speaker complaining that the Vice President should have spoken in minority languages in Chipinge district rather than using Shona. The commentator probed

Figure 1. Web capture of drug use and abuse event (Disseminated by Vemuganga FM)

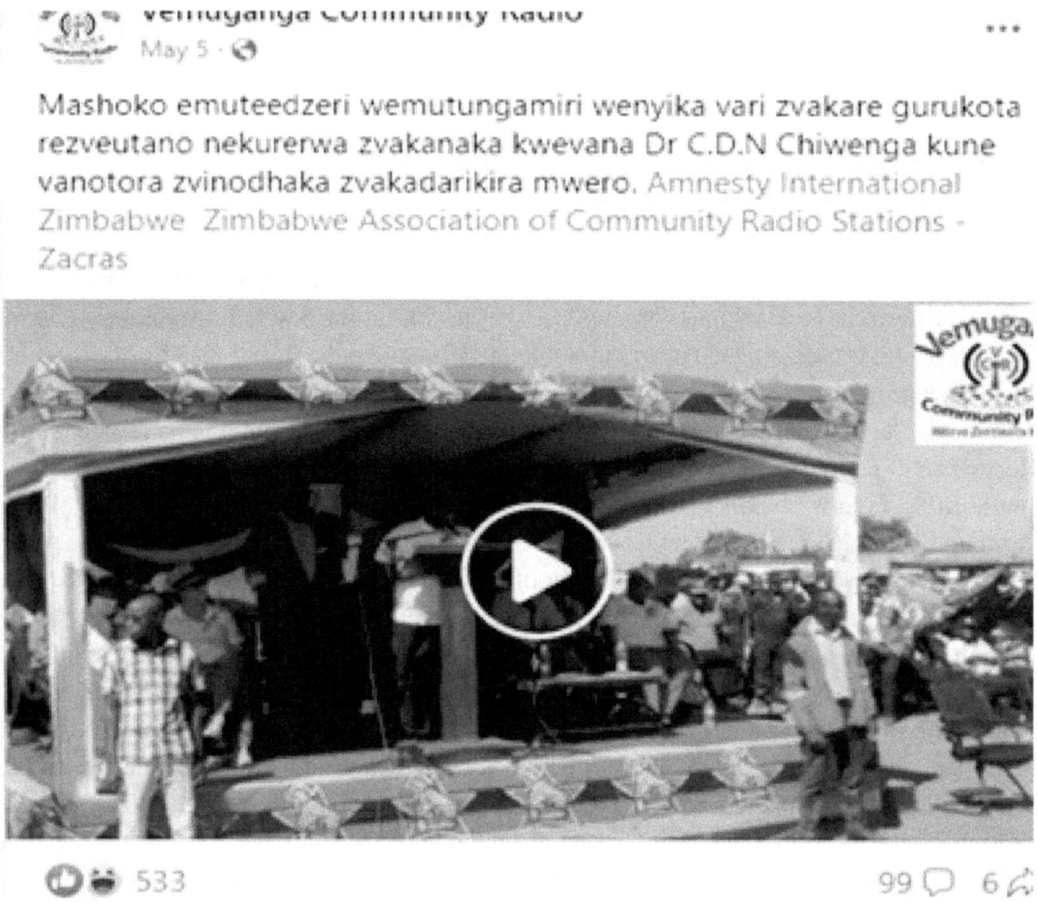
May 5
Mashoko emuteedzeri wemutungamiri wenyika vari zvakare gurukota rezveutano nekurerwa zvakanaka kwevana Dr C.D.N Chiwenga kune vanotora zvinodhaka zvakadarikira mwero. Amnesty International Zimbabwe Zimbabwe Association of Community Radio Stations - Zacras
533
99
6

Figure 2. Commentary forum to video in Figure 1

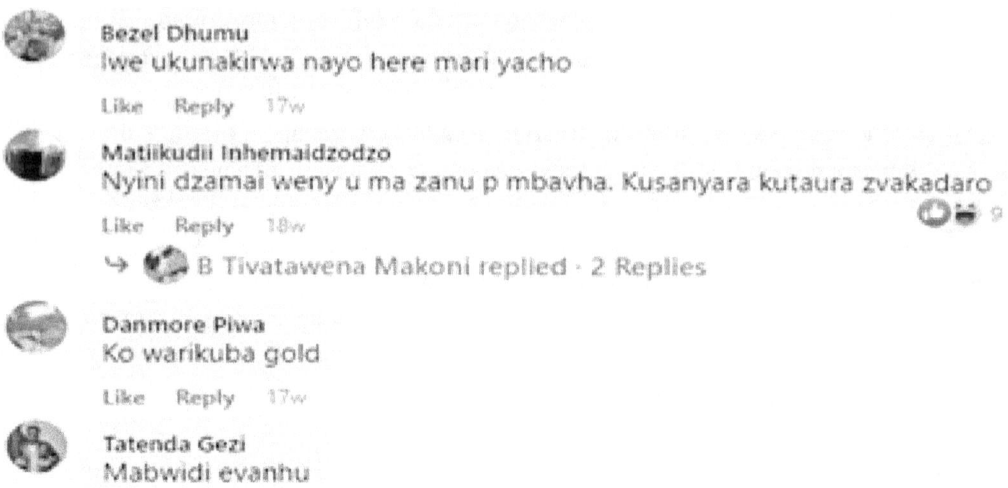
Bezel Dhumu
Iwe ukunakirwa nayo here mari yacho
Like Reply 17w
Matiikudii Inhemaidzodzo
Nyini dzamai weny u ma zanu p mbavha. Kusanyara kutaura zvakadaro
Like Reply 18w
B Tivatawena Makoni replied · 2 Replies
Danmore Piwa
Ko warikuba gold
Like Reply 17w
Tatenda Gezi
Mabwidi evanhu

for the use of English arguing that it is not everyone who understands Shona as shown in the comment "English please some of us speak Nambya and Nyanja". Nambya and Nyanja are minority languages in Zimbabwe. Nambya was recognised in the 2013 Constitution but Nyanja was considered under the category of Chewa. It is noteworthy that government officials in Zimbabwe largely communicated in major indigenous languages namely Shona and Ndebele with English as a common denominator. Literature has shown that Shona and Ndebele enjoy dominance in government although other scholars argue that Shona is more dominant than Ndebele. The underlining statement is that public health communication in Zimbabwe was largely communicated in these major indigenous languages and English as the overriding language. Minorities remain excluded in public health communication as it assumed that they understand major languages (Piller, Zhang & Li, 2020).

The politicisation of language goes as further as promoting mistrust among minorities. The lack of trust in government health authorities has been worsened by poor governance and pitiable health infrastructure (Mathe & Motsaathebe, 2023d). We argue that minority communities have been marginalised not only in terms of language but also in community development and infrastructure just as shown by Avineri et al. (2018) and Piller (2016) that marginalisation of minority communities is common. Thus, lack of trust is also reinforced by histories of political marginalisation and stigmatisation by minorities. According to the Crisis and Emergency Risk Communication (2014) public health communication in local languages should be accompanied by local styles of delivery to promote audience' trust. The findings reflect health authorities used untrusted government officials at the center of public health communication. The heath authorities did not utilise an open collaborative network outside the political reach to work with community leaders and other social actors in the campaign against drug use and abuse.

Figure 3. Further comments to Figure 1

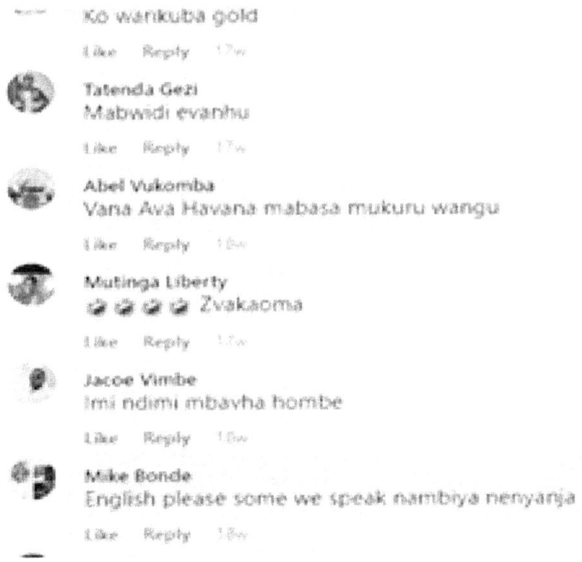

THE DOMINANCE OF ENGLISH IN PUBLIC HEALTH COMMUNICATION

Other findings from the study reflect the dominance of English in health awareness campaigns. The dissemination of content on community radio platforms for public health communication was largely visible in posters and captions. Given that Facebook posts can be utilised in text, video and print posters, the findings reflect English phrases in public health communication. This reflects lack of interpretation and language translation for minorities in their minority languages. The problem as shown by literature emanates from the language use in writing and speeches for example, English as the first language of WHO and the language of the educated in the former British colonies. Literature has shown that the COVID-19 was largely communicated in English ("Coronavirus disease (COVID-19) pandemic," 2020). This applies to every health crises or health communication that it mainly received in English, then translated to majority indigenous and with time limitations, minorities always suffer language exclusion (Avineri et al., 2018; Piller, 2016). For instance, the term Drug Abuse is an English phrase always used in the language mix with indigenous languages. Figure 4 shows public health awareness campaigns on COVID vaccinations in English.

COVID-19 was mainly centralised by the Ministry of Health and community radio was used for communication by health authorities. However, we argue that media was supposed to translate COVID-19 messages from English to minority languages just as shown by literature that member states of the United Nations were supposed to translate COVID-19 public communication from English to various indigenous languages including "linguistic minorities within those states -whether indigenous or migrant

Figure 4. COVID-19 awareness campaign in English on Avuexeni community radio

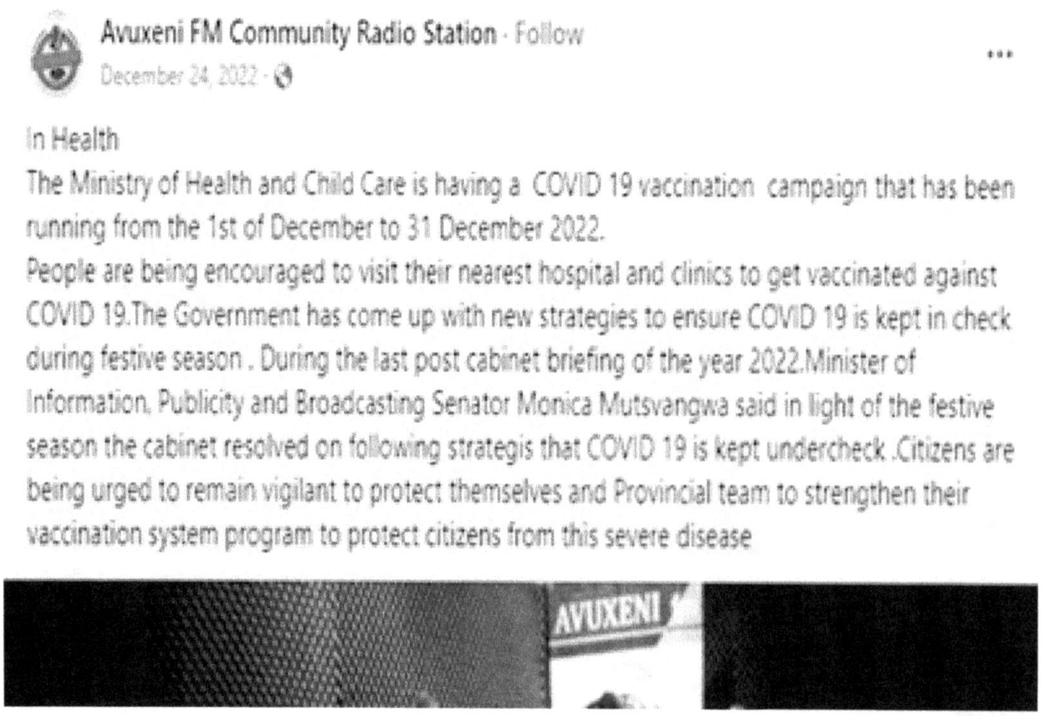
Avuxeni FM Community Radio Station · Follow
December 24, 2022 ·
In Health
The Ministry of Health and Child Care is having a COVID 19 vaccination campaign that has been running from the 1st of December to 31 December 2022.
People are being encouraged to visit their nearest hospital and clinics to get vaccinated against COVID 19.The Government has come up with new strategies to ensure COVID 19 is kept in check during festive season . During the last post cabinet briefing of the year 2022.Minister of Information, Publicity and Broadcasting Senator Monica Mutsvangwa said in light of the festive season the cabinet resolved on following strategis that COVID 19 is kept undercheck .Citizens are being urged to remain vigilant to protect themselves and Provincial team to strengthen their vaccination system program to protect citizens from this severe disease
AVUXENI

Figure 5. Covid-19 focus on women and children

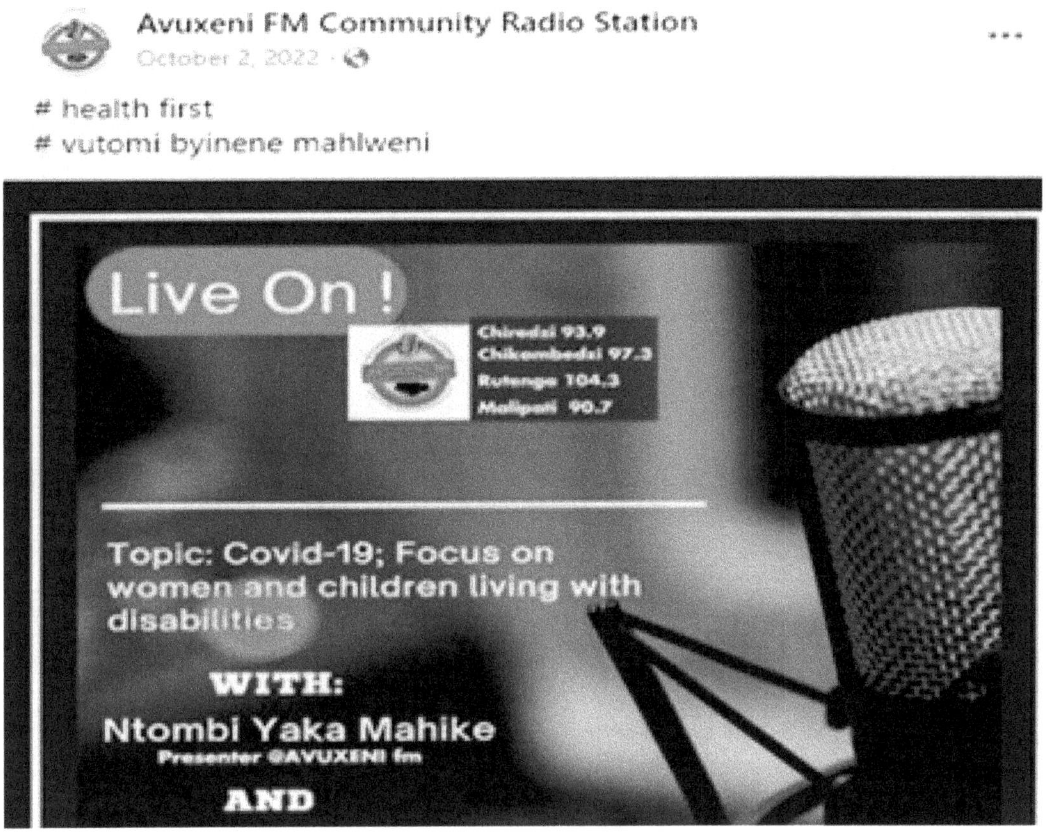
Avuxeni FM Community Radio Station
October 2, 2022
health first
vutomi byinene mahlweni
Live On !
Topic: Covid-19; Focus on women and children living with disabilities
WITH:
Ntombi Yaka Mahike
Presenter @AVUXENI fm
AND

-face significant language barriers" (Piller, Zhang & Li 2020, p. 505). The dominance of English was not only evident in captions but also in posters such as reflected in Figure 5.

Figure 5 shows a mix of minority language in Shangani and English. The caption reads "vutomi byinene mahlweni" meaning Health First. The topic of the programme was, however, in English as seen in the poster "Covid-19; Focus on the women and children living with disabilities". The English topic does alienate indigenous population even minorities which the Avuxeni FM should be focusing on. Another example to cement this argument of English in posters is also reflected in Figure 6. This shows that public health communication awareness campaigns were mainly in English. The speakers on these campaigns were government Health Authorities.

We played several recorded live radio videos on Avuxeni FM platform and other on Vemuganga FM platform to ascertain the languages used in the talk on several health campaigns. The findings of the study corroborate with Mathe and Motsaathebe (2023a) that minority language presenters on radio switch to the dominant languages of the guests or speakers in the radio multilingual public sphere. The presenters on health awareness campaigns did some introductions in minority languages but switched to Shona or English whenever engaging Shona or English guests acting as Health Authorities or knowledgeable speakers on the subject issue. The programme became dominant Shona or English languages disadvantaging minorities as audiences of the community radio. Given that Shona and English have certain content percentages as the language of the community radio, they tend to be dominantly used

Figure 6. Integrated measles and COVID-19 campaigns

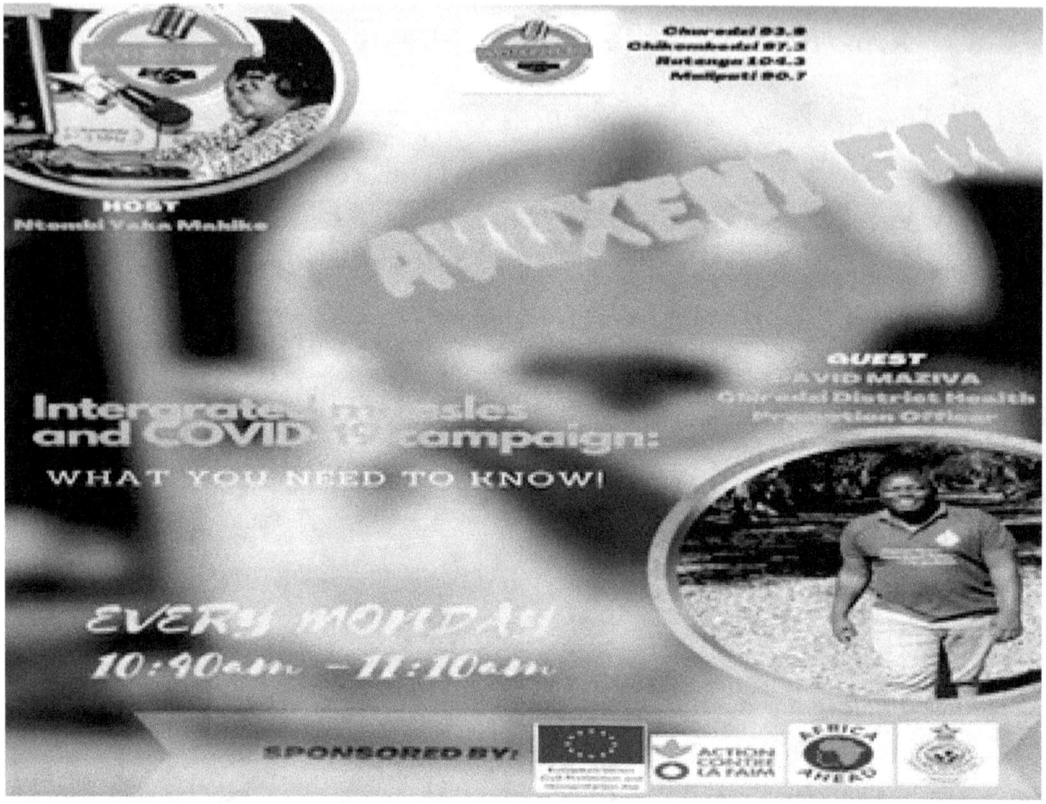

in public health communication. For instance, the Avuxeni FM health awareness shows on drug abuse and COVID-19 were dominated by Shona speaking guests who often switched to English. The minority languages, Shangani and Ndau were only used in introductory sessions by the presenters who switched to Shona to accommodate their guests.

Mathe and Motsaathebe (2023a) have shown that the dominance of major languages in the public sphere of radio reflects their dominance in the African polity. The reflection of health authorities dominantly in major indigenous languages and English shows that minorities are marginalised in the health sector hence the challenges of language translation and recognition. Shona was dominant in the community radio platforms and the guests on awareness programmes spoke largely in Shona and English. Literature has shown that Shona, English and Ndebele were prioritised in government since 1980 disadvantaging minorities. Arguing on multilingualism, Mathe and Motsaathebe (2023a) note that multilingualism (meaning a talk between a minority and majority language speakers) should occur without switching to the language of the majority.

There were several Facebook posts reflecting public health communication in English in most community radio forums. The argument is not necessarily to say English should not be used given that most community radio stations have a mandate of 5% English language content, we note that public health communication should not be entirely disadvantage minorities even through community radio. Figure 7 gives more evidence on COVID-19 updates in English, the news cases and casualties were all in English.

Figure 7. COVID-19 updates on Lyeja FM Facebook platform

LYEJA FM
October 7, 2021

07/10/2021 Covid-19 Update

99 local new Cases of Covid-19 and 1 deaths were recorded by the Ministry of health and child care in the last 24 hours.

The 7 day rolling average for new cases fall to 136 from 183 yesterday

.

Bulawayo Province recorded 5 new cases Matebeleland North 17 while Mat South recorded 3 new cases.

218 new recoveries were reported and the National Recovery rate stands at 95% .

Active cases go down to 2 473.

To date Zimbabwe has recorded 131 434 cases, 124 331 recoveries & 4 630 Deaths.

Meanwhile 11 788 received their 1st dose bringing cumulative for the 1st dose to 3 140 685 while 15 257 received their 2nd dose bringing cumulative for 2nd dose to 2 358 223.

ENDS //

LYEJA FM
October 5, 2021

04/10/2021 Covid-19 Update

76 local new Cases of Covid-19 and 0 deaths were recorded by the Ministry of health and child care in the last 24 hours.

The 7 day rolling average for new cases fall to 183 from 237 yesterday

.

Bulawayo Province recorded 3 new cases Matebeleland North 5 while Mat South recorded 4 new cases.

160 new recoveries were reported and the National Recovery rate stands at 94% .

Active cases go down to 2 631.

To date Zimbabwe has recorded 131 205 cases, 123 947 recoveries & 4 627 Deaths.

Meanwhile 6 101 received their 1st dose bringing cumulative for the 1st dose to 3 117 895 while 10 525 received their 2nd dose bringing cumulative for 2nd dose to 2 322 862.

ENDS //

The terminology was mainly in English as inherited from WHO and the Ministry of Health in Zimbabwe which used mainly English.

Figure 8. Malaria outbreak in Manicaland

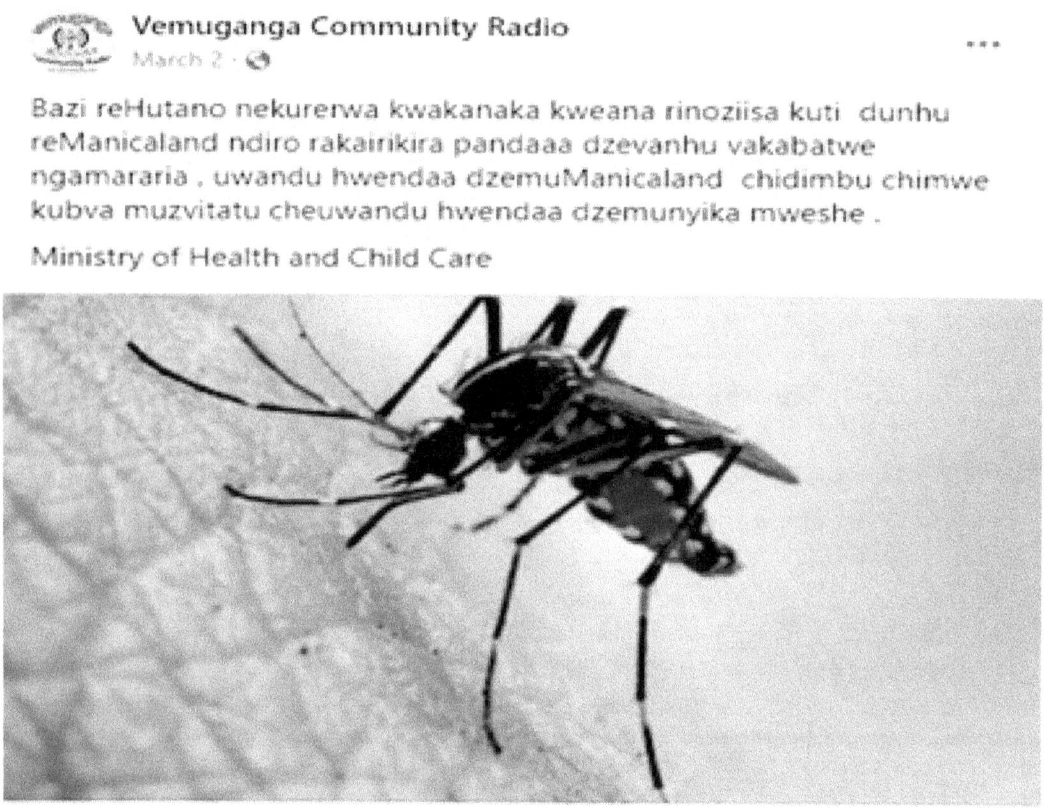

A FEW EXCEPTIONS OF PUBLIC HEALTH COMMUNICATION IN MINORITY LANGUAGES

There were a few exceptions of public health communication or health awareness campaigns in minority languages which we hardly extracted from community radio platforms. Our content extraction through Facebook direct on Community radio platforms did not unveil much content on health awareness campaigns in minority languages. We extracted some few posts on malaria awareness. Zimbabwe has been able to control malaria which was very problematic in the 1990s. The people even minorities understand malaria disease as they were enormous government effort to educate and even include the malaria issue in education. It is therefore not surprising that minorities could now interpret malaria in their own languages as shown in Figure 8. This could mean the necessity of time for response and for language translations.

The Facebook post in Figure 8 written in Ndau informs that there is now a malaria outbreak in Manicaland. This chapter acknowledges the effort by Vemuganga Community and Avuxeni Community radio to communicate in Ndau, a minority language, however English and Shona were more evident. Figure 9 below shows the code-switching from between minority language and English.

Code-switching and mixing is evident in public health communication. The argument in this chapter is that language hybridisation advantages major indigenous languages and English language. Minority languages are always mixed with English or major indigenous language in public health communication.

Figure 9. Drug abuse (marijuana and mukozodo) tops in Chipinge district

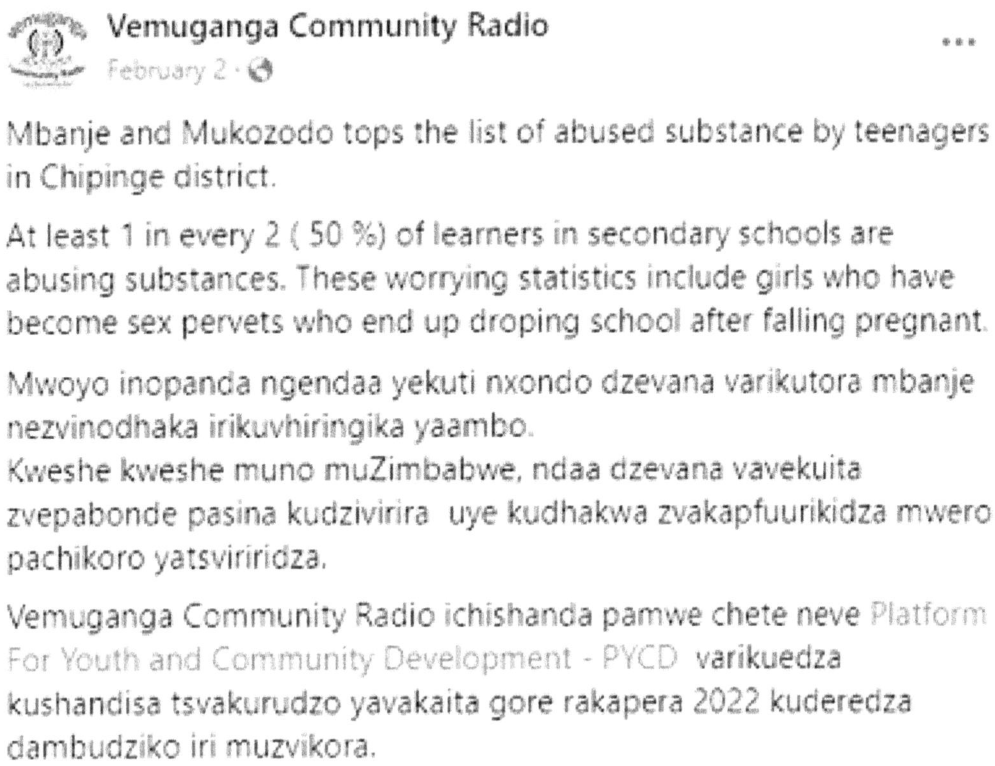
Vemuganga Community Radio
February 2 ·
Mbanje and Mukozodo tops the list of abused substance by teenagers in Chipinge district.
At least 1 in every 2 (50 %) of learners in secondary schools are abusing substances. These worrying statistics include girls who have become sex pervets who end up droping school after falling pregnant.
Mwoyo inopanda ngendaa yekuti nxondo dzevana varikutora mbanje nezvinodhaka irikuvhiringika yaambo.
Kweshe kweshe muno muZimbabwe, ndaa dzevana vavekuita zvepabonde pasina kudzivirira uye kudhakwa zvakapfuurikidza mwero pachikoro yatsviriridza.
Vemuganga Community Radio ichishanda pamwe chete neve Platform For Youth and Community Development - PYCD varikuedza kushandisa tsvakurudzo yavakaita gore rakapera 2022 kuderedza dambudziko iri muzvikora.

DISCUSSION

The findings of the study reflect centralised public health communication by government officials through community radio talk shows. In cases where there was dissemination of health awareness campaigns, administrators made use of posters on Facebook. The posters or textual versions were often more in English than minority indigenous languages. Thus, the findings of the study reflect the use of Shona and Ndebele by government officialised through community radio talk and English through posters. This means public health communication was largely in Shona, Ndebele and English at the expense of minority languages. Theorising public health communication in minority languages, we emphasise multilingualism, open collaborative networks and accessibility of information in various forms of the media for effective communication.

As shown by literature, open collaborative network promotes the utilisation of language and cultural norms among academics, linguists, specialists in health sector, local community leaders and marginalised communities for effective communication (Austin, 2016; Henderson, 2015; Eberhard Simons & Fennig, 2020). Involving local community leaders in the network of public health communication promotes trust rather than making use of government officials especially politicians who represent a history of oppression, misgovernance and corruption. The findings of the study shows that Zimbabwe made use of government officials (health specialists) and politicians in the ruling party to disseminate public health messages yet politicians ate the least trusted in the country as shown by the findings. On the other hand, we emphasise a multilingual approach by health specialists. While the use of community leaders makes public health messages reach the people in their own languages, communication by health specialists or government to minorities should also be in the language of the community. Such an approach, therefore, demands a multingual approach for effective communication. The findings of public health communication during the COVID-19 pandemic in China, notes that the country realised later that there was need to be multilingual after majoring in Putonghua (Grey, 2017; Li, 2020; Li et al., 2019). Last but not least, we emphasise on the utilisation of various forms of media for public health communication in indigenous languages. Communicating in indigenous languages alone without the support of media diversity for information accessibility maybe problematic since the message always needs to reach audiences (O'Brien et al. 2018; O'Brien & Federici. 2019). However, radio remains the most accessible media in Zimbabwe especially community radio for minority languages.

It is important to note that this study is limited to the scope of the study that is community radio and the dissemination of radio content on Facebook. The concept of public health communication on community radio was explored from an angle of health awareness campaigns through various content of radio on Facebook. The limitation of the study remains within the state of language preferences and the speakers of these languages as reflected by the findings of the study.

CONCLUSION

This chapter made use of community radio platforms on social media to analyse the Facebook posts for public health communication. Given that radio content is disseminated in form of text, posters and videos, we perused every available content on health awareness campaigns to analyse how minority languages are used for public heath communication. The heath awareness campaigns communicated issues on Drug use and abuse, COVID-19 and malaria. This chapter unveiled key findings on the subject of public health communication to minorities. In the context of Zimbabwe, the chapter argued that minority languages which are supposed to be exclusively broadcasted on community radio still remain excluded in public health communication on the exclusive media platforms. The findings of the study show that health authorities were mainly the communicators and the educators on the above-mentioned topics. In other section, we note that awareness campaigns were somehow politicised as they were being presided by government officials such as the Vice President who spoke in Shona. We argue that using politicians for health awareness campaigns disrupts the reception of the message, even so in majority indigenous languages. We also argue that the government in Zimbabwe is highly blamed for poor health infrastructure and corruption, therefore public health communication by the same government tends to be less effective. On another note, this chapter reflects the dominance of Shona and English in public health communication. Communication in English and mainly Shona on community radio forums which are meant to also communicate in minority languages undermines the very local languages of the radio. The videos analysed on Facebook show guests or speakers as health authorities communicating mainly in Shona and English while the presenters switches to their main languages abandoning Ndau or Shangani and other minority languages.

Lastly the paper shows that public health communication in minority languages is characterised by code-switching and mixing of health terms borrowed from English and major indigenous languages. In other words, public health communication in minorities is lacking and Zimbabwe has not shown diversity in translating health messages in various minority languages. We argue that lack of public health communication in minority languages reflects lack of minority participation in public health communication. In conclusion, we that the government of Zimbabwe should recognise minority languages not only in education, media and government but is also in public health communication. Language barrier affects communication and minorities are mainly the victims of marginalisation. Minorities should participate in language translation programmes and government must use open collaborative networks to work with community leaders and other social actors in pioneering health awareness campaigns in minority languages.

REFERENCES

Ahmad, R. (2020). Multilingual resources key to fighting. https://www. languageonthemove.com/multilingual-resources-key-to-fighting-covid-19/

Arora, P. (2019). *The Next Billion Users: Digital Life Beyond the West.* Harvard University Press. doi:10.4159/9780674238879

Austin, P. (2016). Language documentation 20 years on. In L. Filipović & M. Pütz (Eds.), *Endangered languages and languages in danger: issues of documentation, policy, and language rights* (pp. 147–170). John Benjamins Publishing Company. doi:10.1075/impact.42.07aus

Avineri, N., Laura, R., Graham, E. J., Johnson, R., Conley, R., & Jonathan, R. (2018). *Language and social justice in practice.* Routledge. doi:10.4324/9781315115702

Benkler, Y. (2006). *The Wealth of Networks.* Yale University Press.

Berry, R. (2014). The future of radio is the internet, not on the internet. In Radio: The Resilient Medium. (pp. 3-15). Sunderland: Centre for Research in Media and Cultural Studies.

Bonini, T. (2012). Doing radio in the age of Facebook. In Radio Evolution: Conference Proceedings. ECREA/University of Minho.

Bosch, T. (2003). Radio, community and identity in South Africa: A rhizomatic study of Bush radio in Cape Town (Doctoral dissertation, Ohio University). http://rave.ohiolink.edu/etdc/view?acc_num=ohiou1079300111

Bosch, T. (2014). Social Media and Community Radio Journalism in South Africa. *Digital Journalism (Abingdon, England)*, *2*(1), 29–43. doi:10.1080/21670811.2013.850199

Burke, F. (2020). The dangers of misinformation and neglecting linguistic minorities during a pandemic. https://horizon-magazine.eu/article/dangers-misinformation-and neglecting-linguistic-minorities-during-pandemic.html

Chan, K. L. R. (2018). Being a 'Purist' in Trilingual Hong Kong: Code-Switching among Cantonese, English and Putonghua. *Linguistic Review*, *35*(1), 75–95. doi:10.17250/khisli.35.1.201803.003

Chonka, P., Diepeveen, S., & Haile, Y. (2023). Algorithmic power and African indigenous languages: Search engine autocomplete and the global multilingual Internet. *Media Culture & Society*, *45*(2), 246–265. doi:10.1177/01634437221104705

Citron, F. M. M., Michaelis, N., & Goldberg, A. E. (2020). Metaphorical language processing and amygdala activation in L1 and L2. *Neuropsychologia, 140*, 107381. Advance online publication. doi:10.1016/j.neuropsychologia.2020.107381 PMID:32061649

Crisis and Emergency Risk Communication. (2014). Atlanta: US Centers for Disease Control and Prevention. https://emergency.cdc.gov/cerc/ppt/cerc_2014edition_Copy.pdf

Croteau, D., & William, H. (2000). *Media/Society*. Pine Forge Press.

Di Carlo, P. (2020). Message- vs. community-centered models in risk communication [internet]. Sydney: Language on the Move. https://www.languageonthemove.com/message-vs-community-centered-models-in-risk-communication/

Di Carlo, P., McDonnell, B., Vahapoglu, J., Good, J., Seyfeddinipur, M., & Kordas, K. (2021). Building climate-sensitive nutrition programmes. *Bulletin of the World Health Organization, 100*(1), 78–80. doi:10.2471/BLT.21.285617 PMID:35017760

Eberhard, D. M., Simons, G. F., & Fennig, C. D. (2020) (eds). Ethnologue: Languages of the World. 23rd ed. Dallas: SIL International.

Endangered Languages Project. (2020). COVID-19 information in indigenous, endangered, and under-resourced languages. https://endangeredlanguagesproject.github.io/COVID-19

Gazzola, M., & François, G. (2013). Is ELF more effective and fair than translation? An evaluation of the EU's multilingual regime. *International Journal of Applied Linguistics, 23*(1), 93–107. doi:10.1111/ijal.12014

Global Preparedness Monitoring Board. (2020). Building trust within and across communities for health emergency preparedness. Geneva and Washington, DC. https://apps.who.int/gpmb/assets/thematic_papers_2020/tp_2020_3.pdf

Grey, A. (2017). How do language rights affect minority languages in China? An ethnographic investigation of the Zhuang minority language under conditions of rapid social change (PhD). Macquarie University. http://www.languageonthemove.com/ wpcontent/uploads/2017/05/Grey_How_do_language_rights_affect_minority_languages.pdf

Grey, A. (2020). How to improve Australia's public health messaging about. https://www.languageonthemove.com/how-to-improve-australias-public health-messaging-about-covid-19/

Haimovich, G., & Márquez Mora, H. (2020). Why it's important to use Indigenous languages in health communication. https://www.languageonthemove.com/ why-its-important-to-use-indigenous-languages-in-health-communication/

Healthy People. (2010). US Dept of Health and Human Services. https://professionals.wrha.mb.ca/old/extranet/publichealth/priorities-communication.php

Institute of Medicine. (2003). *The Future of the Public's Health in the 21st Century*. National Academy Press.

Li, J. (2020). Transnational migrant students between inclusive discourses and exclusionary practices. *Multilingua*, *39*(2), 192–212. doi:10.1515/multi-2019-0125

Li, J., Ai, B., & Zhang, J. (2019). Negotiating language ideologies in learning Putonghua: Myanmar ethnic minority students' perspectives on multilingual practices in a borderland school. *Journal of Multilingual and Multicultural Development*, 1–14. doi:10.1080/01434632.2019.1678628

Lising, L. (2020). COVID-19 health information campaigns in the Philippines. https://www.languageonthemove.com/covid-19-health-information-campaigns-in-the philippines/

Lister, M., Jon, D., Giddings, S., Grant, I., & Kieran, K. (2003). *New Media: A Critical Introduction*. Routledge.

Mano, W. (2012). Why radio is Africa's medium of choice in the global age. In D. Ligaga, D. Moyo, & L. Gunner (Eds.), *Radio in Africa: cultures, publics and communities* (pp. 102–117). Johannesburg Wits University Press.

Mathe, L. (2023). Women's political participation in Zimbabwe: Play and content creation on Twitter. *Information Communication and Society*, *26*(13), 2598–2613. Advance online publication. doi:10.1080/1369118X.2023.2250442

Mathe, L., & Motsaathebe, G. (2023a). African multilingual public sphere: A critical analysis of minority indigenous language(s) representation on Breeze FM talk radio in Zimbabwe. *African Identities*, 1–17. Advance online publication. doi:10.1080/14725843.2023.2251700

Mathe, L., & Motsaathebe, G. (2023b). The political economy of indigenous local media for minority languages in Zimbabwe: A case of Lyeja FM community radio. *Journal of Asian and African Studies*. Advance online publication. doi:10.1177/00219096231160233

Mathe, L., & Motsaathebe, G. (2023c). Dissemination of Community Radio Content in Facebook Posts: Limitations and Opportunities for Indigenous Languages. *Forthcoming in Communicatio*. https://doi.org/10.1080/02500167.2024.2332181

Mathe & Motsaathebe. (2023d). Play on Twitter During a Health Crisis in Non-Democratic Context. Gratification or Dissent? Social Media and Society.

Mignolo, W. D. (2007). Delinking. *Cultural Studies*, *21*(2–3), 449–514. doi:10.1080/09502380601162647

Mohanty, S. N. (Ed.). (2020). *Emotion and information processing: a practical approach*. Springer International Publishing AG. doi:10.1007/978-3-030-48849-9

Motsaathebe, G. (2010). Language, Afrikology and the Tremor of the Political Moment: English as the Main Language of Discourse in Africa. *Indilinga*, *9*(1), 96–109.

Mpofu, P., & Salawu, A. (2020). African language use in the digital public sphere: Functionality of the localised Google webpage in Zimbabwe. *South African Journal of African Languages*, *40*(1), 76–84. doi:10.1080/02572117.2020.1733833

O'Brien, S., Federici, F., Cadwell, P., Marlowe, J., & Gerber, B. (2018). Language translation during disaster: A comparative analysis of five national approaches. *International Journal of Disaster Risk Reduction, 31*, 627–636. doi:10.1016/j.ijdrr.2018.07.006

O'Brien, S., & Federico, M. F. (2019). Crisis translation: Considering language needs in multilingual disaster settings. Disaster Prevention and Management. *Disaster Prevention and Management, 29*(2), 129–143. Advance online publication. doi:10.1108/DPM-11-2018-0373

Pavlik, J. (2001). *Journalism and New Media*. Columbia University Press. doi:10.7312/pavl11482

Piller, I. (2016). *Linguistic diversity and social justice*. Oxford University Press. doi:10.1093/acprof:oso/9780199937240.001.0001

Piller, I., Zhang, J., & Li, J. (2020). Linguistic diversity in a time of crisis: Language challenges of the COVID-19 pandemic. *Multilingua, 39*(5), 503–515. doi:10.1515/multi-2020-0136

Puntoni, S., De Langhe, B., & Van Osselaer, S. M. (2009). Bilingualism and the emotional intensity of advertising language. *The Journal of Consumer Research, 35*(6), 1012–1025. doi:10.1086/595022

Rohloff, P., & Henderson, B. (2015). Development, language revitalization, and culture: the case of Mayan languages of Guatemala, and their relevance for African languages. In J. Essegbey, B. Henderson, & F. Mc Laughlin (Eds.), *Language documentation and endangerment in Africa* (pp. 177–194). John Benjamins Publishing Company. doi:10.1075/clu.17.07roh

Salawu, A., Tsutsa, F., & Mpofu, P. (2022). Adoption of Digital Media by African Language Print Newspapers: The Case of Isolezwe. *Journal of Social Sciences and Humanities, 19*(5), 24–35.

Tkach, B., & Williams, A. A. (2018). Mobile (in) security? Exploring the realities of mobile phone use in conflict areas. *Information Communication and Society, 21*(11), 1639–1654. doi:10.1080/1369118X.2017.1348531

Tyng, C. M., Amin, H. U., Saad, M. N. M., & Malik, A. S. (2017). The influences of emotion on learning and memory. *Frontiers in Psychology, 24*(8), 1454. doi:10.3389/fpsyg.2017.01454 PMID:28883804

Uekusa, S. (2019). Disaster linguicism: Linguistic minorities in disasters. *Language in Society, 48*(3), 353–375. doi:10.1017/S0047404519000150

van Liempt, I., & Mieke, K. (2020). Coronavirus: Misinformation is leading to 'fake news' anxieties in Dutch refugee communities. The Conversation. https:// theconversation.com/coronavirus-misinformation-is-leading-to-fake-news-anxieties-indutch-refugee-communities-141830

Vita, V. (2020). Bridging new and traditional media in the fight against Covid-19. Sydney: Language on the Move. https://www.languageonthemove.com/bridging-new-and-traditional-media-in-the-fight-against-covid-19/

Waisbord, S., & Mellado, C. (2014). De-westernizing communication studies: A reassessment. *Communication Theory, 24*(4), 361–372. doi:10.1111/comt.12044

Wasserman, H. (2005). Renaissance and Resistance: Using ICTs for social change in South Africa. *African Studies, 64*(2), 177–199. doi:10.1080/00020180500355686

Willems, W., & Mano, W. (2016). Decolonizing and provincializing audience and internet studies: Contextual approaches from African vantage points. In W. Willems & W. Mano (Eds.), *Everyday Media Culture in Africa* (pp. 15–40). Routledge. doi:10.4324/9781315472775

World Health Organisation. (2023). Malaria. https://www.who.int/news-room/fact-sheets/detail/malaria

Xiang, Y., Li, W., Zhang, Q., Jin, Y., Rao, W.-W., Zeng, L.-N., Lok, G. K. I., Chow, I. H. I., Cheung, T., & Hall, B. J. (2020). Timely research papers about COVID-19 in China. *Lancet*, *395*(10225), 684–685. doi:10.1016/S0140-6736(20)30375-5 PMID:32078803

Yu, L. (2020). Fighting the coronavirus in local languages. https://www. languageonthemove.com/fighting-the-coronavirus-in-local-languages/

Zarocostas, J. (2020). How to fight an infodemic. *Lancet*, *395*(10225), 676. doi:10.1016/S0140-6736(20)30461-X PMID:32113495

Chapter 9

Public Health Communication and Language Policy at Rhodes University During the COVID-19 Pandemic

Zikhona Mamase
Rhodes University, South Africa

Kealeboga Aiseng
https://orcid.org/0000-0002-5684-9519
Rhodes University, South Africa

ABSTRACT

The COVID-19 pandemic offered unprecedented obstacles to public health communication worldwide. Pandemic revealed disparities and significant gaps in access to public health information for those not proficient in English, potentially leading to the exclusion of indigenous language speakers and minority communities from issues of national interest, including vital COVID-19 updates. This chapter examines the case study of Rhodes University in the Eastern Cape, South Africa and explores the institution's language policies and practices during the pandemic. The institution grapples with linguistic diversity, where English is the primary language of teaching and administration. The study explores language, public health communication, and inclusion at Rhodes University. It seeks to find linguistic and cultural contestations during this time by evaluating the university's response to the pandemic through language. The study uses document analysis to understand how Rhodes University's language practices impacted public health communication during the pandemic.

INTRODUCTION

The COVID-19 pandemic, which emerged in late 2019, disrupted lives, economies, and healthcare systems worldwide. The unprecedented crisis underscored the vital role of effective communication in

DOI: 10.4018/979-8-3693-0624-6.ch009

public health, as timely and accurate information became a critical tool in managing the spread of the virus and mitigating its impact. Language, a cornerstone of communication, was central to disseminating essential health information, ensuring understanding, and fostering community engagement.

The COVID-19 pandemic fundamentally altered the landscape of global health communication, prompting swift and far-reaching responses from governments, organizations, and educational institutions worldwide. Among these, universities faced unique challenges in ensuring the safety and well-being of their campus communities while continuing their core mission of education and research. Public health communication, language choices, and policy were at a crossroads during the unprecedented crisis.

In the wake of the unprecedented global COVID-19 pandemic, the world witnessed a profound transformation in how societies communicated, shared information, and responded to public health crises. At the heart of this transformation lay the crucial intersection of public health communication and language practices – a dynamic and multifaced nexus that demanded innovative strategies, adaptability, and sensitivity to navigate effectively.

Language, as both a medium of communication and a bearer of cultural nuances, plays a central role in the effectiveness of public health communication efforts. During the COVID-19 pandemic, institutions worldwide were confronted with the critical task of crafting appropriate health messages but also ensuring these messages were understood by diverse linguistic and cultural communities.

However, we live in a world where global public communication is conducted only through a few world languages. The COVID-19 pandemic exposed serious challenges with multilingual communication. During the pandemic, the world experienced a large-scale exclusion of minorities from timely, high-quality information (Piller et al., 2020). This was mainly due to the "dominance of English-centric global mass communication; the longstanding devaluation of minorized languages; and the failure to consider the importance of multilingual repertoires for building trust and resilient communities" (Piller et al., 2020, p. 503).

This chapter delves into unique and insightful issues of public health communication, language practices, and language policies at Rhodes University during the COVID-19 pandemic. Within the halls of Rhodes University, situated in the picturesque town of Makhanda, South Africa, a microcosm of the global challenges emerged. The pandemic forced academic institutions like Rhodes to grapple with multifarious public health communication, language practices, and language policy issues.

This chapter examines the nuanced interplay between public health strategies, language choices, and language policy at Rhodes University, comprehensively exploring the challenges, responses, and lessons learned. The chapter illuminates the complex issues surrounding multilingualism, cultural context, educational equity, effective communication of health information, and the university's language policy. Moreover, it underscores the place of indigenous languages in communication and health information during the pandemic in the South African higher education landscape.

RESEARCH QUESTIONS

1. Which language(s) did Rhodes University use to communicate its COVID-19 messages with the university community?
2. How did Rhodes University's language usage impact the university's language policy?
3. What are the potential implications of the university communications' strategies on indigenous languages?

4. In what ways did the COVID-19 pandemic catalyse re-evaluating and potentially revisiting language policies and communication practices at Rhodes University and other South African universities?

LANGUAGE-IN-EDUCATION POLICY: SOUTH AFRICA

In the developed world, language rights protect languages spoken by minority groups (Skutnabb-Kangas, 2006). However, in Africa, language rights are adopted to protect languages most people speak against Indo-European languages and sometimes other dominant African languages (Docrat & Kaschula, 2015; Namyalo & Nakayiza, 2015). In the former, linguistic debates are framed from the language ecology perspective, whereby the primary argument is that languages, endangered languages in particular, need to be supported through inclusive policies in order for them to thrive and live (Hornberger, 2002; Mkhize & Balfour, 2017). However, in the latter instances, language rights are framed from a legal perspective, as evidenced by the articulation of languages in the South African Constitution and other legislative frameworks (Mkhize & Balfour, 2017).

Language-in-education policy in South Africa is a complex and evolving framework that addresses the country's linguistic diversity while promoting equitable access to education. The South African Constitution recognizes 12 official languages, reflecting the nation's rich linguistic heritage. Language policy in education plays a pivotal role in facilitating access to quality education and addressing historical inequalities.

The issue of language policy in South African Higher Education is contentious and involves efforts to create an inclusive system that is transformative and welcoming to every student. Consequently, various policy tools have been developed to steer the higher education system towards a public good, socially inclusive enterprise (DHET, 2017). Cele (2021) states that efforts to transform the linguistic ecology of South African higher education are seen in some of the following documents: the Constitution of the Republic of South Africa Act 106 of 1996, Pan South African Language Board Act 59 of 1995, the 1996 report of the National Commission of Higher Education, the White Paper on Higher Education, the Higher Education Act of 1997, Policy for the Registration of Learners for Home Education, the National Plan for Higher Education, the Language Policy for Higher Education of 2002, the National Policy Framework of 2003, Adult Education Act 52 of 2000, Higher Education Laws Amendment, Act 26 of 2010.

Currently, the Language Policy Framework for Public Higher Education Institutions (LPFPHEI) adopted in 2020 ensures linguistic transformation and the sustainability of indigenous languages in South African universities. The policy recognizes that everyone has a right to learn in their language choice. To give effect to this policy, the LPFPHEI requires universities to develop multilingual language policies and implement multilingualism in their teaching and learning programs.

The LPFPHEI was adopted to address the following:

1. The language of teaching and learning at public higher education institutions, bearing in mind the fundamental right of persons to receive education in the official language or languages of their choice in public education institutions, where it is reasonably practicable to do so, and the duty of the state to ensure adequate access to the implementation of this right (section 29(2) of the Constitution of the Republic of South Africa, 1996)
2. The language or languages of official communication within the higher education institutions

3. The role of higher education in promoting and creating conditions for the development of historically marginalized official South African languages, as well as the Khoi, Nama, San languages, and Sign Language
4. The right of every person to use the language and participate in the cultural life of his or her choice within an educational institution.
5. The role of higher education in preparing sufficient language teachers, interpreters, translators, and other language practitioners to serve the needs of a diverse South Africa's multilingual society.

Arguably, the primary linguistic interests of these policies have always been that of political positioning and social redress, with the primary purpose being to make African languages the languages of teaching and learning in universities (DHET, 2017). This is a response to the Apartheid system of social exclusion, where African languages were marginalized and reduced to non-official communication tools (Cele, 2021). The White Paper on Higher Education and Training of 1998 states that the transformation of universities is broadly conceptualized around principles of equity and redress: democratization and development (Cele, 2021).

Many people in South Africa do not speak English and Afrikaans as their home languages. However, these languages continue to dominate communication in the country, especially in public domains (Mkhize & Balfour, 2017). This hegemony undermines the linguistic rights of other citizens as determined by the Constitution of the Republic of South Africa. Mkhize and Balfour (2017:133) state that "in education, this hegemony circumscribes additive multilingualism as promoted in the Constitution, Language-in-Education Policy, Language Policy for Higher Education and other legislative frameworks."

According to Cele (2021), language policy development for transformation and social inclusion in South African higher education has significantly failed to achieve the ideal order of things. Many students across South Africa entering university find a language foreign to them (Gambushe, cited in Docrat & Kaschula, 2020). Cele (2021) argues that, except for the University of KwaZulu-Natal (UKZN), universities have developed policies to encourage multilingualism but have not fully realized the desired state of such policies. This is partly because language-in-education in South Africa has remained an instrument for reinforcing English supremacy and dominance instead of enhancing the development of indigenous African languages (Cele, 2021). Fleisch (2008) and Moloi and Chetty (cited in Mkhize & Balfour, 2017) state that the continued hegemony of English and Afrikaans in schools has consequences throughout the education sector for African-language-speaking students.

For example, in higher education, academic literacy requirements in English remain challenging and impact throughput rates (Ndebele et al., cited in Mkhize & Balfour, 2017). The English hegemony in South African schools also affects language attitudes (Nkosi, 2014), classroom interaction (Madiba, 2014; Makalela, 2015), and policy implementation (Balfour, 2010; Turner & Wildsmith-Cromarty, 2014). Barnes (2004) argues that this linguistic setup is a result of the education system in South Africa not offering sustained learning and acquisition opportunities for the majority of the population in more than one language throughout the education sector.

However, despite various legal frameworks to promote multilingualism in South Africa's higher education, there is a disjuncture between these legal frameworks and what is happening in universities. Docrat and Kaschula (2020) note that, in universities, English remains the primary language of instruction. Universities encourage using indigenous languages; however, none have adopted indigenous languages as a medium of instruction (Docrat & Kaschula, 2020). This indicates that legal frameworks have not been transferred to reality. Docrat and Kaschula (2020) state that even though this is lawful by the judiciary, it promotes an untransformed exclusionary agenda.

Rhodes University is a public university in Makhanda, Eastern Cape, South Africa. The university was established in 1904 and has a student population of around 8000. Rhodes University's language policy was first reviewed in 2003 and had its last revision in 2021. The policy is predicated on the following principles:

- The university's language of learning and teaching is English, and the university's official business is conducted in English.
- The creation of an environment where language is not a barrier to equity of access, opportunity, and success.
- Promotion of multilingualism and furthering the development of academic languages and literacies of the languages of South Africa where necessary and practicable.
- Creation of conditions for using particularly isiXhosa as a language of learning and teaching.

The policy allows for the development and promotion of multilingualism and prioritizes the main provincial languages for development. Other languages alongside English in translanguaging may be used in teaching and learning, e.g., in the tutorial system. English may or may not be the Language of Learning and Teaching in academic departments where languages other than English are taught as subjects.

The policy also states that all official documentation on campus will be trilingual in isiXhosa, Afrikaans, and English in compliance with the Institutional Transformation Plan's recommendation to transform the institution's identity.

THE ROLE OF LANGUAGE IN PUBLIC HEALTH COMMUNICATION DURING THE COVID-19 PANDEMIC

The role of language in public health communication is a critical aspect of health programs that address disease prevention, health promotion, and quality of life. Language can significantly promote and improve the health of individuals, communities, and societies. Language and health are a sub-discipline of applied linguistics, public health, nursing, linguistic anthropology, and communication studies (Showtack et al., 2019). Applied linguists are well-poised to clarify vital sociolinguistic realities in healthcare communication, explicitly helping to illuminate the relationship between linguistic marginalization and health outcomes for diverse linguistic, racial, and ethnic groups (Showtack et al., 2019). The ideas people have about health, the languages they use, their health literacy skills, and the contexts in which they communicate about health reflect their cultures (Centres for Disease Control and Prevention, 2022).

Communication is essential to any organized response to a crisis (Quinn, 2018). However, the Centres for Disease Control and Prevention (2022) asserts that public health officials belong to professional cultures with their language – such as epidemiological and medical terms. Furthermore, some of these terms are not familiar to the public and hinder the public's understanding of written and spoken health messages. Understanding can be further hindered when other cultural differences exist (Centres for Disease Control and Prevention, 2022).

Language is essential for human beings, for they perceive their reality and self through language (Kokaliari et al., 2013). Kar et al. (2000) state that effective multicultural communication is much more than using a common language or media. Language is vital in representing knowledge systems. Language is also the cornerstone of human communication, a tool that bridges the gap between information and understanding. In public health communication, effective communication is essential for disseminating vital information, raising awareness, and promoting behaviour change. The exploration of the connections between language and health-related information and the progress of the epidemic has implications for the well-being and public communication aimed at indigenous multilingual communities (Chen, 2020).

During public health emergencies, officials develop communication strategies to protect the population from existing or potential threats (Lin et al., 2014). Quinn (2018) alludes to the fact that public authorities' communication during a crisis is essential and indispensable to any response to a situation that may threaten lives. Their capability to effectively communicate risk and recommend preventative behaviours may be the only public health strategy to reduce morbidity and mortality. However, in most cases, a population's social and individual determinants (education, income, race/ethnicity, language) may lead to inequalities in individual or group-specific exposure to public health communication messages (Lin et al., 2014).

Xiang et al. (2020) state that during a disaster, the availability of information becomes even more essential for everyone. However, it has become evident that around the world, the exclusion of linguistic minorities from fair and equitable access to social participation and health is common (Avineri et al., 2018).

Health communications are targeted at the general public, where the source is represented by communicators and journalists (Daniele, 2021). Daniele (2021) further explains that, in health communication, information results from some kind of intra-language translation that transforms the original medical language into a common language. Hence, public health communications emerge from rewritings of a complex medical language that cannot always be modified and acquainted to serve the general public (Daniele, 2021).

Health issues affect all human beings. Consequently, everyone in the world has in some way to cope with the language of medicine (Cappuzzo, 2021). However, Chen (2020) states that the voices of indigenous people have been mainly excluded from top-down efforts and strategies in public health communications. For example, public health communication during the COVID-19 outbreak in Taiwan was initially conveyed mainly in Mandarin Chinese (Chen, 2020), almost disregarding other linguistic groups in China.

During the COVID-19 pandemic, global health knowledge and communication were limited to several languages. For example, the World Health Organization (WHO) made information available in the six official languages of the United Nations (Arabic, Chinese, English, French, Russian, and Spanish) and three additional languages (German, Hindi, and Portuguese). This linguistic setup only reflected the dominant languages in the world. Suffice it also to say that English still predominates UN communications as the language of press conferences and the immediate language of record in a fast-changing information environment (Piller et al., 2020). Piller et al. (2020) argue that this global communication strategy replicated a linguistic hierarchy that disregarded multilingual needs and the reality of our world.

The issue of minority groups' access to COVID-19-related information has been debated (Cappuzzo, 2021). During 'exceptional' conditions, as seen with the COVID-19 pandemic, medical knowledge transmission and spreading are crucial, mainly because people need to be informed and reassured about the facts surrounding their lives (Cloitre & Shinn, 1985). This situation is further exacerbated by the fact that pandemic-related communications are asymmetrically exchanged among many numbers of languages worldwide. This demonstrates that the issue of knowledge and communication in medicine is serious, and during crisis periods, medical and health communications become central.

Kar et al. (2000) stated that available literature on communication theory and practice and health communication is impressive and rapidly expanding. However, it is weak in dealing with multi-ethnic and disadvantaged communities' communication and health promotion issues. While Kar et al. (2000) made this argument more than two decades ago, not a lot has changed. This chapter attempts to fill this gap by examining the use of language for health communication at a public university in South Africa.

METHODOLOGY

The qualitative approach used in this study involved document analysis. The investigation discovered that only 23 public health communication emails were received at Rhodes University between March 2020 and December 2022. These emails were sourced directly from key university officials and departments, including the Vice Chancellor's office, the Deputy Vice Chancellor for Academic and Student Affairs, the Communications and Advancement Division, and the Coronavirus Response Task Team. However, as a sample for the study, five emails will be utilized for data analysis. Language consistency has been observed, and the results will be evident in the findings.

The selection of these documents was purposeful, driven by their relevance to the research objectives, which focused on examining public health communication within the university during the COVID-19 pandemic. The analysis of these documents involved a systematic examination of their content to gain insights into various aspects of public health communication. This included assessing language use, message clarity, and the presence of translations or adaptations for different language groups.

Document analysis was a crucial methodological choice for this study on public health communication at Rhodes University during the COVID-19 pandemic. Document analysis allowed the researchers to tap into an existing archive of public health communication emails and related content. Given the study's focus on a specific time frame (March 2020 to December 2022), relying on these documents provided a comprehensive and historical perspective on the university's communication practices during a critical period. The selection of documents received from key university officials and departments, including the Vice Chancellor's office, the Deputy Vice Chancellor for Academic and Student Affairs, the Communications and Advancement Division, and the Coronavirus Response Task Team, ensured access to authoritative and pertinent communication materials. This approach facilitated the examination of communication from the highest levels of the institution, providing valuable insights into official university policies and practices.

Document analysis was purposefully chosen because it aligned closely with the study's objectives. Analysing official emails and supplementary website content allowed for a focused exploration of communication strategies, language use, and policy adherence within this context. The study could shed light on whether the university's communication practices addressed or exacerbated language-related barriers during the pandemic by examining a sample of emails. Lastly, document analysis allowed for evaluating the university's adherence to its language policies throughout the pandemic. This was critical in assessing whether the institution's stated commitment to linguistic diversity and inclusivity was reflected in its communication practices.

FINDINGS

Email 1: Dated Fri, 13 Mar 2020 at 12:17 (first email released for students about Coronavirus at Rhodes University) Subject: Staff and student travel advisory and declaration form in the context of COVID-19.

The email is written entirely in English. There was no alternative email provided in isiXhosa or Afrikaans.

Email 2 dated Thu, 26 Mar 2020 Subject: Update on teaching and learning during and after recess and National Lockdown.

The email is written entirely in English. There was no alternative email provided in isiXhosa or Afrikaans.

Email 3 dated Sat, 19 September 2020 Subject: VC letter on level 1 arrangements.

The email is written entirely in English. There was no alternative email provided in isiXhosa or Afrikaans.

Email 4 dated Tue, 24 August 2021 Subject: COVID-19 UPDATE | Vaccines open for 18+ age group.

The email is written entirely in English. There was no alternative email provided in isiXhosa or Afrikaans.

Email 5 dated Wed, 31 March 2022 Subject: Update on COVID-19 protocols and awareness.

The email is written entirely in English. There was no alternative email provided in isiXhosa or Afrikaans.

Rhodes University's language policy states, "The official language of record at Rhodes University will be English except when other language needs arise, and where necessary and practicable. All signage and official documentation on campus will be trilingual in isiXhosa, Afrikaans, and English" (Rhodes University, 2019, p.2).

However, per the university's language policy, none of the analysed email communications appear trilingual. They are all written in English. It is inevitable from these emails that English dominated public health communication during the COVID-19 pandemic at Rhodes University. This also demonstrates that the multilingualism that the university advocates for in its language policy was suspended during the pandemic.

DISCUSSION

Rhodes University has a rich academic history and a solid commitment to embracing diversity and inclusivity. It was founded in 1904 (119 years ago) and is gearing up for a special celebration in 2024 when it marks its 120th anniversary, highlighting its enduring dedication to education and knowledge.

One of the most unique features of Rhodes University is its diverse community. The university's stakeholders come from different backgrounds, including various languages, cultures, and ethnicities. This diversity reflects the rich cultural fabric of South Africa, with a particular focus on the importance of indigenous languages. The university's language policy recognizes the importance of being inclusive and wants to embrace the various languages and cultures within its community, particularly emphasizing indigenous languages.

The chapter aimed to assess the status of languages at Rhodes University in communicating health information during the challenging COVID-19 pandemic. This was done to understand how languages were utilized to ensure everyone could access and understand crucial health information regardless of their language background. Another crucial objective was investigating whether Rhodes University's language policy effectively encouraged the use of indigenous languages during the pandemic. The study aimed to evaluate how well the university included different languages in its communication, particularly emphasizing the importance of indigenous languages, especially in the context of public health information.

The role of language in public health communication is multifaceted and pivotal. Language is a primary medium through which health information is conveyed to individuals and communities. Its effectiveness can significantly impact public health initiatives' understanding, adherence, and success. Language is a cornerstone of effective public health communication. It determines how well diverse populations understand, receive, and act upon health information. Acknowledging linguistic diversity, considering cultural context, and delivering messages with inaccessible, empathetic, and trust-inspiring language are crucial elements of successful public health communication. Ignoring the role of language can hinder the effectiveness of health campaigns and may contribute to health inequalities.

Bamgbose (2011) asserts that many African countries have attempted to enhance the status and use of indigenous languages, but their endeavours have remained unsuccessful. English remains an unchallenged language of communication in South African universities. Rhodes University's language practice when communicating its COVID-19 information inevitably imaged English as a solution to any intercultural communication problems due to the COVID-19 pandemic. Li et al. (2020, p.531) refer to this linguistic situation as "English-mediated multilingualism." Li et al. (2020) state that English-mediated multilingualism is rarely challenged but widely assumed to be the only legitimate and most equitable form of embracing linguistic diversity. This linguistic situation legitimizes English as an elite form of multilingualism (Martin Rojo, 2010; Preece, 2019), naturalizes English as a medium of instruction (Piller & Cho, 2013), and accepts English as a source of authority and an index of academic excellence (Piller, 2016a, 2019).

These English-centric ways of approaching multilingualism have resulted in many negative social consequences for non-English-speaking people (Li et al., 2020). Li et al. (2020) further assert that English-mediated multilingualism does not contribute to the common good and global justice; it has entranced social inequality by erasing diversity and paying tribute to the Anglophone center (Piller, 2016b, 2016a).

Bunyi (1999) argues that African education systems must be liberated from the Eurocentric colonial legacy and create a space for African indigenous cultures in African education. However, Kamwangamalu (2003) suggested that using the English language in some African contexts is more than reasonable. This is because it stunts efforts to nurture and grow the use of indigenous languages. It also prevents some parts of the population from participating in essential civil society discourse and affairs in African countries (Cele, 2021).

The chapter's findings resonate with Mkhize's (2020) assertation that, even though South Africa has been decolonized, its many institutions of higher learning remain systematically unchanged and, thus, do not reflect and valorise a multicultural and multilingual society that honours all people. The chapter's findings demonstrate that Rhodes University's health communication during the COVID-19 pandemic was untransformed and alienating towards non-English speaking stakeholders. This shows that the non-English speaking university stakeholders were not catered for; they are in a linguistic space not designed for them.

Mwaniki (2012, p. 214) states that in this context, language "has effectively been used to serve the ends of social exclusion for some and social inclusion for others" and "deployed to serve ends that neither entrench nor deepen social justice." The Rhodes University's monolingual communication in this period was an act of linguistic discrimination. The university inevitably operationalized language in complex situations to exclude and include its stakeholders, empowering and disempowering its community.

Nkoala (2022) explains that, in post-colonial contexts in South Africa, with a deep history of a systematic attempt to deintellectualize the use of indigenous languages through linguistic discrimination, the systems of thinking vested in indigenous languages continue to be marginalized, as Indo-European languages such as English continue to dominate prestigious spaces such as universities.

Given the linguistic and cultural diversity of university students in South Africa, English alone is far from being an effective medium of crisis communication. This demonstrates an urgent need to understand and address the real linguistic needs of students in combating health crises and call attention to new ways of seeing multilingualism in the context of the shifting paradigm of South African universities.

English is an undisputed lingua franca in South African universities. To understand the English hegemony in all South African universities, one has to comprehend the ideologies that underlie the policies and practices in these institutions (Mkhize & Balfour, 2017). Garcia (2009) states that ideologies about language, language policies, and use are linked to socio-historical processes. Pluddemann (2015) asserts that policy is more than text; it is a process that carries an ideological load and is subject to interpretation by competing interest groups in ways that reflect power relations between them. According to Mkhize and Balfour (2017), language rights debates and realizing these rights in South African universities are informed by historical and socio-political processes.

CONCLUSION

The COVID-19 pandemic has brought essential changes in all spheres of life, and the global communities had to adapt. Part of these changes were linguistic, where people had to rely primarily on global dominant languages for health communication. As the medium of international communication (Cappuzzo, 2021), English dominated the COVID-19 discourse at Rhodes University. This linguistic setup contradicted the university's language policy, which promotes multilingualism.

REFERENCES

Avineri, N., Graham, L. R., Johnson, E. J., Riner, R. C., & Rosa, J. (2018). *Language and Social Justice in Practice*. Routledge. doi:10.4324/9781315115702

Balfour, R. J. (2010). 'The long walk…' in a special issue on Languages in Higher Education in South Africa. Language Learning Journal, 37(3), 249-251.

Bamgbose, A. (2011). African languages today: The Challenge of and prospects for empowerment under globalization. *Selected Proceedings of the 40th Annual Conference on African Linguistics,* 1–14.

Bunyi, G. (1999). Rethinking the place of African indigenous languages in African education. *International Journal of Educational Development, 19*(4-5), 337–350. doi:10.1016/S0738-0593(99)00034-6

Cappuzzo, B. (2021). The importance of multilingual information and plain English in Response to the COVID-19 pandemic. *European Scientific Journal, 17*(30), 37–52. doi:10.19044/esj.2021.v17n30p37

Cele, N. (2021). Understanding language policy as a tool for access and social inclusion in South African Higher Education: A critical policy analysis perspective. *South African Journal of Higher Education, 35*(6), 25–46. doi:10.20853/35-6-3730

Centres for Disease Control and Prevention. (2022). *Culture and language*. https://www.cdc.gov/healthliteracy/culture.html

Chen, C. M. (2020). Public health messages about COVID-19 prevention in multilingual Taiwan. *Multilingua, 39*(5), 597–606. doi:10.1515/multi-2020-0092

Cloitre, M., & Shinn, T. (1985). Expository practice: social, cognitive and epistemological linkages. In T. Shinn & R. Whistler (Eds.), *Expository Science: Forms and Functions of Popularization* (pp. 31–60). Reidel. doi:10.1007/978-94-009-5239-3_2

Daniele, F. (2021). The centrality of language in health communication. *European Scientific Journal, 17*(30), 24–36. doi:10.19044/esj.2021.v17n30p24

Department of Higher Education and Training. (2017). *Language Policy for Higher Education*. Department of Higher Education and Training.

Docrat, Z., & Kaschula, H. (2015). Meaningful engagement: Towards a language rights paradigm for effective language policy implementation. *Southern African Linguistics and Applied Language Studies, 5*(1), 1–9.

Docrat, Z., & Kaschula, R. H. (2020). Transformative power of language policies in higher education: A legal English approach or a linguistic African language approach. In R. H. Kaschula & E. Wolff (Eds.), *The Transformative Power of Language: From Postcolonial to Knowledge Societies in Africa* (pp. 85–108). Cambridge University Press. doi:10.1017/9781108671088.006

Fleisch, B. (2008). *Primary Education in Crisis: Why South African School Children Underachieve in Reading and Mathematics*. Juta and Co.

Garcia, O. (2009). *Bilingual Education in the 21st Century: A Global Perspective*. Wiley-Blackwell.

Hornberger, N. H. (2002). Multilingual language policies and the continua of biliteracy: An ecological approach. *Language Policy, 1*(1), 27–51. doi:10.1023/A:1014548611951

Kamwangamalu, N. M. (2003). Globalization of English, language maintenance and shift in South Africa. *International Journal of the Sociology of Language, 2003*(164), 65–81. doi:10.1515/ijsl.2003.056

Kar, S. B., Alcalay, R., & Alex, S. (2000). *Health communication: A multicultural perspective*. Sage publications.

Kokaliari, E., Catanzarite, G., & Berzoff, J. (2013). It is called a mother tongue for a reason: A qualitative therapists' perspective on bilingual psychotherapy – Treatment implications. *Smith College Studies in Social Work, 83*(1), 97–118. doi:10.1080/00377317.2013.747396

Li, J., Xie, P., Ai, B., & Li, L. (2020, September 25). Multilingual communication experiences of international students during the Covid-19 pandemic. *Multilingua, 39*(5), 529–539. doi:10.1515/multi-2020-0116

Lin, L., Savoia, E., Agboola, F., & Viswanath, K. (2014). What have we learned about communication inequalities during the H1N1 pandemic: A systematic review of the literature. *BMC Public Health*, *14*(484), 1–13. doi:10.1186/1471-2458-14-484 PMID:24884634

Madiba, M. (2014). Promoting concept literacy through multilingual glossaries: A translanguaging approach. In Multilingual Teaching and Learning in Higher Education in South Africa. Multilingual Matters. doi:10.21832/9781783091669-007

Makalela, L. (2015). Moving out of the linguistic boxes: The effects of translanguaging strategies for multilingual classrooms. *Language and Education*, *29*(3), 200–217. doi:10.1080/09500782.2014.994524

Martin Rojo, L. (2010). *Constructing Inequality in Multilingual Classrooms*. Walder De Gruyter. doi:10.1515/9783110226645

Mkhize, D., & Balfour, R. (2017). Language rights in education in South Africa. *South African Journal of Higher Education*, *31*(6), 133–150. doi:10.20853/31-6-1633

Mkhize, T. (2020). The role of African languages in decolonizing South African universities. In R. H. Kaschula & E. Wolff (Eds.), *The Transformative Power of Language: From Postcolonial to Knowledge Societies in Africa* (pp. 33–42). Cambridge University Press. doi:10.1017/9781108671088.003

Mwaniki, M. (2012). Language and social justice in South Africa's higher education: Insights from a South African university. *Language and Education*, *26*(3), 213–232. doi:10.1080/09500782.2011.629095

Namyalo, S., & Nakayiza, J. (2015). Dilemmas in implementing language rights in multilingual Uganda. *Current Issues in Language Planning*, *16*(4), 409–424. doi:10.1080/14664208.2014.987425

Nkoala, S. (2022). Educators' experiences of using multilingual pedagogies during emergency remote teaching: A case study of South African universities. *International Journal of Multilingualism*. Advance online publication. doi:10.1080/14790718.2022.2074012

Nkosi, Z. P. (2014). Postgraduate students' experiences and attributes towards isiZulu as a medium of instruction at the University of KwaZulu-Natal. *Current Issues in Language Planning*, *15*(3), 245–264. doi:10.1080/14664208.2014.915456

Piller, I. (2016a). *Linguistic Diversity and Social Justice*. Oxford University Press. doi:10.1093/acprof:oso/9780199937240.001.0001

Piller, I. (2016b). Monolingual way of seeing multilingualism. *Journal of Multicultural Discourses*, *11*(1), 25–33. doi:10.1080/17447143.2015.1102921

Piller, I. (2019). On the conditions of authority in academic publics. *Journal of Sociolinguistics*, *23*(5), 521–528. doi:10.1111/josl.12393

Piller, I., & Cho, J. (2013). Neoliberalism as language policy. *Language in Society*, *42*(1), 23–44. doi:10.1017/S0047404512000887

Piller, I., Zhang, J., & Li, J. (2020). Linguistic diversity in a time of crisis: Language challenges of the COVID-19 pandemic. *Multilingua*, *39*(5), 503–515. doi:10.1515/multi-2020-0136

Pluddemann, P. (2015). Unlocking the grid: Language-in-education policy realization in post-apartheid South Africa. *Language and Education*, *29*(3), 186–199. doi:10.1080/09500782.2014.994523

Preece, S. (2019). Elite bilingual identities in higher education in the anglophone world: The stratification of linguistic diversity and reproduction of socio-economic inequalities in the multilingual student population. *Journal of Multilingual and Multicultural Development*, *40*(5), 404–420. doi:10.1080/01434632.2018.1543692

Quinn, P. (2018). Crisis communication in public health emergencies: The limits of 'legal control' and the risks for harmful outcomes in a digital age. *Life Sciences, Society and Policy*, *14*(4), 1–40. doi:10.1186/s40504-018-0067-0 PMID:29404722

Rhodes University. (2019). *Language Policy*. Accessed on 22nd September 2023 from World Wide Web < https://www.ru.ac.za/media/rhodesuniversity/content/institutionalplanning/documents/Language_Policy_2019.pdf>

Showtack, R., Santos, M. G., Feuerherm, E., Jacobson, H., & Martinez, G. (2019). *Language as a social determinant of health: An applied linguistics perspective on health equity*. https://www.aaal.org/news/language-as-a-social-determinant-of-health-an-applied-linguistics-perspective-on-health-equity##

Skutnabb-Kangas, T. (2006). Language policy and linguistic human rights. In T. Ricento (Ed.), *An Introduction to Language Policy: Theory and Method* (pp. 78–94). Blackwell.

Turner, N., & Wildsmith-Cromarty, R. (2014). Challenges to the implementation of bilingual/multilingual language policies at tertiary institutions in South Africa (1995-2012). *Language Matters (Pretoria)*, *45*(3), 295–312. doi:10.1080/10228195.2014.961525

Xiang, Y. T., Li, W., Zhang, Q., Rao, W. W., Zeng, L. N., Lok, G. K. I., Chow, I. H. I., Cheung, T., & Hall, B. (2020). Timely research papers about COVID-19 in China. *Lancet*, *395*(10225), 684–685. doi:10.1016/S0140-6736(20)30375-5 PMID:32078803

KEY TERMS AND DEFINITIONS

Communication: A required tool used by individuals, organisations, families and even animals to carry out a message.

COVID-19: A deadly virus that spread across the globe which affects one's respiratory system.

Crisis: An unavoidable situation which can have a negative impact should one not pay attention and find solutions.

English-Centric: A situation where everything is revolving around and promoting English without consideration of the existence of other languages.

Health: A state of purity in one physical body, emotional state, and spiritual being.

Indigenous Language: A native language of a certain ethnic group.

LPFPHEI: Language Policy Framework for Public Higher Education Institutions.

Multilingualism: An ability to communicate in more than just one language, verbal or nonverbal.

WHO: World Health Organisation.

Chapter 10
Amplifying the Health Concerns of Minoritized Groups in Nigeria Using Documentary

Abigail Ogwezzy
https://orcid.org/0000-0002-3281-1647
University of Lagos, Nigeria

Akpan Samuel Unwana
https://orcid.org/0000-0003-0862-6377
University of Lagos, Nigeria

Ogechi Okanya Cookey
Edwin Clark University, Nigeria

Iniobong Courage Nda
University of Uyo, Nigeria

ABSTRACT

Several studies have shown that most highly placed government officials in the Ministry of Health in Africa do not bother to get to the hinterlands, slums, or inner cities where there are poor people, and socially excluded people, because according to them, these are hard-to-reach areas; and additionally due to the spate of insecurity in the continent. In the case of Nigeria, it has also been revealed that these top government health officials prefer a situation where they are briefed by their media aids who must have gone to have a one-on-one encounter with these minority groups, by capturing their plights on camera, especially in this era of rising insecurity in the country. This chapter explores the role of documentaries in amplifying the health concerns of these minority groups in Nigeria. The study uses social shaping theory in explaining concepts, themes, and constructs. Findings are shared.

DOI: 10.4018/979-8-3693-0624-6.ch010

INTRODUCTION

When properly packaged, documentaries can be a catalyst for social change and social inclusion especially in the realms of health inequalities and policies (Shaw and Robertson, 1997; Nichols, 2001; Parr, 2007; Dobson, 2007; de Lange, Olivier & Wood, 2008). Some documentaries are intentionally designed to showcase from a health perspective the life of the poor and socially excluded around the world, and especially in Nigeria; to draw the attention of decision makers to their plight and challenges in accessing health care services. This article draws from one of the authors' work on "Partnership for Transforming Health Systems Phase Two" (PATHS2), which was a six-year development initiative that aims to ensure Nigeria achieves important health-related Millennium Development Goals which ran from 2002 to 2008. PATHS2 was designed to use the art of documentary to draw the attention of policy makers to the plights of minoritized groups in Nigeria; and one of the authors was involved in the media production and report. PATHS2 documentaries were designed to showcase the life of unusual people and draw the attention of decision makers to the plight and health challenges facing this group of people in Nigeria. This strategy was informed by two National Strategic Health Development Plan (NSHDP) priorities: to strengthen accountability, transparency and responsiveness of the national health system and to attain effective gender inclusive community participation in health development and management, as well as community ownership of sustainable health outcomes. So, as a catalyst for change and social inclusion, PATHS2 used documentaries to reach the unreached in the nooks and crannies of Nigeria, find their voices and bring such voices into public discourse to influence health planning and policy. Our camera waded through rivers to get to the forgotten masses in the slums of Makoko in Lagos State, climbed the quarry to find women labourers in Ebonyi State, staggered through the deserts to find the Nomads in Jigawa state, stooped under the rocky bridge of Wuse in Abuja to reach the abandoned pensioners, prostrated before Mai angua's (community heads of Hausa communities in urban cities) and even escaped being destroyed in an attempt to reach the almajiris.

Definition of Terms

This section presents definitions of some key terms in respect of how they are used in this paper.

Social Exclusion

Social exclusion (SE) is a process by which certain groups are systematically disadvantaged because they are discriminated against on the basis of their ethnicity, race, religion, sexual orientation, caste, descent, gender, age, disability, HIV status, migrant status or where they live (Koshoedo, Paul-Ebhohimhen, Jepson, Watson, 2015). People who are excluded are not 'just like' the rest of the poor. They are also disadvantaged by who they are or where they live and as a result are locked out of the benefits of development. Some of the socially excluded groups include the rural and urban poor women and men; young people, physically challenged, old people/retirees and other less privileged service users. Social exclusion is a multidimensional process of progressive social rupture, detaching groups and individuals from social relations and institutions and preventing them from full participation in the normal, normatively prescribed activities of the society in which they live (Lashko, 2006; Gohagan, 2008; Pinsky, Ford, Gamito, Higgins, Jenkins, Lamerato, Tenorio, Marcus, Coleman, 2010).

Social Inclusion

- Ensuring the marginalized and those living in poverty have greater participation in decision making which affects their lives; and allowing them to improve their living standards and their overall well-being.[3]

The Hard-to-Reach People

- Hard-to-reach audiences have been called obstinate, recalcitrant, chronically uninformed, disadvantaged, have-not, illiterate, malfunctional, and information poor'. These adjectives used to describe such audiences make the term potentially stigmatizing (Freimuth and Mettger, 1990). It is sometimes used to describe those sections of the community that are difficult to involve in public participation.

It is a common knowledge that the voices of the socially excluded are hardly heard in policy formulation and implementation, which is not unconnected with the challenge of gender inequality.

Health Policy

A set of organizational rules (including but not limited to laws) intended to promote health or prevent disease.

Voice

Voice is the process of citizens making public their needs and concerns and placing pressure on policy makers, politicians and service providers to improve governance and service provision. This could be through media advocacy; campaigns; engagement with local service providers; in policy making, lobbying for new laws; participation in public hearings; citizens' involvement in service provider management; citizens' use of complaints mechanism, etc.

Gatekeepers

Gatekeepers as used in this technical brief refers to religious leaders, traditional rulers, husbands or members of institution/organization's senior management team, whose consent and support are needed for successful community engagements, but it does not always come easy.

Theoretical Grounding: Understanding Social Shaping Theory

Social shaping theory was initially developed by Brian Winston in the 1980s, and it posits that technology and media are not entirely neutral tools but actively shape and are continually shaped by society (Mackay and Gillespie, 1992). It rethinks the notion that technology is deterministic, emphasizing that societal forces, values, and interests play a crucial role in shaping the development and use of technology and media (Anderson, 2008). This theory underscores that technologies and media are products of human decisions and, consequently, have significant impacts on our lives, culture, and values. Social shaping has been grounded in technological usage for communicative social change (Payne, 1989). The concept of social shaping theory therefore focuses on themes within the field of sociology and media studies that explores how technology and society mutually influence and shape each other (Edge, 1988). The theory suggests that technological development is not entirely determined by technical factors, but is also greatly influenced by social, traditional cultural, economic, and political forces shaping the society. Similarly, these technologies, once introduced into the society can have enormous impacts and influence on social norms, behaviors, and structures, as in the case of minority groups in Africa. This theory, though it challenges the concept of technological determinism, which suggests that technology drives a series of social changes independently of human agency or input, it also takes into cognizance the indwelling power and contributions of sociocultural concepts in shaping technological advancement for human consumption. Unlike technological determinism theory, instead, social shaping theory emphasizes the role of human choices, norms, values, and societal factors in the development and adoption of technology, such as the deployment of documentary to capture the plights of minority groups. According to Mackay and Gillespie (1992), social shaping theory underscores the idea that technology is a product of human decisions and reflects the values and interests of those who create and use it. Social shaping theory highlights the dynamic relationship between technology and society, emphasizing how they co-evolve and mutually influence each other.

Documentaries as Agents of Social Change

Documentaries are specially and specifically packaged with their appealing capacity to inform, educate, and emotionally engage audiences, and when well produced are powerful instruments for bringing about social change. They can play pivotal roles in drawing attention to the experiences, struggles, and aspirations of minority groups in Africa. By applying social shaping theory, we can analyze how documentaries both reflect and influence societal perceptions, behaviors, and policies especially in health related issues. These are discussed below:

Reflecting Society: Documentaries often serve as mirrors, reflecting existential realities such as the existing societal attitudes and biases towards minority groups in Africa. Their storyline using pictures and narratives capture the lived experiences, challenges, and triumphs of these communities, providing a platform for their voices to be heard by the authorities and policymakers. In doing so, documentaries highlight the need for societal awareness and change that can benefit minoritized groups.

Shaping Public Opinion: Documentaries have the communicative power to shape public opinion by presenting compelling narratives and evidence that can evoke empathy. When skillfully and aesthetically crafted, they evoke empathy and compassion among viewers and policymakers, challenging preconceived notions and prejudices that are repugnant to the social justice of the minority groups. This emotional engagement can lead to increased support for the rights and welfare of minority groups.

Influencing Policy: The power of documentaries can extend to influencing policy decisions and international involvement. When policymakers and advocacy groups recognize the significance of a documentary's message, it can lead to the implementation of policies aimed at addressing the specific issues faced by minority groups. Documentaries can thus be catalysts for legislative and social change in any society.

Social Shaping Theory and the Power of Documentary in Advocating for African Minority Groups

In media and communication studies track, social shaping theory has emerged as a significant framework for understanding how technology and media influence society and culture, by deploying technological products such as documentaries to attract attention. This theory is particularly key when examining the role of documentaries in bringing to light on the plights of minority groups in Africa. Documentaries, as a form of media, have the potential to shape and reshape societal perceptions, policies, and attitudes towards marginalized communities (Barnes, 1974; Mackay and Gillespie, 1992). This article uses the social shaping theory as its theoretical framework, and its application in using documentaries as a powerful tool for advocating for the rights and issues of minority groups in Africa.

Select Examples of Documentaries in Africa That Provoked International Attention and Empathy

Under this section, we will consider several notable documentaries that have harnessed the principles of social shaping theory to advocate for African minority groups:

"The Act of Killing" (2012): This documentary was directed by Joshua Oppenheimer, which showcased the Indonesian mass killings of 1965-66. While not set in Africa, it demonstrates how powerful documentaries can be in revealing hidden histories and shaping societal discourses that dig out silences.

"The Supreme Price" (2014): Joanna Lipper, directed this documentary which examines the struggle for women's rights and democracy in Nigeria, focusing on the lived experiences of the late Nigerian politician and activist Kudirat Abiola. It went further to highlight the intersectionality of gender and minority rights in Africa.

"God Loves Uganda" (2013): Directed by Roger Ross Williams; the documentary explores the influence of American evangelical missionaries in Uganda, particularly concerning LGBTQ+ rights. It reveals the impact of external forces on minority groups' lives in Africa.

Social shaping theory provides a valuable epistemological lens through which scholars can uncover and understand the dynamic and symbiotic relationship between media, technology, and society (MacKenzie, 1981). When applied to the use of documentaries, it becomes evident how these films can both reflect and shape public opinion, policies, and societal values, particularly in the context of advocating for the rights and plights of minority groups in Africa. Documentaries serve as vital tools in amplifying the voices of marginalized communities, driving awareness, empathy, and action, ultimately contributing to positive social change.

Promoting Health Equalities Through Social Inclusion: The Logic

The socially excluded are everywhere, in rural and urban areas. These millions are victims of a 'social rupture', disadvantaged because of 'who they are or where they live' or both. The gap consistently gets wider and drags them away from social participation and services. (Hudnall & Higson-Smith, 2004; Hudnall, Stamm, Hecht & Choi, 2012;

Pascucci, Chu, Leasure, 2012; Brown, 2015). Since they are often the hardest "hit" of general misfortunes, this group of people bears the burden of poor health systems the most. The health status indicators for Nigeria are among the worst in the world. Nigeria's overall health system performance was ranked in the 187 position among 191 member States of the World Health Organisation (WHO) in 2000 (WHO Commission on Social Determinants of Health, 2008). Among others, the country has one of the highest numbers of HIV infected people in the world and the fourth highest TB burden. Maternal, newborn and child mortality rates are still high, though decreasing. Life expectancy at birth has been reported to be 44 years by the 2009 UNICEF State of the World's Children report (WHO, 2015).

The above have led to a paradigm shift in health promotion approaches, especially to include the socially excluded. In order to ameliorate the impact of a less satisfactory health system, attention has been on strengthening the process of participation, especially by the socially excluded and to have poor people exercise their voice through new forms of inclusion and consultation designed to inform and influence larger institutions and policies. As Dockery et all (2001, p. 36) captured it, "reducing health inequalities and improving local people's quality of life requires public service to take a more holistic and innovative approach in health development activities and to listen and act upon local people's voices and concerns." Realizing the importance of inclusion in governance, the British government created the Office of the Minister for Social Exclusion in 1999 and it became a full cabinet position between May 2006 and June 2007. Although the office has become redundant as it is no longer a position in the government.

Even, the government of Nigeria cannot be described as being indifferent to the new thinking of social inclusion. Hence, the National Health Promotion Policy (NHPP), 2005 provided "guidelines to assist in creating positive outcomes such as empowerment for health action and increased community involvement." PATHS2 use of documentary as a tool for policy advocacy is a classical example of actualising the participation of the socially excluded in decisions about health policy development and implementation in Nigeria.

Past Health Documentaries and Health Advocacy in Nigeria

Documentaries are a powerful tool in drawing attention, and studies have proven this (Chio, 2009; Quinn, Shulman, Knifton, & Byrne, 2011; O'Flynn, 2012, Aston & Gaudenzi, 2012; Villanueva, 2015; Brown, Michie, Walmsley & West, 2016; Mendes, Dos Santos & Ichikawa, 2017). Obviously, documentaries can play a vital and pivotal role in health advocacy in Nigeria by raising awareness, educating the public, and promoting positive behavioral change among the people. Below are a few examples of documentaries and health advocacy initiatives in Nigeria:

"93 Days" (2016): This Nigerian drama film tells the story of the Ebola outbreak in Nigeria in 2014 and the heroic efforts made by healthcare workers to contain the virus. The film highlights the importance of early detection, effective healthcare systems, and community involvement in managing public health crises.

"Silent Tears" (2019): This documentary sheds light on the issue of mental health in Nigeria, focusing on the challenges faced by individuals living with mental illnesses and the need for improved mental health services and support. It aims to reduce stigma and promote understanding of mental health issues in the country.

"Pink Ribbon" (2017): This documentary addresses breast cancer awareness in Nigeria and the importance of early detection and regular screening. It emphasizes the need for improved access to healthcare services, particularly for underprivileged women, and encourages self-examination and awareness campaigns.

"Fueling Poverty" (2018): This documentary explores the impact of environmental pollution caused by oil exploration in the Niger Delta region of Nigeria. It highlights the health consequences faced by local communities, such as water contamination, air pollution, and its association with respiratory and other diseases. The film advocates for environmental justice and sustainable development.

"Beneath the Skin" (2021): This documentary focuses on the issue of albinism in Nigeria, raising awareness about the discrimination and health challenges faced by individuals with albinism. It highlights the need for inclusive healthcare, sun protection, and societal acceptance.

These documentaries, among others, electronically contribute to health advocacy in Nigeria by creating a platform for discussion, challenging social norms, and calling for action to address health issues. They engage audiences, inspire change, and encourage policymakers to prioritize healthcare initiatives and improve health outcomes in the country.

Documentaries: A Social Inclusion Model

It is a common knowledge that only distinguished personalities are invited when stakeholders' meetings targeted at creating a common consensus for securing a better health care delivery system are being planned. Normally at such meetings, health statistics with graphs and diagrams are presented; while Nigerians and especially the poor were seldom consulted in planning, implementing and monitoring health service provision supposedly put in place for them by the government. Sadly, the poor, vulnerable and marginalized persons are however not commonly considered as 'stakeholders', and their views missing during such meetings; yet they are end users of the health system, they have health needs and future health aspirations and would live with the consequences of the consensus to be agreed on at such meetings.

Presenting health statistics with graphs and diagrams during planning sessions is good but not enough. The real life presentations of the perceptions, opinions and facts by the socially excluded about their health should be brought to the fore, in addition to "mere" health indices to add sight and sound of the public to health planning. Against this background, PATHS2 supported the Federal Ministry of Health (FMoH) to go, search and get the voices of this group from different parts of the country. lPATHS2 documentary films combine the strength of audiovisual and motion to present real stories of the socially excluded. Since documentaries are audiovisual, they brought to the fore the reality of the perceptions, opinions and facts about the state of Nigerian health care service delivery; challenged the old status quo on poor leadership, governance and community engagement; and made proposals for positive change especially for the socially excluded.

The documentaries gave various stakeholders the opportunity to articulate the complex social processes which impact on the health delivery system at their level in a participatory way, allowing people's viewpoints and assumptions about their local health system and economy to be brought to light, challenged and tested and jointly proposed a mechanism for achieving positive change in health, especially for the socially excluded. On the supply side, the documentaries highlighted a lot of softer issues that politicians had largely ignored, especially in the area of quality of care. For many of the socially excluded, this did not just mean the technical quality of treatment, it meant waiting time, being listened to; talked with rather than talked at (Lenaghan, 2001). These voices were synthesized into documentaries that were previewed in different fora as captured in the findings of this paper. The perspectives captured in PATHS2 documentaries has been quite influential in the various fora they were previewed and has/would further inform various health policies and interventions in Nigeria as this paper showed amongst others that it led to resolutions in favour of the socially excluded in an attempt to make health care services accessible to all Nigerians.

As a result, it might be concluded that PATHS2 use of documentaries is a real opportunity for the socially excluded to be involved in the shaping of Nigerian health policy as the proposals contained in the documentaries would likely work towards making quality health care services accessible to the socially excluded in Nigeria, which is the concept of participation in Health sector governance by the socially excluded.

THOUGHT PROVOKING VOICES FROM THE DOCUMENTARIES

The story of a woman in Kawo, Kaduna in the PATHS to Health documentary who helplessly watched her sister die following about 48 hours of labour pains will make one shiver at what the socially excluded people suffer as a result of poor access to health care services! There was no health worker or health facility close to her village and no form of transportation whatsoever for emergencies. Although it may sound primitive, but Kawo residents have taken their destiny in their hands, they assist each other in times of emergencies.

Another documentary - State of the health, captured the story of a farmer in Jigawa. Since there was no means of transportation, he bravely saddled his cattle to carry his sick son to the nearest health facility which was about one hour thirty minutes journey. It exposed the plight of the socially excluded in accessing health care services. View it, then you will appreciate further the concept and implication of 'inaccessibility to health care services.' In PATHS to Health, among others, you will empathize with a retiree who was hypertensive and diabetic and could not afford the cost of prescribed drugs. "...they gave me a prescription to buy two capsules (drug) for N2, 000", he lamented, "I kept the prescription (showing) because I don't have the money." Only providence knows what would have become of the gentleman as one reads this brief.

Again, a lady sand parker and widow wept bitterly while narrating her plight to the production team. She complained of serious chest pain due to the nature of her work, but who will feed her many children if she stops working? "…will I allow my children to die for nothing"? Says she.

The above cases are pitiable, aren't they? This group of people requires more than just sympathy but an urgent action to make health care service delivery available to them. Whenever these thought provoking PATHS2 documentaries were previewed at meetings, on several occasions, individuals were reportedly unable to hold back tears after viewing some of the documentaries. In the rooms, you could hear a pin drop after the end of a viewing. The realities were gripping! The issues raised were thought provoking leading to critical questions that require urgent and unambiguous answers. Leaderships and their stewardship roles were challenged. Roles and expectations were defined. Above all, the films were studded with socially excluded views and opinions. They proposed ways forward and in an unprecedented manner which has propelled policy makers across all levels to seek a common solution to issues in sober soaked sessions. So, the resources, professionalism and energy that went into the production of the films with the subsequent mobilization and advocacy to policy makers to see them have been yielding fruits. Subsequent sections will discuss the process of finding the voices of the socially excluded captured and presented in the form of documentary films, various platforms where they have been used and the outcomes.

WHY PATHS2 DOCUMENTARIES?

PATHS2 documentary films were produced to capture the views of the Nigerian public on health issues. Special attention was paid to getting the voices of people that are not usually heard in public discussions. The aim is to get such to the attention of the policy makers who in turn are expected to use the information as a guide in the planning and implementation of health policies. These needs alongside the overall PATHS2 purpose informed the use of documentaries for health policy advocacy.

IN THE BEGINNING

A concept note for each production is developed by the production working group. The concept note guides the theme and defines the style of the documentary. The note provides further details about field schedule, post production, budget and other production logistics required. The production manager then briefs the production crew on the objectives, strategy and locations; and the team sets out to the agreed and approved locations to reach specific clusters of targets, which have been identified through PATHS2 inception phase formative research and social mapping in the communities.

FINDING VOICES

Travels to the interior can sometimes take several hours by road with expectedly bad terrains. Even when there is no road, the journey continues by foot. Crew members climbed hills, waded through the waters on many occasions and traveled in boats with equipment to reach targets. Sometimes, late recording may require crew members to return to the base very late in the night amidst security challenges. Honestly, it is not a task for the faint hearted! Going by the array of socially excluded targets they need to reach without depriving one from the other, the versatility of the PATHS2 production crew in terms of skills cannot be glossed over. Engaging the various groups require top interpersonal communication skills which may be more challenging when the camera is rolling and the boom microphone is pointing.

In order to make access to these groups of people easy, the team worked with 'Fixers' or Community Liaison Officers whose specific job description is community mobilization. They travel ahead of the entire crew to seek permission oftentimes from community gatekeepers (religious leaders, traditional rulers) husbands or members of institution/organization's senior management team. The consent and support of these groups of people are key to the success of the team but it does not always come easy. What will you do when the gatekeepers themselves become the barriers to accessing voice? What about the voices who were reluctant to talk due to lack of trust in the process? A classical example was a respondent who had something to say but due to the fear of "authorities that be" kept mute. Some of them later approached the crew members to explain the true situation 'off record.' Some of the challenges and barriers faced by the crew members in reaching some of the groups identified above and how they were surmounted are discussed in the next section.

HOW DATA WERE GATHERED AND UTILIZED

Basically, since it was a media production set at finding hard-to-reach people, interviews were conducted using professional cameras in the remotest parts of rural communities in some select states across the country (North, South, East and West). The footage gathered was used for the health documentaries. Using the data gathered from the production crew members, key PATHS2 technical officers and staff of the Federal Ministry of Health (FMoH), this technical brief appraises the production processes of PATHS2 documentaries, and documents the experience and lessons learned while reaching the socially excluded; shares the lessons learnt for future social inclusion approaches in health planning and policy; and highlights issues for planning and implementation of PATHS2 documentary production for sustainability of the documentary communication strategy. It provides details of various platforms PATHS2 documentaries have been used for health policy planning and advocacy. They include CSO forum on health in Kaduna, November, 2008; the Future Search Conference in Enugu, March, 2009; the Abuja Presidential Summit on Health, November, 2009; the development of National Strategic Health Development Plan (NSHDP), March, 2010; and the 2nd Annual Health Promotion Conference, Abuja, September, 2010. The documentaries were well accepted in these fora and contents formed input into health planning and policy formulation. Also, they are being used for health policy advocacy by different stakeholders in PATHS2 focal states and beyond. These findings are now discussed thematically.

CHALLENGES OF FINDING VOICES AS TOLD BY PRODUCTION CREW MEMBERS

Gatekeepers Could Be a Barrier

There are two sides to the coin when it comes to engaging gatekeepers in getting access to our targets – the poor, the socially excluded and the vulnerable. Gatekeepers can be very helpful in respect of access, but they can equally be hurdles.

Association Executives:

"They brought an albino woman who was well placed, she worked, she could afford health care from private hospitals or wherever, she wasn't the kind of person we were looking for. Later they presented their general secretary, financial secretary, vice president and so on who were educated and looking well fed and said we should interview them. Meanwhile, we were looking for albinos on the street, those that are not empowered." -Emmanuel Brymore, Assistant Producer, PATH to Health, What of my future?

There was a village we went to in Jigawa State. In this village, this man was dying of this particular ailment but yet, when we wanted to talk to his wife to find out the condition of things she declined speaking on camera unless with the king's permission. And I asked them a simple question: "If her life was dependent on the question, would we have to seek permission from the king first ?" She said, "yes"; and that it is a very sad situation." -Eustace Okwechime, Production Manager.

LOCAL GUIDES/OFFICIALS/PARTNER CBOS

"In a hospital in Jigawa, the presence of the health officials prevented the people from saying anything negative for fear of victimization. ...when we noticed that some of the local guides are now sources of distraction. So, we (production crew) had to devise a strategy to shield them from the surveillance posture they wielded on crew and respondents during field interviews. Some of the CBOs were more political than patriotic; they sought to protect the interest of the powers that be, and only provided access to selected places and facilities. Some hovered around the place of interviews and were passing notes to the respondents, telling them exactly what to and what not to say." - Titi Awobode, Development Producer and Fixer.

Husbands

"He (producer) collected my husband's number to call him. He called him and obtained permission from him before we went ahead with the interview." -Aisha, a married respondent, speaking about her engagement with the crew.

Camera Phobia

Some of the respondents found it difficult to express themselves when a camera is rolling and you may not be able to get the best from them.

"A patent drug medicine dealer in Ebonyi state after the recorded interview session asked me to "tell them (the government) that this is what we need", and I said why didn't you say that during the interview because that was where it counts." - Chidi, Producer.

Misconceptions

Community members were generally apprehensive when they saw crew members and their mission was often misinterpreted.

"...aaah! All these Fashola (Lagos State governor) children (referring to the crew team), if una do anythin, way we no like, we will deal with you people. That was how you people came with cameras to Marako before it was demolished." - Residents of Makoko Community, an urban slum in Lagos.

Knowledge

Ignorance is bliss, they say. The field experience showed that millions of people in Nigerian communities do not even know or expect anything from the government. So, the concept of 'health entitlement' is abstract to them.

"... if a person has never seen a car before and you are asking how it feels like to drive in a car it is going to pose a very big problem. Now some of the community people have not experienced the things we wanted them to talk about as regards health service delivery, some of them had never gone to the hospital in their lives and they were quite elderly. So, asking them what going to the hospital was about

is completely uncalled for because they wouldn't be able to tell you anything useful. Some of them are used to their herbal drugs." - *Emmanuel Brymore, Assistant Producer.*

Few Hopefuls...Many Skeptics

Many people have completely lost faith in the Nigerian system as a whole. They do not think that there can be redemption or a better life because they have been left on their own for far too long.

"The women here (concrete industry) were at first aggressive saying that they were not to be recorded at all. They went as far as putting off their machines and threatening not to work if we are bent on recording them. It took some explanation and promises of not recording them as they work before they went back to their work. From the ones we spoke with, we learnt that the people do not have any faith in the system." - *Titi Awobode, Development Producer, Fixer.*

Insecurity

Security of crew members and equipment was paramount as they visited the communities. Even after a job well done by a "Fixer", some difficult personalities may still throw spanners into the wheel of the process. Meanwhile, no serious security challenge or casualties were reported.

"While we were there in Mpape, an urban slum in Abuja, before we knew it, the whole community was coming out and there was about to be some sort of mob action on us. So, we had to remove our equipment and bags from the vicinity while we tried to keep the situation under control." - *Emmanuel Brymore, Assistant Producer.*

Fear of Stigmatization/ Avoidance by Government Officials

Making a respondent use his or her face was more challenging than finding the voice. This is not unconnected with the fear of intimidation from other members of the community. The crew members therefore had problems with people cooperating with them in some instances.

"There was the case of a lady somewhere in Mpape, Abuja who was living positively with AIDs. She had an issue because her husband and her neighbours, especially her husband, would not like her to talk to people like us and put her on (air it) television and she was also concerned about her neighbours seeing her on TV and getting to find out about her." - *Emmanuel Brymore, Assistant Producer.*

"One of the practicing Medical Doctors working in a public health facility in Lagos volunteered to grant an interview to the crew but chose to be interviewed outside the premises, instead of in the hospital facility where he works. In addition, he insisted that his real identity has to be blocked and protected from public view, if he has to grant the interview and we did just that." - *Titi Awobode, Development Producer, Fixer.*

"The Medical Director for Kogi specialist hospital was very hostile. After much persuasion and delay he agreed to speak with us. When it was time to sign a consent form that he would allow us to use the

material, he refused. Even though it was clear that he would not be implicated in any way." - Mak Kusare, Director.

"The Chief Medical Director (CMD) of a secondary health facility in Lagos insisted that unless he gets a formal letter from the Lagos State Commissioner for Health, he will neither grant interview to anybody nor permit any of the staff working in the facility to be interviewed by the team. Also, at a Teaching Hospital in Lagos, the crew lost a whole day waiting to interview the CMD which also made it difficult to keep an earlier scheduled appointment with an Old People Home in Lagos same day (10th of March, 2009). They all seemed to be afraid of letting out any information. They all said they needed permission to be able to speak to us. And even when they did, it was guided. However, the Public Relations Officers (PRO) of one tertiary health institution in Lagos, made a list of departments and people that we could talk with and made sure that we followed it to the later." - Mariam Mbacha, Fixer.

Give Us Money!

There is widespread poverty in the communities. People sometimes will be willing to give their voices for money which will be unprofessional and against the ethics of getting voices.

"In Lokoja, Kogi State, the production crew wanted to interview some mobilized inmates of a Leprosy Home in the area. They said that they will only talk to us if they give them money; and mentioned that severally in the past similar teams who promised that they were working to improve their health conditions did not because to date, nothing had come out of such interviews and recordings." - Eustace Okwechime, Production Manager.

"I just want food and for God to preserve my life." When PATH2 asked a physically challenged person what he wants from life in Ebonyi.

"We were not allowed to set up our camera at a beach in Lagos, they say it's either we pay or we pack our camera and go." - Mariam Mbacha, Fixer.

Language Barrier

The carefully selected multi-lingual crew lived up to the task in this respect. Regardless of a respondent's language or dialect, there is always someone in the team who has at least a conversational level capacity in the language/dialect to engage such a person.

"I grew up in almost several parts of Nigeria and I speak about 4 Nigerian languages. Luckily for us, the crew consisted of people who could speak several languages in Nigeria." - David Uro, Director of Photography.

TIME CONSTRAINT

In production, time is a luxury. The production crew rushed to catch up with the schedule in order to meet the demands.

"All three productions coincidentally were all rushed, in the sense that normally the crew would have had a bit of pre-production time, but had none. Even after we had promised ourselves that we would never be rushed again, but somehow there is just a way it keeps happening..." - Eustace Okwechime, Production Manager

There were numerous barriers that the crew members faced as a group and as individual professionals in their roles during the production. Generally, the production team used patience, courage, dialogue and wisdom to save challenging situations. Some of them shared their unforgettable experiences. PATHS2 documentaries are expected to make policy makers more responsive to health and give the public reasons to laugh again.

Attention! Critical Issues Raised by PATHS2 Documentaries

Generally, issues raised brought to the fore the deplorable state of the health sector characterized by inadequacy of medical facilities, high cost of drugs, long waiting hours possibly because of poor patient doctor ratio or poor attitude of health care workers leading to neglect of patients by medical personnel, long waiting time for patients and facilities without basic life saving equipment. Some of the issues as captured from the socially excluded in the documentaries are presented in this section.

Accessible Healthcare Services

"My son returned home for the holiday and complained about leg pains, headache, neck pains, that's how I knew it was meningitis. There are no vehicles and motorbikes in our village. So, I saddled my cows and brought him to the hospital here in an hour and thirty minutes." - Farmer, Jigawa.

"When my sister went into labour, we went to get a car from town. There is only one car in this village, once it is gone; it is hard to get another car. While we were searching for a vehicle, her condition deteriorated seriously. We took her to Kawo, they turned her down, and before we got to town, she died." - Housewife, Jigawa.

Affordable Drugs and Services

"Government is not fair; my eyes have been aching for 3 days. I went to buy this drug. It is sold for 250 Naira. If the government were fair, it wouldn't cost more than 60 Naira. I had to suffer and spend a whole day's earnings on it." Commercial motor cyclist, "The only thing that's free here is the registration card, all other things are paid for." Housewife, Lagos.

Alternative Medicine

"A good herbalist is better than queuing up in hospitals. Once you take herbal drugs, you get better." - Trado-medical practitioner, Kaduna.

My people (referring to the production crew) hospital medicines are always very expensive and usually out of the reach of ordinary people like me. Our fore-fathers and fathers survived on them (traditional medicine), why can't we? -An enthusiast of traditional medicine.

Health Versus Religion

"I don't take medicine because our church doesn't take medicine. So, all I do is pray." - A sick student

"Sometimes you find that clerics become a stumbling block in the path of health...because you find a cleric talking about something that he does not know." - Civil Society Leader.

Pro-Poor Healthcare Services Delivery

"Here is where we have the wards (pointing to the direction). It is too congested and we need to expand the wards. At times we admit two people on a bed because of congestion." - A Community Health Extension Worker (CHEW), Jigawa State.

Child Spacing

"My name is Ijeoma Isioge, I am a sand packer, I have seven children and if God wills it, this one will be the eight."

They Were Heard!

PATHS2 exemplifies how the socially excluded voices can be brought into the consultative process for the articulation of health policy objectives. This section presents some of the major platforms where PATHS2 documentaries have been successfully used to contribute to effective health planning at different levels.

They Were Heard at the "CSO Forum on Health", Kaduna - November 2008

Civil Society Organisations (CSOs) contribute to the growing demand for accountability and improved health services in Nigeria. Their roles in policy setting, resource mobilization and health promotion are enormous. PATHS2 as a health governance programme does not only recognize and appreciate their critical roles in improving the health systems but has been consistently consulting and collaborating with these 'partners in progress' for health since inception.

As part of her inception phase activities, PATHS2 engaged the CSOs in Kaduna - a PATH2 supported state, to 'discuss the way forward' with a view to finding common solutions to issues affecting the health systems, particularly towards achieving the health related MDGs in the state. Ivan Lewis, the ex-parliamentarian Under Secretary of State for the UK Department for International Development, was one of the resource persons at the forum that emphasized a 'united call for action'. The *PATH to Health* documentary, which is a robust presentation of the issues and barriers to health in the state captured from the voices of the socially excluded, was effectively used throughout the session to kick off discussions and deliberations on roles and responsibilities of CSOs towards health. Mike Egbo, PATHS2 National Programme Manager anchored the sessions and stressed the fact that the forum was not an avenue for pointing accusing fingers but rather a united call for action.

Participating CSOs rekindled their commitments to improving the health systems in the state after viewing the documentary. The organizations include Pastoral Resolve (PR), Civil Society for HIV/AIDS in Nigeria (CiSHAN), Women in Da'wah, Centre for Advancing Realistic Empowerment (CARE), Inter-Faith, Society for Family Health (SFH), ABANTU for Development, Support Health and Educational Development (SHED), Federation of Muslim Women Association of Nigeria (FOMWAN) and Health Reform Foundation of Nigeria (HEFRON) among others.

They Were Heard at the "Future Search Conference" - March 2009

At the first Future Search (FS) Conference in Nigeria with the theme, *"Securing a Better Future: Transforming Nigeria's Health Care System"*, a total of 110 participants representing various stakeholder groups including the socially excluded worked together 'to create a shared vision for Nigeria's health care system and developed "action" steps to actualize the vision'. More people than those physically present at the conference held in Enugu participated by lending their voices at the conference through *What of My Future?*, produced for the conference by PATHS2 in collaboration with FMoH, funded by DFID.

The way the voices of Nigerians, especially the voiceless across Nigeria were captured and infused into the conference; and the honesty with which the stakeholders present accepted culpability in contributing to the collapse of the health care was awesome. The key priorities identified were ensuring that the product from the conference should be used to contribute to the development of the National Strategic Health Development Plan (NSHDP). - Bahijjatu Bello-Garko, FS Conference participant.

The health crisis situation borne documentary x-rayed the causes and not just the symptoms of an ailing health system with suggested solutions. Above all, it gave voices to the unusual participants at such a high profile and intellectual conference towards improving the health systems.

The concept behind the FS Conference involved bringing the whole system (representatives of all stakeholders in the health care system) into the room to participate in a process of viewing the past, present and future.

They Were Heard at the "Presidential Summit on Health"

Shortly after his appointment as the minister for health in 2010, the former minister, Prof Babatunde Oshintimehin wanted to examine the real state of health and hear real stories in addition to health indices. That was the rationale for making the documentary – *The State of Health in Nigeria*. Having captured the voices and pictures of people from all around the country in a video, the documentary became a potent tool for health advocacy to all stakeholders in health - from development partners to the National Council for Health and finally to the Presidency.

As anticipated, the late President Umaru Musa Yar'Adua was shocked to see the deplorable state of health in Nigeria from the documentary. The aim of achieving the health sector component of vision 20:2020 may be derailed if something was not done urgently. He immediately called for a Presidential

Summit on health in (Abuja – 10th November, 2009), the first of its kind for health in Nigeria. The aim of the summit was to find both short and long term solutions to the challenges in the health sector. At the 'larger house' viewing during the summit, the 36 State governors and the Federal Capital Territory (FCT) Minister with a can-do spirit adopted the Abuja declaration for health in November, 2010. Informed by some of the issues raised by the voices in the State *of Health documentary*, poor community participation and poor utilization was recognized in the declaration. Item 17 of the declaration is committed to improving infrastructure planning and investment targeted at the socially excluded; while item 19 is focused on the agitation for availability of drugs at all government owned facilities.

They Were Heard at the "Development of the National Strategic Health Development Plan" (NSHDP)

The Federal Ministry of Health working with other partners including PATHS2 carefully fed the outcome of the FS Conference into the NHSDP. The report from the FS Conference is a potpourri of stakeholders' voices with special contribution from the documentary *What of My Future?* - A Future Search Film. The Plan was a product of wide consultation and utmost consideration of the need to align with the initiatives of the Federal Ministry of Health; and the national development initiatives including the 7 point agenda, Vision 20:2020, and National Development Plan. It was then rightly described as the 'encyclopedic compilation of health investments' and therefore became the overarching reference health development document for all actors.

The adaptation of the NSHDP in March, 2010 was a landmark success for the health sector in Nigeria and more for PATHS2 quest for social inclusion in the development of health policies. The total estimated costs of the NSHDP for the six year period 2010 / 2015 is USD 26.653.107.239 while health service delivery was allocated over 48 percent of the budget. Now people at the grass roots can have access to affordable pro poor health services.

They Were Heard at the 2nd "Health Promotion Conference", Abuja, September 2010

Another milestone of bringing the health plights of the socially excluded was added at the 2nd Health Promotion Conference held in Abuja in September, 2010 with the theme "Strengthening *Health Promotion Mechanism on Information Dissemination and Achieving Effective Feedback*."About 700 people participated in the event. The '*State of Health in Nigeria*' documentary rose to the occasion again. Introduced by the PATHS2 National Programme Manager, Mr. Mike Egboh before its opening remarks, participants watched the film with rapt attention as they beheld the gripping revelation and the disturbing facts about the pathetic state of health in the country. Against that backdrop, both the presenter and commentators called for a sober review of the attitude of the government and the people of Nigeria to health promotion.

The video was watched by participants from diverse backgrounds, including senior technocrats from the Ministries of Health, Education, Agriculture, Labour and Productivity; NGOs; UN development agencies; other donor agencies and implementing partners; as well as politicians/Supervisory Health Councillors, and various cadres of health officials from all the 36 states Ministries of Health and from the local government health authorities.

CONCLUSION

Experiences shared by the poor and socially excluded; and recorded in the documentaries revealed that gatekeepers sometimes can be barriers to accessing voices and that finding voice is not the same as having voice or wanting to use voices. This is not unconnected with past disappointments in the systems which have created cynicism, hopelessness and despair in the minds of the socially excluded. It suggests the strategies for effectively working with health service providers, planners and policy makers. It is hoped that this technical brief would strengthen PATHS2 internal mechanism for successful achievement of its strategic approach of advocating with leadership at all levels for improved access to affordable health care services for the poor and socially excluded using documentaries and the media; and promote a more open participatory process for designing and implementing health communication in Nigeria.

Apparently, a lot is still required in improving the present state of the health of the nation. The ideal health systems we yearn for still lie ahead. Although past attempts to stop and reverse the trend over the years have recorded less satisfactory results for some reasons not discussed in this paper, PATHS2 has actively provided technical support towards the development of the NSHDP, the new national blueprint for health care in Nigeria.

PATHS2 aims to improve the transparency and responsiveness within the public health system by empowering the ministry to ensure improved availability of information in a form that is accessible and useful. To achieve this, PATHS2 will work with and through the press and information units of the FMOH/SMOHs to develop or strengthen as well as to pilot innovative mechanisms for accessible, accurate, and useful information to key stakeholders of the ministries.

PATHS2 will develop a core group of health systems journalists to monitor priority health issues in the health sector as a means of stimulating improved performance among all stakeholders of health. PATHS2 will, in collaboration with other advocacy groups, also design and implement a political engagement and advocacy strategy on key health issues in support of the health sector reform as a further means of stimulating and monitoring stakeholder performance at federal, state and LGA levels.

Working with different stakeholders, PATHS2 will continue in creatively using documentaries to inform policy and in monitoring the new plan to meet health service delivery needs of the socially excluded groups

RECOMMENDATIONS

With the support of PATHS2, a series of media-led debates on specific health entitlement issues will be held across the states where we work by working with media coalitions and networks. It is expected that the skills of this key stakeholder will be enhanced in health policy advocacy and utilized accordingly to make policy makers more responsive.

As part of the capacity building process, the media partners were trained on special skills required for media capture of community level dialogues and in working with the socially excluded who may sometimes be unreceptive due to some of the reasons discussed earlier. Hands-on-training in the field further enriched their skills in community engagement and in the concept of participation through the production of *Ask Nigeria, a* populist approach to health communication.

REFERENCES

Anderson, C. (2008). *The end of theory: The data deluge makes the scientific method obsolete*. Wired.

Aston, J., & Gaudenzi, S. (2012). Interactive documentary: Setting the field. *Studies in Documentary Film*, *6*(2), 125–139. doi:10.1386/sdf.6.2.125_1

Barnes, B. (1974). *Scientific knowledge and sociological theory*. Routledge & Kegan Paul.

Brown, J., Michie, S., Walmsley, M., & West, R. (2016). An online documentary film to motivate quit attempts among smokers in the general population (4Weeks2Freedom): A randomized controlled trial. *Nicotine & Tobacco Research: Official Journal of the Society for Research on Nicotine and Tobacco*, *18*(5), 1093–1100. doi:10.1093/ntr/ntv161 PMID:26220547

Brown, W. (2015). Examining four processes of audience involvement with media personae: Transportation, parasocial interaction, identification, and worship. *Commun Theor.*

Chio, I. (2009). Interactive Documentary: A Production Model for Nonfiction Multimedia Narratives. *Intelligent Technologies for Interactive Entertainment*, *9*, 44–55. doi:10.1007/978-3-642-02315-6_5

Coleman, D. (2010). Projections of the ethnic minority populations of the United Kingdom 2006-2056. *Population and Development Review*, *36*(3), 441–486. doi:10.1111/j.1728-4457.2010.00342.x PMID:20882702

de Lange, N., Olivier, T., & Wood, T. (2008). Participatory video documentary: Just for whom? *Education as Change*, *12*(2), 109–122. doi:10.1080/16823200809487210

Dobson, M. W., & Ha, D. (2007). Exploring interactive stories in an HIV/AIDS learning game: HEALTH-SIMNET. *Simulation & Gaming*, *39*(1), 39–63. doi:10.1177/1046878107308093

Edge, D. (1988). The social shaping of technology. Edinburgh PICT Working Paper No. 1, Edinburgh University.

Freimuth, V. S., & Mettger, W. (1990). Is there a hard-to-reach audience? *Public Health Reports*, *105*(3), 232–238. PMID:2113680

Hecht, M. L., & Choi, H. (2012). The communication theory of identity as a framework for health message design. Health communication message design. *Theory into Practice*, 137–152.

Hudnall Stamm, B. (2004). Considering a theory of cultural trauma and loss. *Journal of Loss and Trauma*, *9*(1), 89–11. doi:10.1080/15325020490255412

Koshoedo, S. A., Paul-Ebhohimhen, V. A., Jepson, R. G., & Watson, M. C. (2015). Understanding the complex interplay of barriers to physical activity amongst black and minority ethnic groups in the United Kingdom: A qualitative synthesis using meta-ethnography. *BMC Public Health*, *15*(643), 643. doi:10.1186/s12889-015-1893-0 PMID:26164652

Lashko, G. (2006). Meeting the needs of black and minority ethnic communities. *Housing Care Support.*, *9*(1), 2–4. doi:10.1108/14608790200600001

Mackay, H., & Gillespie, G. (1992). Extending the social shaping of technology approach: Ideology and appropriation. *Social Studies of Science*, *22*(4), 685–716. doi:10.1177/030631292022004006

MacKenzie, D. (1981). Interests, positivism and history. *Social Studies of Science*, *11*(4), 498–505. doi:10.1177/030631278101100405

Mendes, L., Dos Santos, H. B., & Ichikawa, E. Y. (2017). Health and safety at work: Analysis from the Brazilian documentary film Flesh and Bone. *Safety and Health at Work*, *8*(4), 347–355. doi:10.1016/j.shaw.2017.01.003 PMID:29276633

Nichols, B. (2001). *Introduction to documentary*. Indiana University Press.

O'Flynn, S. (2012). Documentary's metamorphic form: Webdoc, interactive, transmedia, participatory and beyond. *Studies in Documentary Film*, *6*(2), 141–157. doi:10.1386/sdf.6.2.141_1

Parr, H. (2007). Collaborative film-making as process, method and text in mental health research. *Cultural Geographies*, *14*(1), 114–138. doi:10.1177/1474474007072822

Pascucci, M. A., Chu, N., & Leasure, A. R. (2012). Health promotion for the oldest of old people. *Nursing Older People*, *24*(3), 22–28. doi:10.7748/nop2012.04.24.3.22.c9017 PMID:22567772

Pinsky, P. F., Ford, M., Gamito, E., Higgins, D., Jenkins, V., Lamerato, L., Tenorio, S., Marcus, P. M., & Gohagan, J. K. (2008). Enrollment of racial and ethnic minorities in the prostate, lung, colorectal and ovarian cancer screening trial. *Journal of the National Medical Association*, *100*(3), 291–298. doi:10.1016/S0027-9684(15)31241-4 PMID:18390022

Quinn, N., Shulman, A., Knifton, L., & Byrne, P. (2011). The impact of a national mental health arts and film festival on stigma and recovery. *Acta Psychiatrica Scandinavica*, *123*(1), 71–81. doi:10.1111/j.1600-0447.2010.01573.x PMID:20491719

Shaw, J., & Robertson, C. (1997). *Participatory video: A practical approach to using video creatively in group development work*. Routledge.

Villanueva, S. (2015). Collaborative practices in the contemporary documentary: A proposed analysis and revision of the participatory mode in documentary theory. *L'Atalante. Revista de estudios cinematográficos,* 20.

WHO. (2015). World report on aging and health. Geneva: World Health Organization.

WHO Commission on Social Determinants of Health. (2008). Closing the gap in a generation. Health equity through action on the social determinants of health. Geneva: WHO. https://www.who.int/social_determinants/en/

Chapter 11
Communicating Sexuality and Reporting Reproductive Health Issues Among the Akan:
Questions of Morality, Profanity, and Culture

Kwesi Aggrey
University of Education, Winneba, Ghana

Bismark Odum Sackey
https://orcid.org/0000-0002-7404-6701
University of Education, Winneba, Ghana

Priscilla Aboagyewaa Boateng
University of Education, Winneba, Ghana

ABSTRACT

Societies structure their communication relationships in a variety of ways. The Akan in Ghana have a peculiar way of communicating issues relating to their sexuality. They find it difficult mentioning the real names of the human sex organs; they prefer employing various metaphors to signify these. It is not clear what the reasons are and how feasible this becomes when they (Akan) are confronted with reporting reproductive health since it is usually considered important for patients to indicate specific parts of the body that ail for appropriate diagnosis and healthcare. The study investigated how the Akan communicate sexuality generally, and how this affects their reporting of reproductive health issues. It was grounded on the rhetorical sensitivity theory. A multiple case study was employed for the study. In all, eight respondents were sampled and were categorised into two as cultural respondents and medical respondents. Cultural respondents comprised the Fante ethnic group of the larger Akan group. One respondent each was selected from three Fante traditional communities.

DOI: 10.4018/979-8-3693-0624-6.ch011

INTRODUCTION

In every society, culture has been the bearer of the people's philosophy – thoughts, ideas, beliefs, among others, and shapes their everyday interrelationships and practices (Markus & Kitayama, 2010; Ogbujah, 2017). What people do and say are, therefore, informed by their deeply-held beliefs and understandings about life. Sociologists, in this regard, have long theorised about the twin concepts of "cultural relativism" and "cultural shock" as some traits of culture; implying all cultures have intrinsic worth, yet there is the tendency for first-timers to new cultures to express some feeling of wonderment and surprise. Among the Inuits (Eskimos) and other peoples of Northern North America, for example, where wife sharing is a valued tradition, Hennigh (1970) and Rubel (1978) provide elaborate underlying rationale for such a custom. Hennigh provides scholarly explanations of the practice, and situates it in theoretical contexts, providing economic expediency and the concept of "lost paradise" as the basis for the time-honoured tradition. Similarly, among the Trobriands of New Guinea we learn of a tradition/culture where women virtually rape men during specific periods of their cultural lives, and Malinowski (1947) sheds interesting reasons about that too; indicating that reasons include fertility and agricultural purposes. Much as these examples of the Inuits and Trobriands might superficially sound "weird" to the ethnic Akan in Ghana, perhaps that which may equally appear unusual to a 'first timer' among the Akan of Ghana too is the apparent "strange" way how they (Akan) communicate on issues pertaining to their sexuality. Unlike other cultures, the Akan find it very difficult to call the human sex organs and other related phenomena by their real names, but rather prefer to assuage them by various metaphors.

REVIEW OF LITERATURE

Sexuality Defined

The concept "sexuality" is also perhaps one of the sociological terms that have received various definitions. To some, sexuality simply refers to erotic attractions, identity and practices (Shaw & Lee, 2018), while others situate it in the domain of health and development and therefore suggest that sexuality is part of human life and human development (Macleod & McCabe, 2020; NASW, 2001). But sociologists, (Lindsey & Beach, 2002, p. 161) provide a much broader understanding of the concept; they note, "sexuality is a type of social interaction where we perceive, experience, and express ourselves as sexual beings." The perspective of Lindsey and Beach therefore does not restrict the concept to romanticism and pleasurable life but suggests an all-encompassing phenomenon that denotes everything relating to how humans structure their sexual relationships. In their paper on *...Influences on Responsible Sexual Decision-Making*, NASW (2001) emphasises the importance of the knowledge of good sexual health in particular and reproductive health in general. The paper explains that good sexual health implies not only the absence of disease, but the ability to understand and weigh the risks, responsibilities, outcomes, and impacts of sexual actions, to be knowledgeable of and comfortable with one's body, and to be free from exploitation and coercion. Given the foregoing background on the importance of human sexuality therefore, it becomes a bit intriguing why and how the Akan in Ghana structure their communication relationships with regard to their sexuality in that particular way, especially with regard to how they refer to the human sex organs and related phenomena by various metaphors. Their pattern might not be a case in isolation any way, as Lindsey and Beach (2002), writing from the perspective of the American (US) society, have noted that until fairly recently, beliefs about human sexuality had been shrouded in myth and superstition. Similarly, various reasons appear to be given to this way of life among the Akan too. The interest and motivation of this current paper is, therefore, to find out the underlying reason(s) for such a communicative pattern among the Akan in general and the Fante in particular; it investigates how such communicative pattern affect how the people report issues relating to their reproductive health and how doctors and nurses (also referred to as clinicians or health workers in this paper) especially deal with this issue, inasmuch as doctor-patient interaction thrives on mutual frankness and trust (Anane, 2015).

The Akan and Fante Peoples

In their works, Asante (1995) and Kissi and Van Eck (2017) indicate that Akan is the ethnic name of the Twi-speaking peoples of the Guinea Coast of West Africa. They consist of Ahanta, Akwapim, Akyem or Akim, Agni or Anyi, Asante or Ashanti, Asen or Assin, Bono or Brong, Brusa, Chokosi, Fante, Guan, Kwahu, Nzima, and Wasa or Wassaw. They add that the Akan people occupy practically the whole of Ghana south and west of the Black Volta. With a slight variation, however, Anderson (2015) notes that the Akan include the Bono, Asante, Denkyira, Twifu, Assin, Wassaw, Sefwi, Akwamu, Akyem and Adansi. His categorisation does not include Fante, but nonetheless asserts that the main languages these groups speak are Fante and Twi. On the other hand, Fynn (1987) describes the Fante peoples as those who inhabit the coastlands of the Central Region of Ghana; and whose territory extends the estuary of the river Pra in the west to the borders of Accra in the east. "The Fante, who are part of the Akan ethnic group, may be divided into two broad categories: The BɔrbɔrFante and the non-BɔbɔrFante" (Fynn, 1987, p. 108). According to Fynn, the BɔrbɔrFante lived in Mankessim and later also founded other states like Abora, Ekumfi, Enyanmaim, and Nkusukum. The non-BɔrbɔrFante include Yarbew, Eguafo, Fetu, Asebu, and Agona. Another Perspective of who the Fante are is provided by Crayner (2007). Crayner also puts the group into two, namely the Western Fante and Eastern Fante; he nonetheless also makes reference to one of the groups – the Eastern Fante – as BɔrbɔrFante, as earlier noted by Fynn. Crayner notes that the Western Fante comprise Abrem, Sema (Shama), Esikado and Sekondi, Mfuma (Dixcove), Wassa Mpohor and Wassa Fiase, Asebu and Busua, and Evalue; while Eastern Fante, he indicates are Mankessim, Abora, Nomabo, Ekumfi, Nkusukum, Gomua, Edwumako, and Enyan.

The Akan Concept of the Sacred and the Profane

In Akan thought, certain objects and beings with distinctive characteristics have the potential of affecting life positively or negatively; these include natural phenomena, animals, mediums and spirits. Those, which affect life positively and have pervasive and persuasive characteristics, are what the people conceive as distinctively sacred; whilst those that affect life negatively and have dissuasive characteristics are profane (Ofosuhene, 1993). There is a potential force underlying what is considered to be the sacred and the profane, and this makes them contagious and essentially 'dangerous.' In Akan religious thought, a sacred realm is established wherever there is mystical divine manifestation and consecration. The sacred assumes a superior position to the profane. It is that which is separated from the profane and secular; and it is that which is respected and protected (ibid). Ofosuhene also notes that the two – sacred and profane – represent two poles of a dreadful domain; they are mutually exclusive and contradictory in every sense. He observes,

It is therefore imperative to create water-tight compartments between them [the sacred and profane] since they cannot co-exist without one losing its unique characteristics. The contagious nature of the profane, for example, always causes it to debase, degrade and destroy instantaneously the essence of which the sacred is defined. The sacred is therefore placed outside common usage, guarded and protected by restrictions and prohibitions. (Ofosuhene, 1993)

It is considered that the mysterious power in a being or an object helps differentiate it from the "ordinary". The being or object then becomes a taboo; and what is taboo is what may be conceived as sacred or profane, and which is expressed almost exclusively through taboos (Ofosuhene, 1993). Even though the phenomenon under study – the non-mentioning of the human genitalia by their real names – appears to be given "special" regard and respect by the people, it is wondered whether the phenomenon would merit the status of a taboo, for, as indicated by Ofosuhene, anyone in breach of the cultic and customary precautions of a taboo is believed to suffer automatic and immediate punishment or disaster; and this does not seem to be the case with the issue under consideration, as there have been occasional "breaches" without any disastrous consequences.

The Concept Morality

According to Anderson (2015), the concept of morality derives from the Latin rendition of "mores" which means customs or manners. He notes that the term can be used either descriptive or normative. In the descriptive sense, the term morality would simply refer to a code of conduct put forward by any group, including a society, to govern the attitudes of members. The normative sense of morality refers to a universal guide to behaviour that, in plausible specified conditions, all rational persons would put forward for governing the behaviour of all moral agents (Gert et al, 2020). Wiredu (1992) (as cited in Anderson, 2015) therefore suggests that morality in the strictest sense is universal and essential to culture; it is the observance of rules for the harmonious adjustment of the interests of the individual to those of others in society. Wiredu adds that morality does not just refer to conformity to the requirements of the harmony of interests, but also that conformity to those requirements is inspired by an imaginative and sympathetic identification with the interests of others even at the cost of a possible curtailment of one's own interests. The views of Wiredu (1992) on morality seem to tie in with that of Gyekye (1996). Gyekye notes that morality is a set of social rules and norms intended to guide the conduct of people in a society. He explains that the rules and norms emerge from and are anchored in people's beliefs about right and wrong conduct, and good and bad character. To Gyekye, the core and overriding value embedded in the meaning of morality is the principle of "sense of duty to others" – a social responsibility kind of value. In his contribution, Ibekwe (n.d) notes that morality is the sense and view of what is right and wrong, and that which constitutes an absolute reference for character and behaviour. It is an authoritative code of conduct in matters of right and wrong. He indicates that the African perspective of morality is rooted in tradition; the concept is believed to flow from *God* into the ancestors of the people who are custodians of this tradition. "Tradition in Africa therefore supplies the moral code and indicates what the people must do to live ethically, and also the punishment for defaulters of certain codes of conduct" (Ibid). Reviewing the literature on morality in African thought, Ibekwe critiques Mbiti (1975) apparent paradox of viewing morality in one breath as a divinely sanctioned phenomenon and in the other as a socially inscribed mode of action derived from experiences of what is in the interest and well-being of the community. What appears missing in Ibekwe's analysis is perhaps his lack of understanding for the cosmology of the African moral consciousness. He (Ibekwe) surprisingly indicates elsewhere in his paper that the African conception of the universe is a composite of divine, spirit, animate and inanimate elements hierarchically positioned and always interacting with each other. It is thus a divine process that manifests and is implemented in human society.

THEORETICAL ISSUES

The Rhetorical Sensitivity Theory

Littlejohn, Foss, and Oetzel (2017) indicate that rhetorical sensitivity is the tendency to adapt messages to audiences. The theory was propounded by Roderick Hart and his colleague, Don Burks. These theorists found that effective communication arises from sensitivity and care in adjusting what you say to a listener or audience. Hart and Burks (1972) construct three general types of communicators, namely 1. The Noble Selves, 2. The Rhetorical Reflectors, and 3. Rhetorically Sensitive Individuals.

According to Hart and Burks (1972), the Noble Selves stick to their personal ideals without variation and without adapting or adjusting to others. Rhetorical Reflectors are those who mould themselves to the wishes of others' wishes without following personal scruples. The Rhetorically Sensitive Individuals moderate the extremes. Littlejohn and Foss indicate that Rhetorical Sensitivity embodies concerns for self, concerns for others, and a situational attitude. To Hart, the type that embodies a situational attitude is clearly superior to the other two. Rhetorically adaptive people communicate differently in two different situations. Rhetorically sensitive people are aware of the appropriateness of communicating particular ideas in different situations. An idea can be expressed in many ways and can be adapted to the audience to be effective. The rhetorically adaptive Akan is therefore particularly sensitive to tasks or expectations that his or her cultural values and community place on them, to communicate appropriately and competently as well-bred members of their cultural communities.

Robert Norton (1983) similarly theorises about communicator style and notes that when human beings communicate, not only do they give information, but they also present that information in a certain form that tells others how to understand and how to respond to a message. Norton (1983) as cited in Littlejohn, Foss, and Oetzel (2017) note that for example you might tell a friend about an experience but signal at the same time that your message is to be taken with authority, with or without interest, with or without humour, or with any number of different attitudes. The scholars believe that these signals function as a "style message" by "signaling how a literal (primary) message should be taken, filtered, interpreted or understood." The thesis of Norton (1983), therefore, is that characteristics repeatedly associated with a person's communication constitute their dominant style Littlejohn, Foss, and Oetzel (2017), however note that styles are not totally individual, since cultures affect how people behave and how they perceive others. The cultural dictates of the indigenous Fante/Akan hold quite strongly in their life, and therefore couch peculiar communicator style which conveniently can be described as the metaphorical style of communication in regard to how they communicate issues about their sexuality.

The Competent Communicator Model

Owing to the fact that Hart and Burks (1972) originally set out to distinguish the attitudes of those persons whom they (Hart & Burks) felt maximised communication possibilities, their (the scholars) conceptualisation may eventually prove useful for discriminating between competent and incompetent communicators. Other sources cited by ERIC[1] suggest the likelihood of different strains of thought surrounding the idea of communicative competence. For example, a recent work by DeVito (2014) describes the competent communicator as one who thinks critically and mindfully, is culturally sensitive and listens effectively; and earlier Wiemann (1975) had identified three approaches to defining the competent communicator, namely the *human relations* approach, the *social skills* approach, and the *self-presentation* approach. The *human relations* approach views the competent communicator as one who can successfully manage both the task and socio-emotional requirements placed upon him or her by an identifiable and known group. As highlighted by the work of Argyle (1969), the *social skill* variant sees the competent communicator as one with the knowledge of, and ability to perform the rituals and routines associated with norm-bound transactions. The *self-presentation* school also views the competent communicator as one who can manage the "face requirements" demanded in an interpersonal situation (Wiemann, 1975). Other perspectives that attempt to provide explanation for the competent communicator model are the *sociolinguistic* school and the *gamesmanship* school. The *sociolinguistics* school emphasises that competence in communication derives from the ability to develop and to perform verbal acts which meet the social requirements of a given speech community (Hymes, 1970); while the *gamesmanship* perspective suggests people communicate optimally when: 1, they are able to define the communicative game they are playing, and 2, when they use the "rules of the game" for personal and interpersonal satisfaction (Rosenfield, Hayes, &Frentz, 1976). A careful look at the five communication competency perspectives shows some common inherent features, namely that communication is a communal enterprise. The language vehicle of communication is socially owned and has social expectations of those who participate in it. These are, perhaps, what the five schools have variously captured as task and socio-emotional requirements, norm-bound rituals and routines, verbal acts, "rules of the game," among others.

A more recent dimension to the Rhetsen scholarship is provided by Dilbeck's (2008) work. He notes that under Rhetorical Sensitivity and Communication Competence, two constructs appear conceptualised in almost the same way. He observes that whereas a rhetorically sensitive person balances noble self and rhetorical reflection, a competent communicator balances socio-communicative orientations, assertiveness and responsiveness, with respect to the communication situation. Dilbeck's work showed that though the two constructs appear to be conceptualised virtually the same way, there was not any convergent validity. Dilbeck's work thus provides an ideal framework for assessing this current study.

METHODOLOGY

The study is essentially about how people structure their communication relationships as part of their culture. It aimed at understanding why the Fante communicate the way they do, and whether and how it affected their health reporting. Probing the "hows" and "whys" of a phenomenon falls within the purview of the qualitative approach (Creswell & Creswell, 2023); and in doing so, the best method or design considered effective for data collection and analysis was the case study method. According to Yin (2018) a case study design should be considered when the study, among others, focuses on "how" and "why" questions, and also when it covers contextual conditions that are relevant to the phenomenon under study. Daymon and Holloway (2011) add that a case study enquiry enables a researcher to collect "rich" detailed information across a wide range of dimensions about one particular case or smaller number of cases. The phenomena under consideration in this study are communication issues that manifest in the everyday social relationships of the people. The problem/issue is therefore situated in a cultural context. The population was the entire Akan ethnic community in Ghana. As indicated earlier in this paper, about thirteen (13) – fifteen (15) distinct ethnic groups constitute the larger Akan ethnic group. Among this number, the study purposively selected the Fante ethnic group for reasons of convenience, especially with regard to availability of respondents who were willing to provide information, and their proximity to the researcher (Glesne, 2016). Tongco (2007) avers that personal judgment (purposive sampling) is a non-random technique that does not require underlying theories or set number of subjects. It is a technique where the researcher sets out to find people who can and are willing to provide information by virtue of knowledge or experience (Bernard, 2002; Lewis& Sheppard, 2006). The Fante ethnic group also broadly subdivides into BɔrbɔrFante and non-BɔbɔrFante (Crayner, 2007; Fynn, 1987) which groups, in turn, have several dialectal areas. The study then purposively sampled the following three dialectal areas from the BɔbɔrFante: Mankessim, Ekumfi, and Gomua. Here again, these three ethnic groups were chosen for reasons of convenience and validity purposes. Merriam and Tisdell (2016) have stated that issues of reliability and validity often become problematic, particularly in the social sciences; however, Creswell and Creswell (2023) provide a list of primary verification procedures found to be easy and frequently employed to validate qualitative data. Four of these verification procedures have been applied to validate the study. The four include persistent observation, triangulation, peer review, and "rich" thick description. Observation has been a key aspect of the study because one of the researchers being an ethnic Fante had been observing (perhaps as a participant observer) and informally self-interrogating the phenomenon. Data from the three locations of study – Mankessim, Ekumfi, and Gomua – were variously cross-checked with one another for inherent inconsistencies, peculiarities and unanimity. Again, after data collection and preliminary analysis paper was presented at Faculty Seminar for peer critique and inputs. Respondents who provided data in the study were knowledgeable and experienced in the areas the study required information from, and therefore provided vivid narratives and explanations to the research questions. In all, eight (8) respondents were interviewed. These are categorised, for the purposes of the study as *Cultural Respondents* and *Medical Respondents.* The Cultural Respondents included one respondent each from the three study areas, well-versed in the knowledge and customs of their respective areas; and for the purposes of the study referred to as *JB* (Mankessim), *Nana* (Ekumfi), and *Supi* (Gomua). The Medical Respondents comprised two (2) medical practitioners referred to in this study as MRD1 and MRD2, and three (3) senior nurses – a midwife, a community health nurse, and a family planning specialist and tutor, also referred to as MRN1, MRN2, and MRN3 respectively in this study to protect the identity of the respondents.

FINDINGS AND DISCUSSIONS

RQ1. Why do Akan find it difficult to mention or call the human genitalia by their real names?

Generally, all respondents assign reasons of respect and honour to this communicative pattern; situating it in sacredness.For example, respondent *Supi* (Gomua) provides a tall historical background of the Fante; making innuendoes to some kinship ties with the Hebrews in Christian scripture, specifically to the *Akan* cited in Genesis 36:27 as their forebear. "For this reason, most of our customs and institutions are quite akin to what is found in Old Testament [Biblical] days. The penis has a role to play, and is considered sacred." He ends there like that. But what looks like the continuation of the views of *Supi* is provided by respondent JB (Mankessim). He adds that *Onyame* (God) created the first man and woman; and that these two were to continue with the creation process that he (*Onyame*) initiated."… And so it is a sacred duty," he adds.

Onyame never provided the names of what he created. It was the human being that he created who did… And for the medium or zone in the body of a woman where humans pass through to arrive into the world, it was rightly considered a "natural scar" which translates in Fante as twua, and that of the man, the "erectile organ" – description of its nature during sexual intercourse – which translates in Fante as ɔkɔtsee, literally implying "goes straight." The present rendition of twɛ for the female reproductive organ and kɔtse for that of the male is rather the corrupted form of the original twua and ɔkɔtsee respectively; and it is probably as a result of the passage of time.

Respondent adds that these organs and related activities are therefore specialised phenomena dedicated to the sacred duty of the creation process initiated by *Onyame* and entrusted to the care of the human being for continuation. The God – Human bond factor emphasised in Asante (1995) is somehow re-echoed here. Asante provides a theological analysis of the Akan understanding of the relationship between Onyame and the individual Akan. In this relationship, the Akan believes that the "kra/ɔkra" (soul) residing in him or her comes directly from Onyame. A sacred realm is thus established, for, as indicated by Ofosuhene (1993), in Akan philosophy certain objects and beings affect life positively and have pervasive and persuasive characteristics which make them distinctively sacred. Traditionally therefore, the Fante language has devised various metaphors to depict and preserve the sanctity and honour reserved for this pro/creative activity and related concepts. Some of these metaphors include *m'ewiei*, literally "my end," *m'ammbodzin*, my "unpronounceable part." The concepts (female and male reproductive organs) and related activities therefore appear to have some moral, cultural and religious aura embedded in them, and for which reason(s) must not be disdained.

Questions of Morality, Profanity and Culture

Incidentally all respondents – *JB* of Mankessim, *Nana* of Ekumfi, and *Supi* of Gomua – seem to rule out the question/issue of morality as the underlying factor for why the Fante find it difficult to mention the real names of the human genitalia and related activities. They (respondents) invariably explain that that behaviour and attitude is a tradition that had long been respected and held as such. They however prefer to situate the tradition (non-mentioning of the names of human genitalia) in the realm of sacrality and profanity. *Nana* for example observes that the speaker/user of such words or terms rather pollutes themselves. She adds,

It is not a question of whether it is right or wrong to pronounce them; it is something that has long been respected for the purpose it was made for, and will continue to be like that. Look at where they have been kept; of all the body parts, they are the most hidden. God intended them to be so, and so nobody should bring them to commonness.

On his part, *JB* indicates that in Fante custom the concept of profanity is *kasafi* or *anobow,* dirty words or foul language while taboo is *ekyirwadze*, a forbidden act which generally warrants some sanctions and associated rites. "Profanity, though also abhorred, is considered a bit 'liberal' and sometimes manifests even in the way we dress and the way we speak," respondent JB remarked. Respondent *Supi* on his part only said that there is a difference between taboo and morality. "I would, however, not consider the issue – non-pronunciation of these names – an issue of morality but an issue of profanity." As a sacred phenomenon however, one cannot rule out the commutative tendency of profanity too, for, as noted by Ofosuhene (1993), the two concepts are mutually exclusive, and represent two poles of a dreadful domain. It is not exactly clear why respondents do not seem to see any linkage of this communicative pattern to the issue of morality. Contrary to respondents' view, the study rather finds the responses as having some bearing on the normative view of morality discussed in Anderson's (2015) work; Anderson observes that morality is a universal guide that regulates the behaviour of a people with regard to what is considered right or wrong. Not only that, but also something which community members voluntarily do to identify with the interests of their fellow kinsmen or neighbours for the ultimate good of society. The behaviour – communicative pattern of the Fante – therefore is an unwritten code, as it were, though not rigidly enforced, yet virtually obeyed by everyone in the society. It is a cultural value then, and thus becomes that universal code. The sheer idea that the custom/behaviour is a tradition and anchored in a certain belief – "God intended them to be so…" – reinforces Gyekye's (1996) view on morality indicated above, that morality is about rules and norms that emerge from, and are anchored in the people's beliefs about what is considered right and wrong, and good and bad. All respondents however concede to what they described as a little deviation from the norm of how their compatriots in the coastal communities communicate on issues pertaining to sexuality. They suggest that these people (Fante coastal dwellers) are somehow forthright in these matters, probably owing to the nature of work – artisanal fishing – they do.

RQ2. How the Difficulty in Mentioning Such Real Names Affect Reproductive Health Reporting

All Medical Respondents affirmed that there are diseases and ailments associated with human reproduction. They mentioned some of these diseases as gonorrhoea, syphilis, cervical cancers, HIV/AIDS, and other pelvic inflammatory diseases (PIDs). Respondents note that the inability of patients to mention the human genitalia and related phenomena by their real names affects health reporting. It especially prevents early reporting, and also encourages the resort to unconventional traditional herbs usage, as well as self-medications. These sometimes lead to increased vaginal cancers in women, and prostrate-related problems in men.

With regard to the likely reason(s) accounting for this behaviour or tradition, respondents indicate that it is a certain perception rooted in patients' culture which subsequently manifests and influences their upbringing. This cultural trait appears to cause a kind of unexplained shyness which prevents the indigenous Fante from maligning his or her reproductive organ. It is a cultural value. MRD1elaborately explains as follows:

In referring to their genitals, patients prefer to use various descriptive terms and metaphors. The women would generally say m'ase, [literally "my under,"] m'aserɛmu, [literally "in-between my thighs,"] m'ahemfie, [literally "my palace/court,"] me basia mu, [literally "within my womanhood,"] m'ayerase [literally "my abdomen,"] m'akosua mu,[literally "within my akosua," – a personal feminine name]; while the men would generally use terms such as me dua mu, [literally "within my log,"] me bodua mu, [literally "within my whisk,"] m'adomba mu, [literally "within my bell,"] me banyin mu, [literally "within my manhood,"] among others. It is their culture, and we respect it! According to them, any person who dares to go so "open" and contrary in regard to these terms is considered to have profaned or disgraced themselves.

RQ 3. Whether or Not This Pattern of Communication Affect Quality of Care

Medic Respondents provided a mix-bag of responses. While some think that the phenomenon does not in any way affect the quality of care they dispense, others were of the view that the situation indirectly leads to inaccurate understanding and diagnosis and subsequent inappropriate prescription and treatment. For example, arguing from the perspective that the phenomenon does not affect the quality of care, MRD1 notes that even though the situation affects patients' health reporting generally, it does not really affect the quality of care medics dispense. The reason is that, he notes,

We are Ghanaians, and quite familiar with such situations; you see, though they – patients – wouldn't mention the real names, there are terms such as m'ahanmu, m'ahemfie, m'ammbɔdzin, among others which they prefer to use, and which we understand. However with regard to the specifics, you would have to start treatment before you get to know [that] this is the actual area or zone affected.

This view is similarly reinforced by the comment by MRN3 which said,

We understand them somehow because we are Ghanaians in the first place, and especially because some of us are also Akan working in Fante communities. The situation becomes problematic only when the medic or clinician involved is not Akan. Even in such circumstances when the terms and metaphors used by patients appear incomprehensible, the reported problem could later become clearer owing to the additional physical examination we do as part of diagnosis.

Perhaps the quick follow up to this assertion is whether in matters of health and illnesses "later" scenarios are pleasant experiences to wish for.

But arguing from the perspective of those who consider the phenomenon to have negative consequences on quality of care, MRN2 indicates that the inherent shyness associated with the phenomenon not only encourages the resort to self-medication and use of unconventional herbal medicine but also fraught with the danger of delayed or inappropriate treatment as a result of miscommunication. MRD2 adds:

Sometimes these descriptions and metaphors do not strike the right chord and therefore gets your whole diagnosis wrong and incomplete until further follow ups give you the clue. The incidence of cost in such situations is sometimes phenomenal and not only borne by the individual patient alone but by the medics and state at large.

As an endemic and enduring cultural phenomenon, its crowding-out effect is equally substantial, as more often, medics and clinicians themselves are impelled to communicate with their patients via similar mode – employing similar descriptors and metaphors – sometimes even on one-on-one consulting basis, Family Planning sessions, and or during Public Health Education fora. MRN2 relates an anecdotal incidence of Family Planning session where a husband is reported to have continually worn the condom he was supposed to use, on a piece of wooden penis for the apparent reason that during the counselling session the nurse had stated, *"…ansaana enye no rebedzi ehyia no, fa condom no hyɛ wodua no ho…,"* literally "before having intercourse with her, wear the condom on your log." And actually the nurse had demonstrated how to wear the condom on a miniature penis. Perhaps the husband in this anecdote should not entirely be blamed because the message in the communication was quite clear: the condom was to be worn on his "log," which example was actually shown. The anecdote suggests that because the phenomenon is an endemic cultural trait, even the health workers and medics themselves occasionally swing with its tide as they are found to also use metaphors for the real names of the human genitalia all the same. What this implies is that medics and clinicians are indeed familiar with, and understand the way their patients communicate their sexuality; thus lending credence to the view by MRD1 that the way their patients communicate on their sexuality, though somehow problematic, does not compromise the quality of care they – medical practitioners – dispense.

With regard to how practitioners deal with the phenomenon, medic respondents unanimously concede that it is a challenge but they do their best to understand their patients by probing further to deduce what and where really the problem is. MRD2 for example explains, "we are getting used to it, by and by; it's like a new dialect or vocabulary we are learning. It's time consuming though, because in some cases you virtually struggle to make meaning out of it. For example, a patient tells you, *doctor mokun nnye me nnda bio*, which literally translates "my husband is not sleeping with me any longer." This really is not implying the couple is indeed not sharing the same bed, but implying 'my husband is not having intercourse with me.' The senior and more experienced medics in such (Fante) communities are much acquainted with the phenomenon and know how to deal with it than the younger and less experienced ones.

The future of whether this cultural phenomenon would undergo some changes is also something that respondents were sceptical about. Generally, they appear optimistic but with some reservation. MRD1 for example notes:

We can say yes, because our society is gradually being exposed to outside influences; people are reading a lot of stuff, and therefore can change the trend some day. But again, because it is a deep-seated cultural issue, it is very difficult to tell.

MRD2 shares similar sentiments; he notes "it can get better in the future because more and more people are schooling and reading, and getting to know the essence of some of these things."

Theoretical Implications of Findings

A closer look at the peculiar way the Fante structure their communication relationship, especially with regard to communicating sexuality, shows a bearing on the rhetorical sensitivity theory and sister model the competent communicator model. Analysis of findings shows that even though respondents were unsure whether the phenomenon is a moral issue, they were however sure about the fact that they had been socialised into communicating that way. It is a socio-cultural issue which though infringement does not warrant sanctions on offenders, the social and unwritten rules impel members to take care to adjust what they say to one another. Viewed this way, the typical Fante can be considered to model the rhetorically adaptive individual in Hart's theory. When communicating matters of sexuality, the typical Fante ensures that the message is packaged in a particular cultural sense to be well understood without disdaining the concept involved (Norton, 1983). Aspects of the findings therefore mirror what Hart and Burks describe as the noble selves. These are said to stick to their own ideals without necessarily adapting to others and rules. Perhaps the forthrightness and occasional suggestive disregard for rules of language and norm-bound rituals of the Fante coastal dweller as compared to the other non-coastal Fante rightly places them (coastal dweller) in the category of noble selves.

It looks like findings prominently reflect Hart and Burks' (1975) Competent Communicator Model which is also given credence by DeVito (2014) that the competent communicator thinks critically and mindfully, and is also culturally sensitive and ethical. Views from the sampled *cultural respondents* of the three (3) Fante communities indicate how every "well-bred" Fante prefers to communicate in that particular way – not mentioning the names of the human genitals – when communicating on matters of sexuality; thus, emphasising competence with regard to rules of language, competence with regard to social skills and competence with regard to socio-emotional requirements which include norm-bound rituals and routines, and verbal acts, among others. Note, for example, the view expressed by *Nana* and indicating that the person who goes so "open" in mentioning these names is considered to have polluted themselves rather, which implies that such a person is not "on top" of their cultural values; and put mildly therefore, is considered a "stranger" in their own homeland. Findings in this study also bring to the fore and reinforce Dilbeck's (2008) observation about the rhetorical sensitivity theory and the competent communicator model. According to Dilbeck, the two – theory and model –appear to portray two sides of the same coin; implying that an observed phenomenon can be interpreted from any or both perspectives of the two frameworks. In this connection, whereas the rhetorically sensitive person might be said to be more concerned about the requirements of his or her speech community – whether or not the communicator exhibits the attitude of a noble self or rhetorical reflector, the competent communicator is considered as being concerned about the communicative skills of the given language, namely their control or command over the language. The study revealed that not only are members concerned about communicating according to the cultural dictates of their (Fante) community, but also concerned about being seen as possessing the skills for communicating proficiently in the Fante language. For example, to the extent that the people find appropriate descriptors – metaphors, terminologies, other expressions, among others to convey their messages to the understanding of their audiences underscores their level of competency in the use of their mother tongue. Perhaps buttressing this point is the apparent crowding out effect of this communicative pattern on medical practitioners themselves who, presumably overwhelmed by the adeptness of their clients' way of speaking, also do the same when communicating with them – their clients.

CONCLUSION

The study sought to investigate why the Akan, in general, and Fante in particular, find it difficult to mention or call the human genitalia by their real names; and whether there is any relationship between the non-mentioning of the human genital organs and the concepts morality, profanity, and culture. It also sought to investigate how this communicative pattern – non-mentioning of human genitalia by their real names – affects the Fante people's reproductive health reporting.

Findings showed that the peculiar communicative pattern of the Fante has socio-religious connotations, namely cultural reasons which are firmly rooted in the people's religious philosophy. The Fante believe that the reproductive systems of human beings were created by Onyame for the purposes of procreation – an act which is considered sacred – and for which reason any concepts and related phenomena, by extension become sacred and therefore respected. This idea corroborates the views of Lawler, Wuerl, and Lawler (1996) on the divine origin and sacredness of human sexuality and its purposes. Lawler, et al. note, "the Genesis account of human origins, with much subsequent revelation, proclaims the divine origin and sacredness of human sexuality and its purposes…," (1996, p.72). Respondents do not seem to see any linkage between their communicative pattern on sexuality and the concept morality. They however consider the way they structure their communication on sexuality as influenced by the dual concepts of sacredness and profanity which concepts are rooted in the Fante culture. The study is inclined to consider – though cautiously –that such understanding is rather out of the ordinary given the definitions and meaning of morality, especially as provided for by Wiredu (1992) and Gyekye (1996) and earlier discussed in this paper. Medical Respondents are also unanimous in their view that the difficulty in calling the human genitals by their real names in Fante communities affects their reproductive health reporting. They (Medical Practitioners) were however divided in their opinion on whether or not this communicative pattern affected the quality of care they – Practitioners – dispensed. While some said that they perfectly understood patients' complaints in spite of their peculiar communicative pattern on sexuality, others thought the communicative pattern of patients unduly constrained clear understanding, and therefore engendered a 'trial and error' diagnosis and treatment. This latter category of practitioners laments the associated incidence of social and economic costs of this phenomenon – non-mentioning of human genitalia by real names in Fante culture – which go a long way to affect the human and financial capital of the state. The study also brings to the fore how the typical Fante, always cautious of their cultural demands, structures their communication messages in communication relationships – especially in matters of sexuality – to suit their various audiences; and therefore, by so doing, is considered skillful and adept in their mother tongue. Thus, generally, the study reinforces the twin frameworks of rhetorical sensitivity theory and the competent communicator model as espoused by Hart and Burks (1975) and also reviewed in later scholarly articles by DeVito (2014) and Dilbeck (2008).

REFERENCES

Anane, A. A. (2015). *Doctor-Patient Communication in the Consulting Room: A Study of Two University Health Facilities in Ghana* (Master of Philosophy Thesis, University of Education, Winneba)

Anderson, G. J. (2015). Children, Morality and Abusive Words: The Ghanaian Perspectives. *Humanities and Social Sciences Letters*, *3*(2), 87–93. doi:10.18488/journal.73/2015.3.2/73.2.87.93

Asante, E. (1995). *Towards an African Christian Theology of the Kingdom of God: The Kingship of Onyame*. Mellen University Press.

Bernard, H. R. (2002). *Research Methods in Anthropology: Qualitative and Quantitative Methods* (3rd ed.). Alta Mira Press.

Crayner, J. B. (2007). *Borbor Kunkumfi: History of the Migration of the Fantes to their Present Homes* (2nd ed.). Bureau of Ghana Languages.

Creswell, J. W., & Creswell, J. D. (2023). *Research Design: Qualitative, Quantitative, and Mixed Methods Approaches* (6th ed.). Sage Publications Inc.

Daymon, C., & Holloway, I. (2011). Choosing Between Different Types of Research. *Qualitative Research Methods in Public Relations and Marketing Communication*, *2*, 99–113.

Dilbeck, K. E. (2008). *Rhetorical Sensitivity and Communication Competence: A Test for Convergent Validity* (Doctoral Dissertation, Bangkok University).

Fynn, J. K. (1987). The Political System of the Fante of Ghana during the Pre-Colonial Period. *Universitas*, *9*(1), 108–120.

Gert, B., & Gert, J. (2020). The Definition of Morality. *The Stanford Encyclopedia of Philosophy*. https://plato.stanford.edu/archives/fall2020/entries

Glesne, C. (2016). *Becoming Qualitative Researchers: An Introduction* (5th ed.). Pearson.

Gyekye, K. (1996). *African Cultural Values: An Introduction*. Sankofa Publishing Corp.

Hart, R. P., & Burks, D. M. (1972). Rhetorical Sensitivity and Social Interaction. *Speech Monographs*, *39*(2), 75–91. doi:10.1080/03637757209375742

Hennigh, L. (1970). Functions and Limitions of Alaskan Eskimo Wife Trading. *Open Journal Systems*, *23*(1), 24–34. doi:10.14430/arctic3151

Hymes, D. (1970). Linguistic Method of Ethnography. In P. Garvin (Ed.), *Method and Theory in Linguistics*. Mouton. www.academia.edu/16312703/

Kissi, S., & van Eck, E. (2017). Reading Hebrews through Akan Ethnicity and Social Identity. *Hervormde Teologiese Studies*, *73*(3), a4490. doi:10.4102/hts.v73i3.4490

Lindsey, L. L., & Beach, S. (2002). *Sociology* (2nd ed.). Prentice Hall.

Littlejohn, S. W., Foss, K. A., & Oetzel, J. G. (2017). *Theories of Human Communication* (11th ed.). Waveland Press Incorp.

Macleod, A., & McCabe, M. P. (2020). Defining Sexuality in Later Life: A Systematic Review. *Australasian Journal on Ageing*, *39*(S1), 6–15. doi:10.1111/ajag.12741 PMID:32567178

Malinowski, B. (1947). *Freedom and Civilisation*. George Allen.

Markus, H. R., & Kitayama, S. (2010). Cultures and selves: A cycle of mutual constitution. *Perspectives on Psychological Science*, *5*(4), 420–430. doi:10.1177/1745691610375557 PMID:26162188

Mbiti, J. S. (1975). *The Prayers of African Religion*. SPCK.

Merriam, S. B., & Tsdell, E. J. (2016). Qualitative Research: A Guide to Design and Implementation (4th ed.). Jossy Bass.

Norton, R. (1983). *Communicator Style: Theory, Applications, and Measures*. Sage publications.

Ofosuhene, M. (1993). *Women Traders as Heads of Households in Larteh Akwapim* (Thesis, University of Ghana).

Ogbujah, C. (2017). Ideals and Values: Pivots to Meaningful Intercultural Dialogue. *Dialogue and Universalism*, *1*(1), 67–81. doi:10.5840/du20172717

Rosenfield, L. W., Hayes, L. S., & Frentz, T. S. (1976). *The Communicative Experience*. Allyn and Baycon.

Rubel, P. G. (1978). *Your own pigs you may not eat: A comparative study of New Guinea societies.* Australian National University Press.

Shaw, S. M., & Lee, J. (2018). *Gendered Voices, Feminist Visions: Classic and Contemporary Readings* (8th ed.). Oxford University Press.

Tongco, M. D. C. (2007). Purposive Sampling as a Tool for Informant Selection. *Ethnobotany Research and Applications*, *5*, 147–158. doi:10.17348/era.5.0.147-158

Wieman, J. M. (1975). *An Exploration of Communicative Competence in Initial Interaction: An Experimental Study*. Purdue University.

Wiredu, K. (1992). *Person and Community: Ghanaian Philosophical Studies* (Vol. 1). CRVP.

Yin, R. K. (2018). *Case Study Research and Applications: Designs and Methods* (6th ed.). Sage Publications Incorp.

ENDNOTE

1 ERIC: Education Resources Information Center – of the US Department of Education

Chapter 12
Audience Perception of COVID-19 Vaccination and Its Effect on the Behavioural Responses of Respondents in Oyo West Local Government

Adenike Omotayo Okeya-Olayinka
Ajayi Crowther University, Oyo, Nigeria

ABSTRACT

The COVID-19 disease presents an imminent danger that requires immediate action as it could be deadly. Vaccines against COVID-19 are considered to be of great importance to prevent and also to control, but there are challenges, one of which is uncertainty about public acceptance of the vaccine. The study looked at audience perception of COVID-19 vaccination and its effect on the behavioural responses of respondents in Oyo West Local Government. The study was anchored on the perception theory and the behaviour theory. The multistage probability sampling technique was adopted. The study found out that the COVID-19 vaccination awareness was not enough, thereby making the social media to have the upper hand by passing false rumours about the vaccine in order to get the people discouraged thereby leading to their non-challan behaviour and superstitious beliefs. The study concluded that the masses should be educated on the need to get vaccinated and therefore recommended that there should be more awareness on the COVID-19 vaccination to prevent future infections and deaths.

INTRODUCTION

The world woke up to the report of a novel viral infection, coronavirus (Covid-19), in December 2019 with its first case reported in China's Wuhan territory. The upper respiratory tract virus has since been called a global pandemic after cases were recorded in most continents (Kolawole, 2020). Corona virus also known as Covid-19 is a severe acute respiratory disease that is known to have symptoms such as

DOI: 10.4018/979-8-3693-0624-6.ch012

pneumonia, fever, breathing difficulty and lung infection. The World Health Organization (WHO) used the term 2019 novel coronavirus to refer to a coronavirus that affected the lower respiratory tract of patients with pneumonia in Wuhan, China on 29 December 2019. The WHO announced that the official name of the 2019 novel coronavirus is coronavirus disease (Covid-19). The coronavirus belongs to a family of viruses that may cause various symptoms such as pneumonia, fever, breathing difficulty, and lung. According to Anho and Muoboghare (2021) in Nigeria, the index case was recorded on the 27th February, 2020, when an Italian citizen in Lagos tested positive for the virus while the second case involves a Nigerian citizen who had contact with the Italian citizen was reported in Ewekoro, Ogun State on the 9th March 2020. Researchers noted that in a bid to control the spread of Covid-19 in Nigeria, there was immediate prohibition of social gathering and religious activities and lockdown of the major epicenters of Lagos, Ogun and Abuja and this was later followed by a total lockdown, which lasted for almost two months in the first phase before gradual easing in subsequent phases. Newman (2020) avers that the pandemic has played a significant role in shaping human history throughout the ages by giving the examples of the Antonine plague (165-180AD), the Black death (1346-1353), the Spanish flu (1918-1920), the Asian flu (1956-1958), the HIV (1981-present), the Ebola (2014) among others.

The covid-19 was declared a pandemic by the World Health Organisation on 11th March, 2020. According to worldometers, (2021) in Ajayi, Fatukasi and Asemah (2021) since it broke out, the virus is said to have accounted for about 4,181,853 deaths globally out of a swooping statistics of 195,275,961 positive cases which sadly increases daily. In order to curtail the rate at which people were dying from the disease, it became necessary for vaccines to be created to control the spread of the virus and mitigate the impact of the pandemic on public health systems all over the country.

Scholars have explained that vaccines are an essential tool for stemming the spread of pandemics like Covid-19, influenza, and other infectious diseases while Bhartiya, Kumar, Singh, Murugan, and Wadhwani (2021), revealed that there were approximately one hundred competitors running for the position of delivering the Covid-19 vaccine, stating further that the Covid-19 vaccine was introduced into the market just nine months after the virus was identified. Several Covid-19 vaccines have been given the go-ahead to be used, and their distribution is currently being expanded across the globe. According to Rodrigues, (2020), when a person is immunized against a disease, the body's immune system is prompted to begin developing defenses against that illness. The Immunization Action Coalition (2021) on March 2, 2021, records theworld'sfirst vaccine that can act against the virus. This occurred at the same time that the Centers for Disease Control and Prevention (CDC) published an interim recommendation for the utilisation of the Jassen (Johnson and Johnson) Covid-19 vaccine. This was the first vaccine developed to combat the Covid-19 virus. Following this, the staff at the Mayo Clinic (2021) report that a number of vaccines were eventually granted permission to be used in a variety of countries. Vaccines such as mRNA, Vector, and Protein subunit that were developed by Moderna, Astra Zeneca, and Novavax filled the market. But the issue now is the perception of the people towards the vaccine as majority of the population have not deemed it fit to collect based on their perception of the vaccine and this has actually affected their behavioural responses to the vaccine.

STATEMENT OF THE PROBLEM

Scientists all over the world have been motivated to collaborate, share data, and reach some level of compromise in order to find a cure for Covid-19 by providing a vaccine for that purpose. Scholars have noted that Vaccines are one of the most reliable and cost-effective public health interventions ever implemented that are saving millions of lives each year while research indicated that eleven (11) vaccines were approved by the World Health Oganisation (WHO) in December 2022, with Nigeria receiving approval for seven of those vaccines. Schoch-Spana, Brunson, Long, Ruth, Ravi, and Trotochaud (2021) noted that despite the approval of these vaccines, there have been news about misinformation and anti-vaccine sentiments. Also, there are numerous conspiracy theories surrounding the Covid-19 virus that have been carefully designed which has led to the perception of the people concerning the vaccine, thereby affecting their behaviourial responses to the vaccine.

OBJECTIVES OF THE STUDY

1) To find out the level of exposure of respondents of Oyo West Local Government to Covid-19 vaccination.
2) To examine the perception of Oyo West Local Government residents on Covid-19 vaccination.
3) To determine the extent, of the audience perception of Covid-19vaccination on the behavioural responses of respondents.

THEORETICAL FRAMEWORK

This study is anchored on the perception theory. The theory states that mass communicators want audiences to pay attention to their messages, learn the contents of the messages and make appropriate changes in attitudes or beliefs or produce the desired behavioural responses (Anaeto, 2012). The theory further tells us that the process of interpreting messages is complex and that those goals may be difficult to achieve. The theory is relevant to the study in that perception of the audience on covid-19 vaccination has an effect on their behavioural responses whether to get vaccinated or not.

AUDIENCE PERCEPTION OF COVID-19 VACCINATION AND BEHAVIORAL RESPONSES

The efficacy of the Covid-19 vaccines in preventing the spread of the disease has been established by research (Dinleyici et al., 2020, Munoz et al., 2021). When the vaccine becomes available, the success in preventing the spread of disease will depend on public acceptance of the vaccine (Karlsson et al., 2021). Consequently, numerous studies have been conducted to understand audience perception and behavioral responses to Covid-19 vaccination. Scholars have noted that since the emergence of Covid-19 in Wuhan, China, in December 2019 the disease has been declared a global pandemic and has been associated with the deaths of more than 2.3 million people around the world. Thereby making it to be a dynamic and evolving pandemic. Research has also indicated that the first case in Africa was reported in Egypt on 14 February 2020 and cases have since been reported in all 55 African Union Member States. In addition, Africa faced a second wave, of which Nigeria is one with far more reported cases and deaths than in the early months of the global pandemic. In addition, new virus variants have emerged. Research has also indicated a scarcity of covid-19 vaccines in Africa while according to Adane, Ademas and Kloos (2022), several African countries have discarded large numbers of vaccines doses that expired before they were used due to low demand in the population. They also noted that the low accessibility of covid-19 vaccines and hesitancy to be vaccinated for covid-19, a preference for traditional medicines may constitute another barrier to vaccine acceptance in African countries.

Willingness to receive a Covid-19 vaccine is a challenge in many countries (WHO, 2020) Covid-19 vaccine acceptance rates in the general population were highest in Vietnam (98%), India (91%), China (91%), Denmark (87%), and South Korea (87%) and lowest in Serbia (38%), Croatia (41%), France (44%), Lebanon (44%), and Paraguay (51%) (Wouters, Shadlen, Salcher-Konrad, Pollard, Larson & Teerawattananon (2021). Scholars have noted that negative attitude and mistrust towards covid-19 vaccines are major barriers to increasing vaccine coverage worldwide. According to African News, majority of respondents do not believe in the vaccine as they think that the virus is a sign of God's wrath upon the country while another set of respondents were of the opinion that prayers can solve the problem. Winning the battle against covid-19 requires a significant number of Nigerians to get vaccinated. Scholars have noted that three out of every ten Nigerians still remain unvaccinated with a significant portion of them indicating that they want to "wait and see" what happens after. The fact that covid-19 vaccines have gone through an unusually rapid development process sparked many fears over vaccine safety (Bunch 2021, Chou & Budenz, 2020). These fears are further coupled with anger, sadness and disgust (Wang, Luo, Zhang, Huang & Yan (2021) which are likely fuelled by controversies and disagreements over vaccines between polarized groups.

EMPIRICAL REVIEW

Anho and Muoboghare (2021) in the study titled Newspaper Coverage of Coronavirus Disease (Covid-19) in Nigeria examined media coverage of Covid-19 in Nigeria with a focus on the frequency of coverage, prominence given to the issue, story format, news sources and media tone. The study employed the content analysis method where three newspapers (Guardian, Vanguard and Punch) were content analyzed. Results revealed that the newspapers gave much attention to Covid-19 reportage but did not give much importance to Covid-19 in terms of story placement and space allotment. The study concluded that the newspapers predominantly used straight news reports without pictures to provide information about the pandemic and recommended that pictures should be considered in telling stories for better understanding and media organizations should utilize them more in their reportage of covid-19 in ways that would facilitate believability of the situation.

Onyebuchi, Onwubiko, Anukam and Nwosu (2021). In the study titled influence of radio messages on adoption of covid-19 preventive measures among residents of Owerri Municipality using Hot FM. The researchers examined the impact of radio messages on adoption of covid-19 preventive measures, using residence of Owerri Municipality as a focus. A cross sectional survey research method was adopted for the study. The study was restricted to Hot FM Owerri, its messages through news, jingles and other public enlightenment programmes during the pandemic outbreak in 2019. The researchers adopted agenda setting theory. A sample of 360 residents of Owerri Municipality was used for the study. The simple random sampling technique was used to select respondents for the study. The findings showed that the level of radio listenership in Owerri Municipality was high. It also found out that the messages to a large extent helpfully influenced the adoption of covid-19 preventive measures among residents of Owerri Municipality using Hot FM. The study recommended that radio stations, private and /or state owned, should be proactive and involved in ensuring that the masses are properly and timely updated on pivotal societal issues, especially on health risk situations.

Onwukwe, Onyebuchi, chikwe and Ihekwoaba (2021) in the study titled Owerri residents's perception of the transmission of information via social media during covid-19. The study sought to examine the perception of Imo residents's perception of social media information dissemination amidst covid-19 pandemic era. The technological determinism theory was adopted as the theoretical framework for the study. The survey research design was employed. The Wimmer and Dominick sample size calculator was used to derive 384 as the sample size while the questionnaire was used as the instrument for data collection and the multistage sampling technique was adopted for the study. Findings revealed that at an average of 5% respondents confirmed that to a large extent, social media information and dissemination on covid-19 influenced Imo residents'behaviour towards practicing covid-19 guidelines. The study recommended that, the campaigns on safe practices on covid-19 guidelines should be sustained on the social media where everyone has access, so as to help curtail the spread of the deadly virus.

Cajetan, Jumbo and Etumnu (2021) in the study titled influence of Covid-19 broadcast media campaigns on the health consciousness of Owerri residents. Perception and agenda setting theories served as the theoretical underpin of the study. The researchers employed the survey method. From the population of 555,500 of Owerri urban residents, 384 sample was derived using survey monkey online sample size calculator. The multistage sampling technique was used and questionnaire as instrument for data collection. Findings revealed that an average of 85% the Imo state residents to a large extent are exposed to broadcast media campaigns on covid-19 as it relates to their health. Further findings, indicated that at an average mean of 3.0(N=370) respondents are of the view that broadcast media campaigns on covid-19 have caused a lot of panic, though, through the media campaigns on covid-19 they are made to believe that unhealthy exposure to infected persons they can contract it. It was recommended that given, that large percentage 85% of respondents are exposed to broadcast media campaigns on covid-19, the channel of communication could be a veritable platform where authorities can leverage on in educating the masses on covid-19 and other health issues.

METHODOLOGY

This study employed the descriptive survey design. Residents of Oyo West Local Government, Oyo made up the population of the study. According to Oyo State government in 2017, the population of Oyo West Local Government is 856,988. The local government was chosen because of its bustling and economy activities. A sample size of 400 as derived from Taro Yamane formular. The respondents were reached through the simple random probability sampling method. This method was used to give equal opportunity to all the respondents. Questionnaire was used to collect data from the respondents. The questionnaire contained both close and open ended questions and was administered with the aid of two research assistant. Data gathered from the questionnaire was analyzed quantitatively. Frequency tables was used to present measurements using a five-point scale of which the criterion mean/mean cut off point was 3.00

Table 1. Level of exposure to COVID-19 vaccination

Option	Frequency	Percentage %
High	95	25
Moderate	55	14
Low	225	58
Can't say	10	3
Total	**385**	**100**

DATA PRESENTATION

A total of 400 copies of questionnaire were administered to respondents in Oyo West Local Government, Ibadan, Oyo State but only 385 copies which represent (96%) were retrieved and found usable for the study. The demographic information shows that the majority of the respondents were aged between twenty-two and fifty-five years old, single, male and had at least primary school certificate.

Research Question One: What is the Level of Exposure of Respondents of Oyo West Local Government to Covid-19 Vaccination?

Analysis of data from the above table 1 revealed that 58% of the respondent have low level of exposure to covid-19vaccination. This implies that majority of the respondents level of exposure to the covid-19 vaccine is low.

Research Question Two: What is the Perception of Oyo West Local Government Residents on Covid-19 Vaccination?

Analysis of data from the table above revealed that majority of the respondents have the perception that the vaccine will make them fall sick hence the reason why they are not interested in taking them. In addition, majority of the respondents do not believe that the vaccine works while some are also of the opinion that the vaccine is creating fear in them as a result of the news on social media. This implies that the perception of respondents on covid-19 vaccination is negative.

Table 2. Responses on the perception of Oyo west local government residents on COVID-19 vaccination

Variables	SA	A	D	SD	N
The covid-19 vaccine will make me fall sick hence the reason, why I do not want to take it	255 (66%)	105 (27%)	15 (4%)	10 (3%)	385 (100)
I do not believe in the covid-19 vaccine that it works as a result of what I read on social media	240 (62%)	125 (33%)	15 (4%)	5 (1%)	385 (100)
I know that the covid-19 vaccine is effective	10 (3%)	15 (4%)	255 (66%)	105 (27%)	385 (100)
Covid-19 vaccine is creating fear in me as a result of what I read on the social media	255 (66%)	105 (27%)	15 (4%)	10 (3%)	385 (100)

Table 3. Responses on the extent of the audience perception of COVID-19 vaccination on the behavioural responses of respondents

Option	Frequency	Percentage %
Large extent	235	61
Moderate Extent	85	22
Low Extent	65	17
Not at all	-	-
Total	**385**	**100**

Research Question Three: To what extent is the audience perception of Covid-19vaccination on the behavioural responses of respondents?

Analysing findings of data, it was revealed that 61% of respondent's perception of covid-19 vaccination has an effect on their behavioural responses to a large extent. By implication, majority of the respondents are of the opinion that the covid-19 vaccination has an effect on their behavioural responses to a large extent.

DISCUSSION OF FINDINGS

The findings revealed that majority of the respondents have low level of exposure to the covid-19 vaccination. Based on the data obtained, it was discovered that the level of exposure to the covid-19 vaccine was very low. The findings collaborates with Adane, Ademas and Kloss (2022) who noted that willingness to be vaccinated depends to a large extent on factors beyond the availability of vaccine. Stating further that Low rates may be due to earlier study dates (when prospects of the vaccine rollout were uncertain), limited knowledge about vaccines, lack of trust in government management capacity, and concerns about vaccine safety. This findings also corroborate previous literature showing greater hesitancy among those reporting concerns about vaccine safety and efficacy, low trust in government and the perception that covid-19 is a low risk which might have actually affected the level of exposure. This findings also resonates well with that of Lazarus et al (2022) whose findings revealed that frequent exposure to misinformation increases vaccine hesitancy. Stating further that, misrepresentation of covid-19 vaccine on social media most commonly include misinformation about the medical/health benefits, false content about vaccine development and conspiracy theories. Scholars have also indicated that misrepresentation can derail progress in covid-19 vaccination coverage, particularly if audience choose not to seek covid-19 information from official sources such as World Health Organization and so on.

The data analyzed revealed that majority of the respondents have the perception that the vaccine will make them fall sick hence the reason why they are not interested in taking it. This findings corroborates with Adane, Ademas and Kloss (2022) in there study, they noted that high rates of not intending to be vaccinated when vaccines become available were associated with negative attitude and low perception about Covid-19 vaccine. The low acceptance level of Covid-19 vaccines among the people can be attributed to multi factors, some of which are shared with the wide global community and there is an evident uncertainty clouding the Covid-19 vaccines (Elimat, Abuaisamen, Almomani, Al-sawalha & Alali 2021).

Studies from Rahman, Chisty,Alam,Sakib,Quader,Shobuj (2022) found that positive knowledge and attitude may reflect vaccination hesitancy among people if they have negative knowledge, perception and attitudes. The result of this data is similar to findings from studies in the United States (Islam, Siddique, Akter, Tasnim, Sujan,& Ward 2021 ; Bari,Hossain, Ahmed, Sarker, Khandokar, Charity 2021). In a study conducted in China, more than half of the respondents said they are worried about the vaccine's side effects and would delay the Covid-19 vaccination until the vaccine's safety is confirmed (Zhou, Tian, Zhao, Li, & Yang (2021), reflecting their uncertainty regarding vaccine safety, even though they believe it´s important to stop the pandemic. This may be related to misleading information spread through the media and social media that encourages vaccine resistance and rejection.

Analysis of findings further revealed that majority of the respondent's perception of covid-19 vaccination has an effect on their behavioural responses to a large extent. By implication, majority of the respondents are of the opinion that covid-19 vaccination has an effect on their behavioural responses to a very large extent. This findings corroborates with Adane et al (2022) who noted that negative attitudes and poor perception towards the anticipated covid-19 vaccination were significant factors to refuse to be vaccinated. Further saying that management authorities and stakeholders should promote and improve attitudes, knowledge and perception towards covid-19 vaccination.

CONCLUSION AND RECOMMENDATION

This study revealed low level of exposure to covid-19 vaccination in Oyo West Local Government. It also revealed negative perception of the vaccine and because of this, there was an effect on their behavioural responses to the vaccine. In addition, the masses should be educated on the need to get vaccinated so as to change their perception and behavior. The study therefore recommends that there should be more awareness to change people's perception about the covid-19 vaccine in other to prevent future infections and deaths.

REFERENCES

Adane, M., Ademas, A., & Kloos, H. (2022). Knowledge, attitudes, and perceptions of COVID-19 vaccine and refusal to receive COVID-19 vaccine among healthcare workers in northeaster Ethiopia. *BMC Public Health*, *22*(1), 128. doi:10.1186/s12889-021-12362-8 PMID:35042476

Adejumo, O. A., Ogundele, O. A., Madubuko, C. R., Oluwafemi, R. O., Okoye, O. C., Okonkwo, K. C., Owolade, S. S., Junaid, O. A., Lawal, O. M., Enikuomehin, A. C., Ntaji, M. I., Sokunbi, A., Timothy, A. O., Abolarin, O. S., Ali, E. O., & Ohaju-Obodo, J. O. (2021). Perceptions of the COVID-19 vaccine and willingness to receive vaccination among health workers in Nigeria. *Osong Public Health and Research Perspectives*, *12*(4), 236–243. doi:10.24171/j.phrp.2021.0023 PMID:34289295

Africanews (2021). Ethiopia launches Covid vaccination in Addis Ababa. Available from: https://www.africanews.com/2021/03/14/ethiopia-launches-covid-vaccinations-in-addis-ababa

Ajayi, J.O, Fatukasi, O & Asemah, E. S (2021). Utilisation of WhatsApp for Communicating Covid-19 Messages in Akure, Ondo State. SAU Journal of Management and Social Science, 6(2).

Anaeto, S. Onabanjo, O. & Osifeso .J. (2012*) Models and theories of communication*. United State of America. Africa Renaissance Books Incorporated, Anho, E. J & Muoboghare, N (2021). Newspaper Coverage of Coronavirus Disease (Covid-19) SAU Journal of Management and Social Science, 6(2).

Bari, M. S., Hossain, M. J., Ahmmed, F., Sarker, M. M. R., Khandokar, L., Chaithy, A. P., Aziz, F., Mitra, S., Emran, T. B., Islam, M. S., Islam, M. R., & Mohamed, I. N. (2021). Knowledge, Perception, and Willingness towards Immunization among Bangladeshi Population during COVID-19 Vaccine Rolling Period. *Vaccines*, *9*(12), 1449. doi:10.3390/vaccines9121449 PMID:34960195

Bhartiya, S., Kumar, N., Singh, T., Murugan, S., Rajavel, S., & Wadhwani, M. (2021). Knowledge, attitude and practice towards COVID-19 vaccination acceptance in West India. *International Journal of Community Medicine and Public Health*, *8*(3), 1170. doi:10.18203/2394-6040.ijcmph20210481

Biswas, N., Mustapha, T., Khubchandani, J., & Price, J. H. (2021). The nature and extent of COVID-19 vaccination hesitancy in healthcare workers. J Community Health. https://www.ncbi.nlm.nih.gov/pubmed/33877534

Bunch, L. A. (2021). Tale of two crises: Addressing Covid-19 vaccine hesitancy as promoting racial justice. *HEC Forum*, *33*(1-2), 143–154. doi:10.1007/s10730-021-09440-0 PMID:33464452

Cajetan, I. O., Jumbo, C. N., & Etumnu, W. E. (2021). Influence of Covid-19 Broadcast Media Campaigns on the Health Consciousness of Owerri Residents. SAU Journal of Management and Social Science, 6(2).

Callaghan, T., Moghtaderi, A., Lueck, J. A., Hotez, P., Strych, U., Dor, A., Fowler, E. F., & Motta, M. (2021, March). Correlates and disparities of intention to vaccinate against COVID-19. *Social Science & Medicine*, *272*, 113638. doi:10.1016/j.socscimed.2020.113638 PMID:33414032

Chou, A. B., & Budenz, A. (2020). Considering emotion in COVID-19 vaccine communication: Addressing vaccine hesitancy and fostering vaccine confidence. *Health Communication*, *35*(14), 1718–1722. doi:10.1080/10410236.2020.1838096 PMID:33124475

Dinleyici, E. C., Borrow, R., Safadi, M. A. P., van Damme, P., & Munoz, F. M. (2020). Vaccines and routine immunization strategies during the COVID-19 pandemic. *Human Vaccines & Immunotherapeutics*, *17*(2), 400–407. doi:10.1080/21645515.2020.1804776 PMID:32845739

Ehreth, J. (2003). The value of vaccination: A global perspective. *Vaccine*, *21*(27), 4105–4117. doi:10.1016/S0264-410X(03)00377-3 PMID:14505886

Hajj Hussein, I., Chams, N., Chams, S., El Sayegh, S., Badran, R., Raad, M., Gerges-Geagea, A., Leone, A., & Jurjus, A. (2015). Vaccines Through Centuries: Major Cornerstones of Global Health. *Frontiers in Public Health*, *3*, 269. doi:10.3389/fpubh.2015.00269 PMID:26636066

Hu, S., Wang, S., Luo, W., Zhang, M., Huang, X., Yan, Y., Liu, R., Ly, K., Kacker, V., She, B., & Li, Z. (2021). Wang, W. Luo, M. Zhang, X. Huang, Y. Yan (2021).Revealing public opinion towards COVID-19 vaccines with Twitter data in the United States: Spatiotemporal perspectiveJ Med. *Internet Research*, *23*(9), e30854. doi:10.2196/30854 PMID:34346888

Islam, M. S., Kamal, A.-H. M., Kabir, A., Southern, D. L., Khan, S. H., Hasan, S. M. M., Sarkar, T., Sharmin, S., Das, S., Roy, T., Harun, M. G. D., Chughtai, A. A., Homaira, N., & Seale, H. (2021, May 12). COVID-19 vaccine rumors and conspiracy theories: The need for cognitive inoculation against misinformation to improve vaccine adherence. *PLoS One*, *16*(5), e0251605. doi:10.1371/journal.pone.0251605 PMID:33979412

Islam Md, S., Siddique, A. B., Akter, R., Tasnim, R., Sujan Md, S. H., & Ward, P. R. (2021). Knowledge, attitudes and perceptions towards COVID-19 vaccinations: A cross-sectional community survey in Bangladesh. *BMC Public Health*, *21*(1), 1851. doi:10.1186/s12889-021-11880-9 PMID:34645399

Karlsson, L. C., Soveri, A., Lewandowsky, S., Karlsson, L., Karlsson, H., Nolvi, S., Karukivi, M., Lindfelt, M., & Antfolk, J. (2021). Fearing the disease or the vaccine: The case of COVID-19. *Personality and Individual Differences*, *2021*, 172. doi:10.1016/j.paid.2020.110590 PMID:33518869

Kolawole, O (2015) Social distancing and the coronavirus outbreak in Nigeria: what's the bigger picture? Techpoint Africa Newsletter.

Lyu, J. C., Le Han, E., & Luli, G. K. (2021). COVID-19 vaccine-related discussion on Twitter: Topic modeling and sentiment analysis. *Journal of Medical Internet Research*, *23*(6), e24435. doi:10.2196/24435 PMID:34115608

Onwukwe, A. C, Onyebuchi, A. C, Chikwe, U. O & Ihekwoaba, U. P (2021). Owerri Residents Perception of the Transmission of Information via Social Media during covid-19. SAU Journal of Management and Social Science, 6(2).

Onyebuchi, A. C, Onyebuchi, A. C Chikwe, U. O & Ihekwoaba, U. P (2021). Influence of Radio Messages on Adoption of Covid-19 Preventive Measures among Residents of Owerri Municipality using Hot FM. SAU Journal of Management and Social Science, 6(2).

Rahman, M. M, Chisty, M. A, Alam A, Sakib, M. A, Quader, M. A, Shobuj, I. A, Abdul Halim, M., & Rahman, F (2022). Knowledge, attitude, and hesitancy towards COVID-19 vaccine among university students of Bangladesh PLUS ONE Collection Psychology. doi:10.1371/journal.pone.0270684

Rodrigues, C. M. C., & Plotkin, S. A. (2020). Impact of Vaccines; Health, Economic and Social Perspectives. *Frontiers in Microbiology*, *11*, 1526. doi:10.3389/fmicb.2020.01526 PMID:32760367

Schoch-Spana, M., Brunson, E. K., Long, R., Ruth, A., Ravi, S. J., Trotochaud, M., Borio, L., Brewer, J., Buccina, J., Connell, N., Hall, L. L., Kass, N., Kirkland, A., Koonin, L., Larson, H., Lu, B. F., Omer, S. B., Orenstein, W. A., Poland, G. A., ... White, A. (2021). The public's role in COVID-19 vaccination: Human-centered recommendations to enhance pandemic vaccine awareness, access, and acceptance in the United States. *Vaccine*, *39*(40), 6004–6012. doi:10.1016/j.vaccine.2020.10.059 PMID:33160755

Tobin, E. A., Okonofua, M., & Azeke, A. (2021). Acceptance of a COVID-19 Vaccine in Nigeria: A Population-Based Cross-Sectional Study. *Annals of Medical and Health Sciences Research*, *11*(5).

WHO. (2020). WHO issues its first emergency use validation for a COVID-19 vaccine and emphasizes need for equitable global access. Available from: https://www.who.int/news/item

World Health Organization. (n.d.). WHO Coronavirus (COVID-19) Dashboard. Available online: https://covid19.who.int/

Wouters, O. J., Shadlen, K. C., Salcher-Konrad, M., Pollard, A. J., Larson, H. J., Teerawattananon, Y., & Jit, M. (2021). Challenges in ensuring global access to COVID-19 vaccines: Production, affordability, allocation, and deployment. *Lancet*, *397*(10278), 1023–1034. doi:10.1016/S0140-6736(21)00306-8 PMID:33587887

Zhou, Q., Tian, T., Ni, J., Zhao, X., Li, H., Yang, Y., Zhang, Y., & Pan, J. (2021, November 25). COVID-19 Vaccination Acceptance in China after It Becomes Available: A Cross-Sectional Study. *Vaccines*, *9*(12), 1398. doi:10.3390/vaccines9121398 PMID:34960144

Chapter 13
COVID-19 Messages and High Risk Areas:
Interrogating the Role of Radio in Disseminating Health Information to Refugee Camps in Zimbabwe

Jennings Joy Chibike
Lupane State University, Zimbabwe

Samuel Anesu Muzhingi
https://orcid.org/0000-0003-0138-5080
Daystar University, Kenya

ABSTRACT

This chapter examines the views and perspectives of journalists on the role played by Radio Zimbabwe in informing refugee residents at Tongogara Refugees Camp in Zimbabwe about COVID-19. Also, the chapter examines their views and perspectives on the potential of Radio Zimbabwe and its COVID-19 message in creating a sense of belonging for the refugees. Its theoretical toolkit is drawn from the social responsibility theory and public sphere theory. Empirical data were drawn from in-depth interviews with 12 purposively selected radio journalists from Zimbabwe. The chapter established that Radio Zimbabwe's jingles, news, and announcements on COVID-19 were not directed at refugees; thus, it was argued that the radio station did not adequately inform refugees residing at Tongogara Refugee Camp. Also, the chapter fleshes out Radio Zimbabwe's mediation of COVID-19 failed to fan a sense of belonging in refugees. Instead, the way Radio Zimbabwe handled COVID-19 strengthened the minority and marginalised identity in Zimbabwe.

DOI: 10.4018/979-8-3693-0624-6.ch013

INTRODUCTION

Refugees make up the world's most vulnerable people (Vonen et al., 2021: 27). Their vulnerability stems from the socio-political and environmental quandaries ranging from wars, genocides, climate change, dilapidating economies in their original countries among other things. Due to these consequences, they migrate to other countries where they are placed in refugee camps which are meant to temporality house them. However, in some instances, refugees have stayed in these overcrowded camps for many years (Raju and Ayeb-Karlsson, 2020:515). Consequently, Harmen et al (2017) aver that staying in overcrowded and less-resourced refugee camps has had a toll on the refugees' health. In the same vein, Montegomery et al., (2019) state that by virtue of mostly being a minority and located away from city centres refugees' access to medical care and medical information is restricted. Against this milieu, the chapter grapples with the role of *Radio Zimbabwe* which is the leading radio station in Zimbabwe in terms of listenership and reach, in propagating Covid-19 messages to minority groups, precisely refugees staying at Tongogara Refugee Camp. There is mature scholarship on the interplay between Covid-19 and radio. Some studies have delved into the framing of Covid-19 in radio programmes (Abubakhar et al., 2022), the pivotal role of radio in responding to crises induced by the Covid-19 pandemic (DoSantos and Brasil, 2020), the perceptions of audiences regarding radio-delivered Covid-19 messages (Talabi et al., 2022), the utilization of radio in educational contexts during the Covid-19 pandemic (Ayanwale et al., 2023), and, closely related to the focus of this chapter, the examination conducted by Chibike and Ncube (2023) concerning the mediation of Covid-19 by *Radio Zimbabwe* and its impact on the broader narrative of nationalism in Zimbabwe. In sum, the collection of studies presented above underscores the multifaceted role of radio during the course of the COVID-19 pandemic. These scholarly contributions collectively emphasise the pivotal role of radio in framing the pandemic, responding to crises, conveying critical information, delivering education, and shaping national narratives. The comprehensive examination of these studies offers a nuanced understanding of the intricate dynamics between media, public health, education, and national identity in times of crisis, ultimately contributing to the broader discourse on the role of media in contemporary society. However, the brief overview of the literature exposes the fact that there is a dearth of scholarship on the effectiveness of radio in disseminating Covid-19 messages to refugee camps hence, the study grabs an opportunity to fill this glaring gap. Also, against the background that Zimbabwe is a multi-ethnic, multi-racial and multi-lingual this chapter interrogates the potential of health communication in enhancing the belonging of refugees who have stayed in Zimbabwe for a very long time. In light of this, the chapter, through the views of selected journalists, tackles the following objectives:

- To examine the role of *Radio Zimbabwe* in aiding refugees' understanding of Covid-19
- To examine the role of *Radio Zimbabwe* in helping facilitate a sense of belonging among refugees through Covid-19 messages.

This chapter holds noteworthy significance as it provides valuable insights into the potential of radio as a medium for conveying critical health information to marginalised minority groups. Furthermore, it sheds light on radio's role in engendering a sense of belonging among individuals who often find themselves on the periphery of society. This is against the backdrop that radio in Africa has been celebrated as a penetrative channel of communication reaching a far wide geographic boundary and easily accessible to a lot of people. The chapter's novelty is drawn from the fact it interrogates the interlink between health communication and the issue of belonging and nation-building in Zimbabwe, something prior studies have not looked at. This chapter is also important in that it is an avenue for radio journalists to critically reflect on the role that the cultural products they produce on minority and marginalised societies.

BACKGROUND AND CONTEXT OF THE STUDY

Minority groups often contend with marginalization from the mainstream socio-political and economic dialogues of their respective geographic regions. Their plights and whims are usually ignored by virtue of being a minority. Concurrently, the predicament of refugees worldwide has garnered attention, but governments have often struggled to address their issues, particularly in the context of the Covid-19 pandemic (Vonen et al., 2021). For instance, the Moria Refugee Camp in Greece reported one of the initial cases of Covid-19, revealing the dire consequences of overcrowding and limited access to essential resources, notably water (Stathopoulo et al., 2019). Similarly, in refugee camps in Bangladesh, housing the Rohingya people who fled brutal atrocities in Myanmar, Covid-19 outbreaks occurred due to overcrowding, inadequate water supply, and limited medical resources (Raju and Ayeb-Karlsson, 2020:514). This situation aligns with the findings of Ezeh et al. (2017) and Schwerdtle et al. (2017), who assert that individuals residing in densely populated areas with limited access to water and healthcare services are more vulnerable to diseases and infections.

Raju and Ayeb-Karlsson (2020) also noted that India's first Covid-19 case was recorded in a refugee camp covering less than one square kilometre but accommodating a staggering 23,000 people. Contact tracing in such densely populated facilities became an immense challenge. Kluge et al. (2020) further argue that in these overcrowded environments, implementing the World Health Organization's (WHO) Covid-19 protocols and procedures becomes exceedingly difficult. Additionally, Raju and Ayeb-Karlsson (2020) raised concerns about the spread of Covid-19 misinformation within refugee camps. They provided an example where false information circulated, claiming that anyone found with Covid-19 would be killed. Given this backdrop, it becomes imperative to examine the residents of Zimbabwe's Tongogara Refugee Camp, assessing their access to official Covid-19 information and how this information contributes to their sense of belonging and prioritisation in Zimbabwe, even as foreign nationals.

TONGOGARA REFUGEE CAMP

Tongogara Refugee Camp, the largest refugee camp in Zimbabwe, is located in a secluded, dry, hot and mosquito-infected place situated 488 kilometres outside the capital city, Harare (Chikanda and Crush, 2016). The camp is home to over 13,000 migrants constituting mainly those from the Democratic Republic of Congo, Ethiopia, Kenya, Mozambique and Sudan. According to an international humanitarian organisation World Vision, the situation is dire at the overpopulated Tongogara Refugee Camp. A glimpse at the camp shows the inhuman condition in which the occupants live as the infrastructure is old and there is little access to water and electricity (Mufandauya, 2015). According to Govere (2017), residents at the refugee camp have begun showing symptoms of mental ill health attributed to their traumatic experience and the pity living conditions they live in. The latter is a shortage of water, fuel, food, and health facilities among other things. As a result, they have turned to religious practices as they seek solutions to the dilemmas they face at the Camp. Govere (2017) highlights the issue of the language barrier as being another concern exacerbating the plight of the refugees as they cannot easily communicate with other refugees and service providers. This has consequently left them out of full and proper service delivery, especially from external stakeholders. Against the background of overpopulation, overcrowding and little access to water, eyebrows are raised in relation to the camp's ability to wade off Covid-19. Thus, the chapter is poised at examining the role of *Radio Zimbabwe* in communicating Covid-19 to refugees and how this resultantly gives them a sense of belonging.

LITERATURE REVIEW

Media, Belonging, and Loneliness

The intricate relationship between media consumption, belonging, and loneliness has become a focal point in contemporary literature, underscoring the evolving role of media in shaping interpersonal connections and societal dynamics. Media, spanning social media platforms to traditional media, holds the potential to engender a profound sense of belonging by facilitating social interaction and identification. Scholars such as Dahal and Aram (2013), and Njuguna (2006) support this notion arguing for the significance of radio in creating a sense of national identity and belonging by broadcasting shared cultural events and narratives. As we delve into the role of *Radio Zimbabwe* in aiding refugees' understanding of Covid-19, we must consider how this medium transcends geographical boundaries to convey critical health information and, in doing so, potentially contributes to a broader sense of global community among displaced populations. Amid the challenges posed by the pandemic, examining the role of *Radio Zimbabwe* in helping refugees find a sense of belonging through Covid-19 messages underscores the transformative potential of media not only as a source of information but as a conduit for fostering a collective identity and solidarity in times of crisis.

Media consumption, as demonstrated by Cauwenberg et al. (2014), can both foster and hinder feelings of loneliness and isolation through pervasive social comparison. It is crucial to consider this dual impact when examining *Radio Zimbabwe*'s role in aiding refugees' understanding of Covid-19 and fostering their sense of belonging amid the pandemic. Additionally, excessive media consumption, as highlighted by Marino et al. (2020), can hinder meaningful face-to-face interactions, raising questions about how *Radio Zimbabwe*'s broadcasts may have affected refugees' ability to connect with others in their community. Hence, the media's intricate influence on loneliness and isolation prompts a critical examination of *Radio Zimbabwe*'s impact on refugees' well-being in the context of Covid-19 messaging.

Radio, Health, and COVID-19

Scholars have extensively recognised radio as a potent conduit for disseminating health-related information to diverse audiences (Janes and Marques, 2013:70). The power of radio is also celebrated by Al Hassan et al (2011:2) and Waters et al (2011:2) who attribute this power to the capability of radio to speak to an individual in a community thus making private persons and undermined communities feel empowered. In comparison to other communication platforms, radio stands out for its accessibility (Smith et al. 2011:1), making it an ideal medium for effective communication. Drawing from this argument, this chapter explores the viability of radio in conveying Covid-19 information to refugees at the Tongogara Refugee Camp, with a particular focus on how it fosters a sense of belonging within a displaced population.

The role of radio in churning out information to the minority and the marginalised has been widely documented by scholars (Paravala, 2003). Hinging on this view Sighn et al (2017:365) posit that radio is essential in helping the general populace to be aware of health issues hence helping arrest societal problems birthed by death and illnesses which are aggravated by locals' lack of health knowledge and awareness.

Mediated messages have proven to be effective in inducing behaviours that help curb the spread of health pandemics (Talabi et al., 2022; Ufuophu-Biri, 2017; Leak et al., 2010). Among many communicative platforms, this chapter focuses on radio. Hugelius et al. (2019) underscore the instrumental role of radio messages in raising awareness and disseminating preventive measures during health crises, as exemplified during the Ebola outbreak. Consequently, radio's role in informing citizens about health issues is paramount in the African context. Further, Hugelius et al., (2019) herald not only the importance of radio in informing citizens but in helping those affected by health pandemics to de-stress. This spectacle the importance and centrality of radio as a communicative channel for health-related issues (do Santos and Brasil, 2020). Benefiting from do Santos and Brail's (2020) argument the chapter grapples with the potential of *Radio Zimbabwe* to inform refugee residents at Tongogara Refugee Camp about Covid-19. More so, the chapter goes on to examine if this information creates a feeling of belonging to the refugees who in most cases feel isolated and marginalised in the countries hosting them.

Ankomah et al. (2014) note that active and religious radio listeners often adopt preventive measures during disease outbreaks, based on information they receive through radio broadcasts. In the same vein, Talabi et al., (2022) posit that radio listeners in South-Western Nigeria adopted Covid-19 preventative measures which they heard on the radio. These findings underscore radio's influence on audience behaviour, particularly regarding health-related issues. However, the chapter departs from this established narrative to explore uncharted academic territory, investigating the mediation of health issues and the sense of belonging in Zimbabwe, which has not received sufficient scholarly attention.

Though scholars celebrate the influence of radio in positively influencing health behaviour, Ata-Awaji and Confidence (2021) fail to find the merit of this populist scholarly celebration. Instead, they argue that the consumption of radio and television messages is not directly proportional to desired health behaviours. In fact, their studies revealed that the more the audience consumed Covid-19 messages the more they became reluctant to adopt desire behaviours. This raises thought-provoking questions about whether audiences perceive radio-delivered Covid-19 messages as important and useful. Thus, this chapter aims to provide insights into the role of radio messages in informing refugees about the Covid-19 pandemic, considering the complexities of their response to such information.

Theoretical Framework: Social Responsibility Theory and Public Sphere Theory

The chapter uses the theoretical lens extracted from the social responsibility theory. The theory underscores that the media should be free to play its role in society responsibly and free from any political impingements (Okunna and Omenugha, 2012). It asserts that the media should primarily serve the interests of citizens (Obagwu and Idris, 2019; Ravi, 2012). This responsibility to society according to Abukhar (2012) and Sibert et al., (1956) emboldened the media to provide information to all sects of society, monitoring government activities, flagging government malpractices and emancipating communities among other things. While acknowledging the multifaceted roles of media, this chapter specifically focuses on the media's role in educating minority groups about health-related matters. Therefore, the chapter uses the social responsibility theory of the media theory to examine the effectiveness of *Radio Zimbabwe* in the lives of members of society, especially refugees. The unabated mind-boggling question is what role the radio station plays in empowering refugees through availing information about Covid-19 and how this information creates a sense of belonging to the refugees that have suffered the effect of being 'homeless.' This is of importance because this theory has often been overlapped to issues to do with media ethics while little scholarship in the realm of health communication has tested the practicability and applicability or potential extension of this theory within the confines of Covid-19 communication.

The chapter also draws from the Public Sphere Theory. As articulated by Lubenow (2012:229), a public sphere is characterized as an accessible platform featuring diverse viewpoints and a wealth of information, fostering rational discussions on societal issues. Therefore, this chapter epitomises the media as a public sphere in the sense that it should be easy to access, carry divergent views and be a communicative platform of rational debates. The public sphere theory then in this chapter is used to examine *Radio Zimbabwe* as a public sphere with regards to availing Covid-19 information to refugees and affording them the platform to engage on issues around the pandemic. However, the public sphere has been criticised for not being 'public' enough and only benefiting the elite (Asen, 2000). The minority, marginalized, women, and uneducated among other marginalized groups are usually excluded from the public sphere (Asen, 2000:437, Squaires, 2002). By examining *Radio Zimbabwe* in the context of the Public Sphere Theory, this chapter not only evaluates the radio station's viability as a public sphere but also addresses concerns of exclusion, particularly with regard to refugees and other marginalized groups, shedding light on their inclusion in the public discourse surrounding the Covid-19 pandemic.

Having discussed the theoretical thrust of this chapter the next section offers a discussion of the methodological stance adopted.

METHODOLOGY

This qualitative study relies on in-depth interviews conducted with radio journalists drawn from six carefully selected radio stations in Zimbabwe, including *Radio Zimbabwe*. Qualitative studies are bent on examining a social phenomenon through a subjective approach entailing human understanding of it (Cresswell, 2014; Hannock et al, 2013; Merriam, 2002; Shank, 2002). Therefore, the qualitative approach is suitable for this study since it seeks to examine journalists' views and perspectives of *Radio Zimbabwe's* Covid-19 programmes precisely their role in informing refugees at Tongogara Refugee Camp about Covid-19 and whether the Covid-19 messages illuminated a sense of belonging in Zimbabwe against the background that they originate from other countries. A total of 12 journalists were purposively selected to participate in this study. Purposive sampling entails the section of research participants who possess certain attributes which make them ideal for the research (Atkins & Alkassim, 2016; Jones et al., 2009). The choice of journalists as participants stems from their unique insight into the information disseminated about Covid-19 on radio. Each of the 12 journalists represented one of the six local radio stations, ensuring that two journalists were selected from each station. This deliberate selection strategy aimed to capture a rich array of perspectives from journalists with varied editorial biases and orientations, enhancing the depth and diversity of insights gathered. The journalists were subjected to in-depth interviews which Ncube (2018) and Fox (2009) define as a conversation between the researcher and the participants in the study bent on unearthing participants' views and perspectives on a particular subject. The aim here was to unearth their perspectives on the role of *Radio Zimbabwe* in informing refugees about the Covid-19 pandemic and also the implications of Covid-19 messages in fanning fames of belonging in Zimbabwe.

ANALYSIS AND DISCUSSION OF FINDINGS

Overview of the Findings

The chapter is poised at examining the role of *Radio Zimbabwe* in informing refugees about Covid-19 and also to interrogate whether the Covid-19 messages disseminated by the radio station aided refugees in cultivating a sense of belonging in Zimbabwe. Against this background, some diverse views and perspectives were drawn from data gathered from in-depth interviews with journalists on the role of *Radio Zimbabwe* in informing refugees about Covid-19 and also cultivating in them a sense of belonging through the messages. Most participants in this study were of the view that *Radio Zimbabwe* was not a robust public sphere and did not play its social responsibility role of informing refugees at Tongogara refugee camp about Covid-19. Consequently, they are spectacled that *Radio Zimbabwe's* failure to inform refugees about Covid-19 further dampened refugees' sense of belonging in Zimbabwe.

The Role of *Radio Zimbabwe* in Aiding Refugees' Understanding of COVID-19

Empirical data gathered through in-depth interviews with journalists suggests that *Radio Zimbabwe* failed to contribute to refugees living at Tongogara refugee camp's understanding of Covid-19. The participants reiterated that the fact that *Radio Zimbabwe* did not use languages that some refugees understand in conveying Covid-19 messages was a major hindrance in its quest to adequately inform them. As such, respondent two said:

Most Covid-19 messages and adverts that were circulated by Radio Zimbabwe were mainly in English, Shona or isiNdebele. Radio Zimbabwe failed to take into consideration that some of these refugees do not understand those three languages.

Adding to this assertion was Participant Six who said:

Radio Zimbabwe only uses mainly Shona and Ndebele in its programming and dissemination of Covid-19 information. They failed to acknowledge that there are people in refugee camps coming from other countries who speak Portuguese, French and other African indigenous languages. This automatically means that they were left uninformed even though the radio stations claimed to inform everyone about Covid-19.

The participants' views and perspectives reinforce the idea that *Radio Zimbabwe* failed to cater for refugees living in Tongogara Refugee Camp. This is because it failed to disseminate information which they could easily understand, crafted in languages that they are familiar with. Against the background that Al Hassan et al (2011:2) and Waters et al (2011:2) argue that radio empowers minoritised communities the chapter's findings are of the notion that, *Radio Zimbabwe* failed to empower refugees who are a minority group in Zimbabwe with important information on Covid-19. Thus, challenges the populist scholarly view cemented by Sighn et al., (2017:365), Smith et al. (2011:1) and Paravala (2003) which celebrates radio as a communicative medium empowering the marginalised communities. The fact that *Radio Zimbabwe* failed to empower citizens with information in a language that they understand translates to the fact that it failed to play its societal role of serving citizens in particular the minoritised citizens against the background that Obagwu and Idris (2019) and Ravi (2012)'s argument that the media must be liable to the society. Consequently, this further underscores *Radio Zimbabwe's* failure to be a robust public sphere. This is so because it has failed to provide information to refugees in languages that they understand. This is in sync with the postulation of Asen (2000:437) and Squaires (2002) that public spheres have failed to accommodate minority groups in society. All in all, it can be seen that *Radio Zimbabwe* was blinded to the fact that Zimbabwe is a country in which refugees from various nations who speak different languages live. As such in its mediation of Covid-19 the station failed to consider refugees as all its programming was mainly done in Ndebele and Shona and in some instances, English was used thus side-lining those who do not understand the three languages.

Other participants articulated that the language used in the dissemination of Covid-19 messages was problematic to audiences in Tongogara Refugee Camp, but they also lamented the absence of tailor-made programming for refugees. This is against the background that the station carried out tailored programmes for other high-risk people such as those suffering from underlying chronic illness, women, school children and toddlers. In light of this Participant Ten said:

There was no Covid-19 program which specifically addressed those staying in overcrowded places such as refugee camps. This shows that the producers and presenters at Radio Zimbabwe did not have refugees in mind. They did not say anything about the spread and consequences of Covid-19 in refugee camps.

Reinforcing this thought was Participant One who said:

Zimbabwe's Covid-19 communication spoke to many vulnerable groups for example those with chronic illness. It also spoke to those who spend most of their time in high-risk areas such as school children and workers. So, this shows that it tried to communicate Covid-19 to those who are at risk of contracting the virus and those susceptible to serious sickness. However, the station was quiet when it came to refugees. Refugees also stay in high-risk areas and some even have underlying conditions.

Participant 7 also added:

No information was directed at officials manning high risk areas such as refugees' camps. We see that communication was directed to other officials responsible for other areas such as workplaces and schools. The radio station did not do much to availing adequate information to refugees and officials at those camps.

The participants here lament the lack of official communication targeting refugees and authorities that are responsible for the Tongogara refugee camp. They point out the total exclusion of refugees as people who are at a high risk of catching the Covid-19 virus and subsequently suffering its implications. This is against the background that *Radio Zimbabwe* carried information which was tailor-made for other people who are at a high risk of catching the virus. This therefore glaringly exposes the blatant exclusion of refugees in Covid-19 communication by *Radio Zimbabwe*. Consequently, while Hugelius et al. (2019) are of the notion that radio helps in raising awareness about health issues *Radio Zimbabwe* in this case failed to raise awareness of Covid-19 among refugees because it did not have any information targeting them. This raises concerns about the power of radio to speak to different multitudes of people for purposes of social change. This concern is further drawn from do Santos and Brasil (2020) who argue that radio is the main source of health-related information which speaks to different people from diverse backgrounds. Based on the views and perspectives of the participants in this chapter *Radio Zimbabwe* did not cater for people of diverse backgrounds heifer among them refugees who did not get information directly linked to them, thus in the process highlighting the minority and subaltern status in Zimbabwe. While Sibert et al (1956) posit that the media must represent every member of society, *Radio Zimbabwe* in its mediation of Covid-19 failed the minority and subaltern in the form of refugees regardless of the fact that they made up a group of those at a high risk of contracting the virus. This goes on to show that refugees as a minority are not a priority when it comes to global disasters such as the outbreak of health pandemics, in Zimbabwe. This also goes against Lubenow's (2012:229) view that a public sphere is pregnant with diverse views speaking to a diverse population. It can therefore be argued that *Radio Zimbabwe* failed to recognise refugees despite the fact that they were people at high risk of contracting Covid-19 and chose to focus on other groups of people thus leaving refugees on the fringes with regard to Covid-19-related information.

Though *Radio Zimbabwe* carried Covid-19 programmes, jingles and news updates the study's participants are of the view that these proved worthless to refugees. They attribute this to a lack of radio reach and access. In this respect participant 12 said:

It is unfortunate that Tongogara refugees do not have access to radio. They stay in a place where they do not have the necessary gadgets that allow them to access the station. With such a problem at hand, it is clear that Radio Zimbabwe's mediation of Covid-19 was not effective at all for refugees.

Participant Three also highlighted that in some instances radio waves are not easily accessed at the refugee camp. The participant said:

Looking at the area in which Tongogara is located we should also consider the fact that radio transmission is generally poor. You will discover that even if there are people who want to listen to the radio, they fail to access it due to restricted bandwidths.

Participant Eleven also brought in a different perspective in line of the issue to do with accessibility and reach by stating that refugees lack access to equipment that allows them to listen to the radio. In light of this the participant said:

We should take into consideration that people who stay in the Tongogara Refugee Camp do not have equipment that makes it possible for them to access information. For example, they do not own any radio sets because they do not afford them. Most of them are unemployed, school-going and the elderly there is no way they can afford buying radio sets.

The views of the participants therefore show that besides the fact that *Radio Zimbabwe* had totally overlooked refugees in its Covid-19 content the challenge that also remains is that of reach. The participants make it clear that due to the area in which Tongogara Refugee Camp is located there is no guaranteed 24/7 access to radio waves. This is against the fact that *Radio Zimbabwe* is one of the leading radio stations in Zimbabwe when it comes to reaching precisely remote areas. Also, the participants make it clear that the majority of residents at Tongogara Refugee Camp do not have access to radio sets thus further complicating efforts aimed at making sure they have access to Covid-19 news and information. This then makes it difficult to take Covid-19 preventative measures since Talabi et al., (2022) argue that receivers of Covid-19 information from the radio were more likely prone to adopt measures that were aimed at curbing the spread of the virus. Thus, it can be argued that the lack of stable radio waves in the Tongogara Refugee Camp coupled with the refugees' failure to get access to radio sets resulted in them lagging when it comes to Covid-19 news and information. This argument ultimately speaks to Asen's (2000) argument that public spheres only benefit the elite. In this case, the elite are the majority social groups in urban areas who enjoy access to radio waves and radio sets. This also problematizes the fact that radio is a powerful communication space and tool which reaches marginalised communities as refugees in post-colonial Zimbabwe still struggle to have access to mediated information about Covid-19 on radio.

Against the background that refugees have their families in other countries, they need to know the effects of Covid-19 in their home areas. However, most participants noted that *Radio Zimbabwe* failed to adequately inform refugees about the ravaging effects of Covid-19 in different countries. In this respect, Participant Five said:

For people to be able to understand something there is a need to make reference to conditions and social settings that they are used to. However, in its reportage of Covid-19 Radio Zimbabwe was silent about what was happening in other African countries such as the Democratic Republic of Congo, Somalia and Rwanda which happen to be the home countries of some of the refugees. To them the absence of this information creates information gaps on whether Covid-19 affected Zimbabwe only, the state of their families among other important thing. This lack of information can induce stress on refuges.

This view exhibits the fact that *Radio Zimbabwe* failed to adequately and comprehensively inform refugees about what is taking place in other countries particularly those from which the refugees come. Thus, it can be shown that *Radio Zimbabwe* failed to serve the communicative interests of refugees against the background that Obagwu and Idris (2019) and Ravi (2012) state that the media must carry information which is of interest to people of diverse backgrounds facing different consequences. Thus, this translates to the fact that refugees are seen as the subaltern in the media. They are not prioritised as evidenced in how *Radio Zimbabwe* crafted its Covid-19 messages which seemingly left out refugees as a minority group.

Having discussed the role of *Radio Zimbabwe* in mediating Covid-19 information to refugees the next section explicates whether this mediation created a sense of belonging in refugees.

THE ROLE OF *RADIO ZIMBABWE* IN HELPING FACILITATE A SENSE OF BELONGING AMONG REFUGEES THROUGH COVID-19 MESSAGES

Issues of belonging are pertinent, especially to displaced, minority, marginalised and peripherised groups. With regards to the perspectives and views of journalists who happen to be this study's participants, *Radio Zimbabwe* failed to cultivate a sense of belonging among refugees resident at Tongogara Refugee Camp. This is because of the fact that *Radio Zimbabwe* has failed to include them linguistically in its coverage and dissemination of Covid-19 information. This was said by participant seven who stated that:

I do not think that Radio Zimbabwe's messages created a sense of belonging to the refugees. This is simply because of their failure to get Covid-19 information from the station that they could easily understand. The fact that everything was done in English, Ndebele, and Shona rubberstamped to them that they are not Zimbabweans since English, Shona and Ndebele are the main languages in the country.

Adding to this view was Participant Six who stated that:

There was no attempt to use other languages that were easily understood by foreigners precisely refugees. This meant that they were left out of the government's efforts in the fight against Covid-19. This mere act of linguistically eliminating, them furthers the sense of them being foreigners and not being important in the country.

These views and perceptions point to the fact that *Radio Zimbabwe* neglected other languages which are understood by refugees in its mediation of Covid-19. This is against the background that *Radio Zimbabwe* only used English, Ndebele and Shona languages in its Covid-19 messages, announcements and jingles while ignoring the fact that there are refugees who do not understand those languages. This problematizes the argument by Waters et al (2011:2) that radio speaks to every individual in any community. *Radio Zimbabwe* failed to speak to refugees in refugee camps. This then translates to the fact that refugees are either not taken into consideration or muted in the health, socio-political and economic discourse of Zimbabwe. Thus, this underline, in them, that they are foreigners and discourses in Zimbabwe are not for them. In sum, *Radio Zimbabwe*'s Covid-19 communication excluded refugees and this spectacle of the refugee status of refugees consequently failed to create a sense of belonging in Zimbabwe. Thus, the failure of *Radio Zimbabwe* to be an inclusive public sphere keeps the minority and marginalised communities within their status of marginality and minority especially refugees residing at Tongogara Refugee Camp.

Furthermore, participants Seven and Six's views align with the literature review's exploration of the relationship between media, belonging, and loneliness. They emphasize the critical role of language in media communication, particularly in the context of *Radio Zimbabwe*'s role in aiding refugees' understanding of Covid-19 and fostering a sense of belonging among them. Participant Seven rightly points out that *Radio Zimbabwe*'s failure to provide Covid-19 information in languages accessible to refugees may have contributed to a lack of belonging. Language plays a crucial role in fostering a sense of belonging, and when communication is primarily in languages that are not understood by refugees, it can create a sense of exclusion and reinforce their outsider status. This aligns with the findings of Dahal and Aram (2013) and Njuguna (2006), who argue for the significance of radio in creating a sense of national identity and belonging by broadcasting shared cultural events and narratives.

Also, Participant Six further underscores the impact of linguistic exclusion on refugees' sense of belonging. The absence of efforts to use languages that refugees easily understand not only hinders their access to critical information but also sends a message that they are not considered a significant part of the community. This act of linguistic exclusion can perpetuate feelings of being foreigners and not being valued in the host country. This resonates with the literature's emphasis on the transformative potential of media in fostering a collective identity and solidarity, particularly in times of crisis.

Journalists lamented that the fact that there was no specific program, advert or jingle speaking directly to refugees and the dire conditions they live in dented the sense of belonging among refugees at Tongogara Refugee Camp. Accordingly, Participant Four had this to say:

Radio Zimbabwe's programming showed that it took a blind eye towards issues to do with refugees. Totally the producers/presenters at the station forgot that Zimbabwe had marginalised and minoritised groups such as refugees since there was no information directly addressing refugees. This problematizes refugees' sense of belonging as they see themselves as muted in the media, their plights not making it into the main communicative spaces in Zimbabwe.

This view and perspective exhibit the crucial issue of exclusion and the failure of *Radio Zimbabwe* to address the needs and concerns of marginalised groups, such as refugees. This exclusion from media content can profoundly impact refugees' sense of belonging. It resonates with the literature's exploration of how media can either create a sense of community and identity or, conversely, exacerbate feelings of isolation and loneliness. The critique raises concerns about how this exclusion problematizes refugees' sense of belonging. When refugees perceive that their experiences and plights are ignored or muted in the media, it reinforces their outsider status and can intensify feelings of isolation. This situation directly relates to the literature's discussion of media's potential to shape interpersonal connections and societal dynamics. Additionally, the statement points to the broader implications of media representation for collective identity. The absence of information directly addressing refugees within *Radio Zimbabwe*'s programming can hinder the formation of a collective identity for refugees within the broader Zimbabwean community, as discussed by Dahal and Aram (2013) and Njuguna (2006) in the context of creating a sense of national identity. In essence, this critique emphasizes the importance of media inclusivity, especially in the case of marginalized groups like refugees. It aligns with the literature's recognition of media's dual potential to foster belonging or contribute to isolation, prompting a critical examination of *Radio Zimbabwe*'s role in addressing the needs and sense of belonging of refugees during the Covid-19 pandemic.

Another issue raised is the fact that refugees in Tongogara do not have any means to get mediated radio messages about Covid-19. In light of this Participant Eight stated that:

The fact that refugees residing at Tongogara Refugee Camp do not have access to communicative platforms such as Radio Zimbabwe is interpreted as a sign that they are seen as unimportant within the health discourse of Zimbabwe, further translating to the fact that they are mere refugees who should return to their homeland.

Participant Eight here exhibits that refugees at Tongogara Refugee Camp lack access to communicative platforms like *Radio Zimbabwe* raises concerns of exclusion and underscores the potential impact on their sense of belonging, resonating with the literature's exploration of media's role in shaping belonging and loneliness. This exclusion from mainstream media implies that refugees are considered unimportant within Zimbabwe's health discourse, reinforcing their outsider status and undermining their access to crucial health information during the Covid-19 pandemic. This issue underscores the significance of equitable media access, particularly during crises, and prompts a critical examination of *Radio Zimbabwe*'s role in addressing refugees' information needs and fostering their sense of belonging.

CONCLUSION

The chapter has demonstrated the fact that social responsibility theory and the public sphere theory are product prisms enabling the interrogation of the role of *Radio Zimbabwe* in informing refugee residents at Tongogara Refugee Camp about Covid-19, through the views and perspectives of sampled journalists. The chapter also grappled with the impact of *Radio Zimbabwe's* handling and mediation of Covid-19 in infusing a sense of belonging in refugees. The chapter showed the complex understandings brought by journalists but chief among them was that *Radio Zimbabwe* failed to comprehensively and adequately inform refugees about Covid-19. This is because they did not craft Covid-19 messages in languages that the refugees understand, there was no specific information targeting refugees. This raises questions with regard to the populist scholarly postulation that radio has proved to be an effective communication platform for the marginalised communities as it in this case failed to serve the information interests of refugees at Tongogara Refugee Camp. In reference to the second objective, the chapter concludes that the way *Radio Zimbabwe* constructed its Covid-19 messages failed to inspire a sense of belonging in refugees. This is attributed to the lack of inclusive language and information directly speaking to them. Therefore, the argument here is that *Radio Zimbabwe*'s failure to be an ideal public sphere and serve the interests of diverse people in Zimbabwe led to its failure to adequately inform refugees at Tongogara about Covid-19 in the process failing to ignite a sense of belonging on refugees. Against this background, there is a need for more studies focusing on refugees to modify or strengthen the arguments made in this chapter. Also, there is a need for scholars to interrogate the views of the refugees themselves on their take on how radio is including them in discussions not only about Covid-19 but other important issues in Zimbabwe.

REFERENCES

Abubakhar, A., Jibrin, R., & Umar, M. A. (2022). Radio stations framing of the Covid-19 pandemic in Borno State radio stations. *Nigerian Journal of Communication*, *18*(1), 138–151.

Al-Hassan, S., Andani, A., & Abdul-Malik, A. (2011). The Role of Community Radio in Livelihood Improvement: The Case of Simli Radio. *The Journal of Field Actions*, *5*(19).

Ata-Awaji, A. R., & Confidence, O. S. (2021). Exposure to broadcast media messages and knowledge of Covid-19 pandemic among residents of Port Harcourt, Nigeria. *Media Communication Currents*, *5*(1), 19–37.

Atkinson, R., & Flint, J. (2016). *Accessing Hidden and Hard to Reach Populations: Snowball Research Strategies*. Available at: https://www.sru.soc.survey.ac.uk/SRU33.PDF

Ayanwale, M. A., Adewuyi, H. O., & Afolabi, O. (2023). Learning through radio and television during Covid-19: Perspectives of K12 stakeholders. *Social and Humanities*, *2*(1), 61–72. doi:10.21303/2504-5571.2023.002663

Berger, A. (1991). *Media research techniques*. Sage.

Cauwenberg, J. V., Donder, L. D., Clarys, P., Bourdeaudhuij, I. D., Owen, N., Dury, S., Witte, N. D., Buffel, T., Verté, D., & Deforche, B. (2014). Relationships of individual, social, and physical environmental factors with older adults' television viewing time. *Journal of Aging and Physical Activity*, *22*(4), 508–517. doi:10.1123/JAPA.2013-0015 PMID:24231688

Chibike, J. J., & Ncube, B. J. (2023). Local radio, Covid-19 and nationalism: The role of Radio Zimbabwe in the Zimbabwean project of nationalism. In Communicating Pandemics Globally [Work in progress].

Chikanda, A., & Crush, J. (2016). The geography of refugee flows to Zimbabwe. *African Geographical Review*, *35*(1), 18–34. doi:10.1080/19376812.2014.933706

Creswell, J. W. (2014). *Research design: Qualitative, quantitative and mixed methods* (4th ed.). Sage.

Dahal, S., & Aram, I. A. (2013). Empowering Indigenous Community through Community Radio: A Case Study from Nepal. *The Qualitative Report*, *18*(41), 1–26. doi:10.46743/2160-3715/2013.1456

Do-Santos, F. O., & Brasil, A. (2020). Broadcasting the Covid-19 pandemic in Central Africa: A content analysis of United Nations Peacekeeping Radio. *Radiofonas*, *11*(2), 89–128.

Ezeh, A., Oyebode, O., Satterthwaite, D., Chen, Y.-F., Ndugwa, R., Sartori, J., Mberu, B., Melendez-Torres, G. J., Haregu, T., Watson, S. I., Caiaffa, W., Capon, A., & Lilford, R. J. (2017). The history, geography, and sociology of slums and the health problems of people who live in slums. *Lancet*, *389*(10068), 547–558. doi:10.1016/S0140-6736(16)31650-6 PMID:27760703

Fox, N. (2009). *Using Interviews in Research Projects*. National Institute for Health Science.

Govere, E. (2017). *Exploring the perception of refugees and asylum seekers regarding access to mental health service in Zimbabwe: A case study of Tongogara Refugee Camp*. Unpublished Master's Thesis. University of Witwatersrand.

Hallin, D. C., & Mancini, P. (2004). *Comparing media systems: Three models of media and politics*. Cambridge University Press. doi:10.1017/CBO9780511790867

Hannock, B., Ockleford, E., & Windridge, K. (2013). *An Introduction to Qualitative Research*. Available at: https://www.rds-yh.nihr.ac.uk/wpcontent/uploads/2013/05/05/introduction-to-qualitative-reserch.pdf

Hermans, M. P. J., Kooistra, J., Cannegieter, S. C., Rosendaal, F. R., Mook-Kanamori, D. O., & Nemeth, B. (2017). Healthcare and disease burden among refugees in long-stay refugee camps at Lesbos, Greece. *European Journal of Epidemiology*, *32*(9), 851–854. doi:10.1007/s10654-017-0269-4 PMID:28597126

Hugulius, K., Adams, M., & Romo-Murphey, E. (2019). The Power of Radio to Promote Health and Resilience in Natural Disasters: A Review. *International Journal of Environmental Research and Public Health*, *16*(14), 2526. doi:10.3390/ijerph16142526 PMID:31311142

Jones, S., Torres, V., & Arminio, J. (2009). *Negotiating the complexities of qualitative research in higher education: Fundamental Elements and Issues*. Routledge.

Kluge, H. H. P., Jakab, Z., & Bartovic, J. (2020). Comment refugee and migrant health in the COVID-19 response. *Lancet*, *2019*, 2019–2020.

Leask, J., Hooker, C., & King, C. (2010). Media coverage of health issues and how to work effectively with journalists: A qualitative study. *BMC Public Health, 10*(535), 1–7. doi:10.1186/1471-2458-10-535 PMID:20822552

Lubenow, T. A. (2012). The public sphere 50 years later: Public Sphere and Mass Media in Jurgen Habermas. *Revista Transformacao, 35*(3), 229–274. doi:10.7443/15110

Marino, I. M., Adogba, O., & Tilli, N. (2020). Mental health interventions: Reflections on a radio program as alternative for stigma reduction and social integration. *Frontiers in Communication, 5*, 550912. doi:10.3389/fcomm.2020.550912

Merriam, S. (2002). *Qualitative research in practice: Examples for discussion and analysis*. Jossey-Bass.

Montgomery, J., Stathopoulou, T., & Eikemo, T. A. (2019). Asylum-seeking parents' reports of health deterioration in their children since fleeing their home country. *Journal of Refugee Studies, 32*(Special_Issue_1), 52–62. doi:10.1093/jrs/fez018

Mufandauya, R. (2015). *Effectiveness of the refugee encampment policy in Zimbabwe; a study of Tongogara Refugee Camp (2013-2014).*

Ncube, B. J. (2019). *Radio Mthwakazi and the Construction of Ndebele Ethnic Identity*. Doctoral Thesis. Johannesburg: University of Johannesburg.

Njuguna, C. (2006). Globalisation, media and culture: The role of the broadcast media in promoting a national identity in Kenya, MA thesis, University of Nairobi.

Obagwu, P. U., & Idris, K. M. (2019). Social responsibility theory of the press: A critique of it application and constraints. *International Journal of Innovative Research and Development, 8*(12), 26–35. doi:10.24940/ijird/2019/v8/i12/DEC19010

Okunaa, C. S., & Omenugha, K. A. (2012). Introduction to Mass Communication (3rd Edition). Enungu: New Generation Books.

Paravala, V. (2003). Building solidarities- A case of community Radio in Zharkhand. *Economic and Political Weekly, 37*(22), 2188–2197.

Raju, E., & Ayeb-Karlsson, S. (2020). Covid-19: How do you isolate in a refugee camp. *International Journal of Public Health, 65*(5), 515–517. doi:10.1007/s00038-020-01381-8 PMID:32385541

Ravi, K. (2012). Media and Social Responsibility: A critical Perspective with Special Reference to Television. *Academic Research International, 2*(1), 306–325.

Schwerdtle, P., Bowen, K., & McMichael, C. (2017). The health impacts of climate-related migration. *BMC Medicine, 16*(1), 1–7. doi:10.1186/s12916-017-0981-7 PMID:29301536

Shank, G. (2002). *Qualitative Research. A Personal Skills Approach*. Merrill Prentice Hall.

Siebert, F., Peterson, T., & Schramm, W. (1956). Four theories of the papers. The authoritarian, libertarian, social responsibility and soviet community concepts of what the press should do. Urban: University of Illinois.

Smith, M. L., Menn, M., Lisako, J., & McKeyer, J. (2011). Effectiveness of Radio as a Health Information Source. *Journal of Radio & Audio Media*, *18*(2), 196–211. doi:10.1080/19376529.2011.615776

Stathopoulou, T., Avrami, L., Kostaki, A., Cavounidis, J., & Eikemo, T. A. (2019). Safety, health and trauma among newly arrived refugees in Greece. *Journal of Refugee Studies*, *32*(Special_Issue_1), 22–35. doi:10.1093/jrs/fez034

Talabi, F. O., Oyedeji, K. A., Adelabu, O., & Bernice, O. (2022). Public perception of radio campaign messages in managing COVID-19 pandemic in selected states. *Human Vaccines & Immunotherapeutics*, *18*(5), 1–6. doi:10.1080/21645515.2022.2085958 PMID:35714340

Ufuophu-Biri, E. (2017). Relationship between exposure to media campaigns on family planning and adoption of family planning methods among women in delta state. *Journal of Social Management Science*, *12*, 153–162.

Vonen, H., Olsen, M. L., Eriksen, S. S., & Eikemo, T. A. (2021). Refugee Camps and Covid-19: Can we prevent a humanitarian crisis. *Scandinavian Journal of Public Health*, *49*(1), 27–28. doi:10.1177/1403494820934952 PMID:32522120

Waters, D., James, R., & Darby, J. (2011). Health promoting community radio in rural Bali: An impact evaluation. *Rural and Remote Health*, *11*(2), 1555–2011. doi:10.22605/RRH1555 PMID:21375357

Chapter 14
Framing of Opinion Leaders' COVID-19 Stance(s) on society:
The Case of Oppah Muchinguri-Kashiri's Comments in Studio 7 and Zim Eye

Witness Roya
https://orcid.org/0000-0002-1394-4428
Mangosuthu University of Technology, South Africa

ABSTRACT

Using framing as a springboard and critical discourse analysis as the methodology, this chapter aims to conduct a thoroughgoing exegesis of two speeches that were made by Oppah Muchinguri between the 14th of March 2020 and the 16th of January 2021. This chapter seeks to critically explain the influence of social, political, religious, and cultural factors on opinion leaders' attitude to COVID-19 and show the extent to which they represent perceptions of Zimbabweans regarding the virus and what should be prioritized between privacy of journalists' sources and the public interest. The chapter also adds to the huge corpus of studies on society's conceptualization of COVID-19 and urges stakeholders to avoid unsubstantiated claims and to use their influence to rally behind experts' advice in dealing with the pandemic.

INTRODUCTION

From time to time, the world has been ravaged by pandemics such as smallpox, human immunodeficiency virus (HIV), Ebola and severe acute respiratory syndrome (SARS). However, COVID-19 was so severe that it popularized descriptors such as 'the novel virus'[1] and 'superspreader'[2]. Also identified as coronavirus or euphemistically as 'the virus', COVID-19 became the first new disease to be declared a pandemic (Van Damme, Dahake, Delamou, 2020). COVID-19 spawned an 'infodemic', huge volumes of information (Lee1, Kanji, Wang, Mamuji, Rozdilsky & Chu, 2021) which sometimes resulted in conflation of truth, myths, misinformation and disinformation. Sheikh (2016, Paragraph 19) defines the

DOI: 10.4018/979-8-3693-0624-6.ch014

'post-truth era', as "when lies replace the truth, emotions replace honesty, personal analysis replaces verified information and one opinion replaces multiple opinions". A joint study by the Digital Forensic Research Lab (DFRLab) and the Associated Press in 2020 found that countries like the United States and China accused each other of manufacturing the virus as a bioweapon. Hawthorn (2021) refutes claims by Chinese and Russian media that the virus was created by the United States to fight its foes. After results of the Scientific Advisory Group for the Origins of Novel Pathogens (SAGO) which was set up in 2021 by the WHO to investigate claims that the COVID-19 was manufactured in a Chinese laboratory obtained inconclusive results, the WHO accused Chinese authorities of stalling further investigations by not providing required data (Furlong, 2023).Even though COVID-19 is widely regarded as originating in China, some Chinese authorities made black people scapegoats, subjecting them to racial profiling even when there was no known COVID-19 case involving black people at the time. Many Africans were denied access to accommodation, shops, restaurants and public facilities. A black woman was prevented from entering a McDonald's franchise which displayed a sign barring black people, yet a white woman was allowed (Human Rights Watch, 2020).

Social, cultural, religious, spiritual and political leaders greatly influence social behaviour; they can cultivate tolerance or promote prejudice due to racial, ethnic and geographical differences. As cultural institutions, the media's projection of people and issues influences social perceptions. African footballers, Samuel Eto'o, Demba Ba and Didier Drogba expressed dismay over suggestions made by two French doctors, professors Jean-Paul Mira and Camille Locht, on French television station La Chaine Info that pilot tests for COVID-19 should be conducted in Africa (France, 2020). The media emerged as having the potential to fuel or mitigate stigmatization of COVID-19 patients. A report on the coverage of COVID-19 by Zimbabwean newspapers revealed that on the 16th of April 2020, state-controlled newspaper, The Chronicle alleged that a COVID-19 positive patient had exposed residents to the virus by violating lockdown rules yet the violator did not have the virus.

Similarly, Energy Mutodi, then deputy minister of information erroneously claimed that sex workers were "at high risk of person-to-person transmission" (Tapfumaneyi, 2020). It was also noted that newspapers heavily relied on politicians "for expert comments, leaving out other views which can bolster the understanding of the COVID-19 narrative in Zimbabwe" (Musitini, 2020). Musitini cites a story in The Chronicle just before the government rolled out its vaccination programme which had one source, Gibson Mhlanga, the permanent secretary in the ministry of health and childcare. State controlled newspapers like The Herald and The Sunday Mail did not cover claims by the Makamba family that Zororo's death from COVID-19 was caused by the absence of a ventilator at Wilkons hospital (see also discussion below).

The fact that most of the reliable information on social media platforms is produced by large media outlets and influential public figures who mainly use indigenous minimally means a significant number of people were excluded from conversations. Nick Mangwana, Zimbabwe's government spokesperson was forced to delete an X (formerly Twitter) post in which he accused health workers of being "medical assassins" suggesting that they had "eliminated" ministers who died in quick succession (BBC, 2021a).

One of the misconceptions about COVID-19 vaccines is that they cause sterility (Willingham, 2021). However, probably the most common COVID-19-related myth in Africa was that the virus only affects white people, especially the elderly[3]. This was debunked when Zororo Makamba, a youthful journalist and son to prominent ZANU PF member, James Makamba became the first person to die from COVID-19 complications on the 14th of March 2020, three days after its declaration as a pandemic by the World Health Organisation (WHO). Zororo's elder brother Tawanda told private newspaper, Daily News that the government was lying that it had provided his late 30-year-old brother with medical attention. Tawanda revealed that among other things, the family had to source a ventilator since there was none at Wilkins Hospital but realized that there was no socket in the room that Zororo was admitted (Nyoka, 2020).

In 2020, former United States president Donald Trump referred to COVID-19 as 'Chinese virus'. Trump's then challenger for the presidency, Joe Biden allegedly used a soundbite of Trump's speech which was edited out of context to create the impression that Trump had said COVID-19 is a 'hoax' (Lybrand, 2020).

From the foregoing, one can deduce that distortion of information can have serious implications. To assist the media in fulfilling their role as conduits of accurate information and crusaders of responsible behaviour as called for by the crisis, the United Nations, governments and non-governmental organisations provided COVID-19 information online and printed copies free of charge in different languages. Holtez, a physician-researcher argues that the term 'misinformation' masks the fact that "it's an organized, well-financed, politically motivated campaign that's meant to tear down the fabric of science (Holtez, 2023, p. 681)." He suggests adoption of 'anti-science' which has been applied to situations in countries like Brazil, 'democracies' and 'dictatorships' like the United States and Hungary whose operations resemble Joseph Stalin's government treatment of scientists as enemies of the state in the 1930s.

BACKGROUND

Zimbabwe has faced numerous crises since the turn of the 21st Century. These included droughts, floods, economic decline among others. Besides establishing a government of national unity in 2009 which was characterized by constant bickering, Zimbabwe's leadership has often failed to inspire hope among citizens. COVID-19 brought challenges and lessons to opinion leaders. Due to an avalanche of sources of information due to technology, the media ought to consider ethical ways of disseminating information. Oppah Muchinguri's comments about COVID-19 as a challenge for western countries only and her outbursts regarding vaccinations to Zim Eye's Simba Chikanza who disguises himself as her acquintance show that public officials should learn from mistakes and behave responsibly because they are role models.

FOCUS OF THE STUDY: THE IMPACT OF LEADERSHIP DURING THE COVID-19 PANDEMIC

Since a crisis is a culmination of an unsolved problem, leadership is required to deal with the situation. A leader should motivate everyone to work together towards a positive turnaround. Leadership entails "putting the collective good ahead of business or political goals" and quickly adopting to the new situation (UN Global Compact Media, 2020). Samad, Al Jerjawi and Dadich observe that political leaders represent their constituencies, making decisions at local, national, and/or international levels that significantly impact citizens' lives. COVID-19 "created a greater focus on leadership, increasing the burden on leaders to make decisions for the public in an uncertain time" (2023, p.1). Instead of leading from the front, leaders were found wanting on numerous occasions. Davies (2020, p.1) avers that during crises, political leadership can improve or worsen the situation though "more often than not, politics is presented as an ignoble irritant in contrast to the public health domain".

Similarly, Shilts, (2011) observes that in the early 80s society initially dismissed HIV/AIDS as a disease for gays and was only taken seriously after the death of Rock Hudson, a movie actor in 1985. He argues that "the federal government viewed AIDS as a budget problem, local public health officials saw it as a political problem, gay leaders considered AIDS a public relations problem, and the news media regarded it as a homosexual problem that wouldn't interest anybody else. Consequently, few confronted AIDS for what it was, a profoundly threatening medical crisis" (Shilts, 2011, p.3).

PERFORMANCE OF WOMEN IN LEADERSHIP POSITIONS

Studies found that countries with women in leadership positions recorded six times less COVID-19-related deaths than male-led countries (Coscieme & Skodowska-Curie, 2020). Female leaders such as New Zealand's Jacinda Ardern and Germany's Angela Merkel swiftly implemented ways of dealing with the pandemic as opposed to male leaders like Brazilian president Jair Bolsonaro and US president Donald Trump. By 1 June 2020, Germany had recorded 10 deaths per 100 000 people and New Zealand had a total of 22 deaths whilst mortality rates increased in the US and Brazil (Piscopo & Och, 2021). Studies noted differences in structures which restrict women's executive powers in some countries and the limited nature of the sample size; there were only eleven female heads of state by March 2020. Kelly and Johnson (2020) observe that twenty-five years after the Beijing Conference, women's participation in leadership positions has improved though more needs to be done. Henley (2020) and UN Women (2020) note that despite Merkel, Ardern, Mette Frederiksen of Denmark, Finland's Sanna Marin and Taiwan's Tsai Ing-wen's prominent media coverage, little research has been conducted on how they dealt with the pandemic.

AFRICAN WOMEN IN LEADERSHIP POSITIONS

Contributions made by women in leadership positions have received less recognition than their white counterparts in western countries. They may as well be described as 'unsung heroes'. In a major policy shift from her COVID-19 denialist predecessor, John Magufuli, Tanzania's first female president, Samia Suluhu Hassan saved many lives by implementing vaccination, inspiring other public office holders like health minister, Dorothy Gwajima to do the same. In a show of professionalism, Gwajima instructed the police to arrest her relative for trying to influence Tanzanians to reject vaccines, "Gwajima is my brother, he definitely is my brother-in-law, but I'm a minister and I have taken an oath to serve my country, not my brother" she said (The Chanzo Reporter, 2021, Paragraph 5). This was a remarkable policy shift from the minister. During Magufuli's presidency, Gwajima was one of the few female public officials who opposed vaccination: "In the glare of cameras, Gwajima and the health officials drank a herbal concoction including ginger, garlic, and lemons, and inhaled steam from herbs, promoting them as natural means of killing the virus" (Makoni, 2021, p.566).

Like her health minister, Hassan chose to follow ethics over political loyalties when she chastised Gwajima, a fellow Chama cha mapinduzi MP for his opposition to vaccination (BBC, 2021b). At the height of COVID-19 in 2020, South Africa's minister of cooperative governance, Nkosazana Dlamini-Zuma, a medical doctor by training, vigorously campaigned against the sale of cigarettes to mitigate effects of the virus. When she reinstated the ban after President Cyril Ramaphosa's announcement that cigarettes could be sold under lockdown level 4 restrictions, there was speculation that Dlamini Zuma had contradicted Ramaphosa but he defended her (Mavuso, 2020). After initially failing to provide reliable updates, the appointment of Agnes Mahomva as Chief National Coordinator, Zimbabwe emerged as one of the countries with the best COVID-19 responses in Africa (Pindula, 2023).

Despite the fact that some religion were opposed to observing COVID-19 protocols and prescriptions, some female congregants exhibited traits of transformative leadership. Gladys Mapondera, leader of a sect under Johanne Marange Apostolic, one of Zimbabwe's most popular apostolic churches, broke ranks by getting vaccinated (Nyati, 2021). She disclosed that (their) "church doctrine says we don't go to the hospital when we are sick or get vaccinated, but with COVID-19 it is a new ball game altogether and I have to take matters into my own hands". She retained her position in the church after her confession. In a further demonstration of progressive changes within these churches, Apostolic Women's Empowerment Trust (AWET) partnered UNICEF, the Health Development Fund (UK Aid, EU, SIDA-Sweden, Irish Aid and GAVI) and the Ministry of Health and Childcare to promote the uptake of vaccines (Nyati, 2021).

THEORETICAL FRAMEWORK: FRAMING THEORY

This paper invokes framing to provide theoretical lenses to examine the influence of opinion leaders on society. Framing is premised on the notion that selection, presentation (framing) and frequency of texts is meant to influence readers' perceptions. Since Lippmann (1922), discussed the influence of opinion leaders on public opinion, many scholars have reinforced his assertion. Goffman, in his 1956 work, *The Presentation of Self in Everyday Life,* is credited with popularizing framing theory by focusing on the way messages are communicated (the frame) to the receivers by the senders. He asserts that the sender of a message uses a framework to structure the message. Therefore, for this study, Covid-19 is the framework around comments made by opinion leaders, represented by Oppah Muchinguri-Kashiri. Using metaphors of theatre like 'dramaturgy' to real life conversations to stage performances, Goffman defines a frame as "an arbitrary slice or cut from the stream of ongoing activity" (Goffman, 1974, p. 10). Goffman's concept resembles a theatre concept which regards "a play as a slice of life", a phrase that was coined by French playwright Jean Jullien in his 1892 book, *The Living Theatre*. Shakespeare's characterization of life as a stage was another inspiration.

Apparently influenced by Lippmann[4], Goffman opines that people's experiences provides them with "schemata of interpretation" which they use "to locate, perceive, identify, and label" incidents or events (1974, p.21). Scheufele notes that "framing emphasizes specific aspects of reality (2004, p.405) echoing Entmann (1993, p.52) who asserts that framing involves "salience", giving prominence to some issues whilst downplaying (silence) others. This implies that, through silence and salience, the media respectively downplay and emphasize certain aspects to influence public opinion. Entmann clarifies the objective of framing *as* "to promote a particular interpretation, evaluation, and/or solution" (2003, p. 417).

Goffman observes that during interactions, people may have different thoughts but agree on key issues for the sake of unity: a "veneer of consensus is facilitated by each participant concealing his own wants behind statements which assert values to which everyone presents is likely to give lip service (Goffman,1959, p. 9). Unlike theories like the magic bullet theory which fall under the effects tradition which view media consumers as passive recipients, framing avers that the media cannot foist information on consumers but presents messages to them and re-presents their perspectives (Crandell, 2013). Framing recognizes the audience's ability to offer opposing views through "confrontational framing and counterframing" (Wood, Stoltz, Van Ness & Taylor, 2018, p.252). The media, however, seek to influence the audience through "a frame (which) can obscure or highlight elements of a story, depending on what message the audience should receive" (Wood et al, 2018, p.252). Gamson and Modigliani describe a frame as "a central organizing idea or storyline that provides meaning to an unfolding strip of events" (1987, p.143).

THE RELATIONSHIP BETWEEN AGENDA SETTING AND FRAMING THEORY

The relationship between agenda setting and framing has generated different conceptualizations. Entmann (1993) contends that agenda setting is "the first function of framing: defining problems worthy of public and government attention" which outlines issues that need to be addressed and priming is "the goal, the intended effect, of strategic actors' framing activities" (p. 165). On the other hand, Weaver (2007, p. 142) views framing as, a "second level" of agenda setting. In the same vein, Melkote (2009) considers framing a subgroup of agenda setting and regards the media's attempt to influence audience how to think and feel as a 'second level' or 'attribute'agenda-setting. However, some scholars consider agenda setting and framing as similar but autonomous fields of study (Maher, 2001; Scheufele, 1999; Tewksbury & Scheufele, 2009). Agenda setting is focused on the relative salience (usually operationally defined as perceived importance) of issues or subjects, the ''second level'' examines the relative salience of attributes of issues. Entmann (2007, p164) dismisses Cohen's statement ''the media may not be successful much of the time in telling people what to think but is stunningly successful in telling its readers what to think about'' as an "oft-quoted but misleading phrase" because "what to think" cannot be separated from "what to think about" unless it is induced through physical means. This implies that instead of pitting framing with agenda setting, what is important is to recognize them as complementary.

ASPECTS OF FRAMING THEORY

Priming is central to both agenda setting and framing. In describing the concept, Iyengar and Kinder assert that: "By calling attention to some matters while ignoring others, television news influences the standards by which governments, presidents, policies, and candidates for public office are judged" (1987, p. 63). Frequency and placement of stories is meant to influence opinions of the audience by projecting the issues associated with the stories as more topical than others.

Iyengar (1991) distinguishes between episodic frames and thematic frames whereby the former is often a feature of an ordinary person and a specific event whilst the latter offers a panoramic view of wider issues, explaining patterns or trends over an extended period and providing contextual information. Thematic framing places "public issues in some more general or abstract context and takes the form of a 'take out,' or 'backgrounder,' report directed at general outcomes or directions" (p.14). On the other hand, episodic framing involves narratives that appear as "a case study or event-oriented report and depicts public issues in terms of concrete instances" (p.14). Presentation of media content indicates whether producers of such content believe it requires individual or collective attention. For instance, episodic frames provide cues to solving a problem whereas thematic frames proffer possible solutions to causes of the problem. Episodic frames basically regard the audience as receivers of information whilst thematic frames treat them as active participants to the narrative. As solutions, episodic frames require more information and thematic frames need better policies. Thematically framed news elicits more public involvement than episodic news. Media, especially from commercially oriented outlets, often use episodic frames to explain broader issues in humanizing ways (De Swert & Kuypers, 2020). However, the importance of background information cannot be overemphasized (Iyengar, 1992); it is "important to consider cultural context" (Scheufele & Iyengar 2012, p. 8).

Framing is also split between equivalence and emphasis framing (Krishnatray & Shrivastava, 2021). In equivalence framing, the same information is presented in different ways, for instance, 95% employment or 5% unemployment is technically the same. On the other hand, emphasis framing involves manipulation of information by focusing on contrasting perspectives, for example, weighing advantages of using nuclear technology with its risks for workforce and the environment (Liu & McLeod, 2019). Critics argue that "frame" and framing have different meanings, including the frame as a framework and the frame as a shaping mechanism, contribute to its vagueness as a theoretical concept (Van Gorp, 2007).

Framing's strength, however, lies in its facilitation of analysis using different methodologies and "and not just assuming that the powerful are able to set and naturalize those definitions unproblematically (Reese, 2007, p.148). D'Angelo (2002) and Reese (2007) credit framing for generation of theoretical and methodological perceptions. Scheufele opines that a single news item may contain two different frames (2004, p. 5). There is the largely oral discourse used by officials who are directly involved in decision- making roles on the issue and by those who attempt to influence them. There is the challenger discourse...media discourse dominates the larger issue culture, both reflecting it and contributing to its creation. Journalists use ideas from other forums in a language understood by their audience and contribute their own frames and invent their own clever catchphrases, drawing on a popular culture that they share with their audience (Gamson & Modigliani, 1987, p.2).

LITERATURE REVIEW

Framing is widely used in areas like sociology, psychology, political science communication and anthropology (Reese, 2007; Cacciatore, Scheufele, & Iyengar, 2016). The theory's popularity transcends academic circles: "framing, unlike many more esoteric research concepts, has gained remarkable popularity in both the scholarly literature and the public imagination" (Reese, 2007, p.148). In his 2003 track entitled "Step in the name of love", R'n'B singer, R Kelly's states that, "you can change the frame but the picture remains the same". Framing also occupies prominent space in political discourse; it "plays a major role in the exertion of political power, and the frame in a news text is really the imprint of power - it registers the identity of actors or interests that competed to dominate the text" (Entman, 1993, p. 55). Cohen (1963) acknowledges that the audience's interpretation of media text is determined by "the map that is drawn for them by writers, editors, and publishers of the papers they read" (p.13). New media are also a key influence of influencing opinions. Technological affordances enable integration of content produced by traditional media and bloggers (Riebling & von der Wense, 2019). Measures such as verification badges provide checks in gauging reliability and authenticity of sources.

INFORMATION, PANDEMICS, AND PROPAGANDA

Pandemics often bring desperation which usually culminates into untested claims and conspiracy theories (Pieri, 2019, p.73). Conspiracy theorists allege that bird flue is a hoax that is meant to reduce supply and fuel inflation (CBS, 2022) whilst others claim that it is just covid for chicken. During the 2014-2016 Ebola outbreak, the British mainstream media insinuated that the virus would only affect far flung (African) countries (Pieri, 2019). Pieri adds that western countries only developed an interest in covering stories related to the virus when its devastating impact reached their shores proving that to them, diseases and deaths in western countries are more 'equal' than others. Pandemics often expose the unequal playing field in medical terms. Herbal remedies are extracted from developing countries and combined with a few western supplements and tested on people from these countries. Not only do developing countries miss out in acknowledgement and financial benefits such as intellectual property rights, but they also struggle to access medication as western countries stockpile the drugs (Pieri, 2019, Benyera, 2021). COVID-19 became synonymous with words such as "vaccine nationalism" (Murhula, & Singh, 2022, p.93) and "vaccine apartheid" (Brown & Rosier, 2023, p.535) to describe how rich countries hoarded vaccines at the expense of poor countries.

Davies and Wenham note that COVID-19) "is a political problem as much as it is a public health tragedy" (2020, p.1227). Pieri (2019) justifies the withdrawal of some countries from WHO initiative, blaming the organization for enabling multinational companies to profiteer at the expense of the developing countries by sharing viral samples from developing countries with foreign owned pharmacies. Wald observes that COVID-19 resulted in "a contradictory but compelling story of the perils of human interdependence" (2008, p.3). Developed countries were initially interested in their safety, procuring safety equipment for their citizens but later realized that they could be infected by people who have no protection. UN Secretary-General António Guterres noted that "none of us is safe until we all are" (UN News, 2020). Wald notes that COVID-19 resulted in "a contradictory but compelling story of the perils of human interdependence" (2008, p.3). Developed countries were initially interested in their safety, procuring safety equipment for their citizens but later realized that they could be infected by people who have no protection. UN Secretary-General António Guterres noted that "None of us is safe until we all are" (UN News, 2020) (compare with how Rock Hudson's death influenced responses to HIV in the discussion in the next segment).

A HISTORY OF SEGREGATION

Referring to it as the "outbreak narrative" Wald (2007, p.1), notes that in the mid-80s, stories of epidemics emerged in scientific publications and the mainstream media worldwide and were consolidated in popular novels and films in the mid-1990s. This topos "in its scientific, journalistic, and fictional incarnations—follows a formulaic plot that begins with the identification of an emerging infection and chronicles the epidemiological work that ends with its containment". xenophobia, racism, gender stereotyping and classicism are some of the inherent stereotypes of the outbreak narrative which apparently has an early provenance.

René Girard observes that every plague story needs a scapegoat, and since the early twentieth century when Typhoid Mary became a household name, women and racialized "others" have filled that role (McGuire, 2021, p.55). The most popular monicker is "Typhoid Mary" which was assumed by Mary

Mallon, an asymptomatic cook who infected different households with typhoid. George Soper, a self-proclaimed engineer who was hired to test Mallon for typhoid described Mallon as "an Irish woman about 40 years of age, tall, heavy, single" (Foss, 2020). In 1987, the National Review referred to Gaetan Dugas, a gay French-Canadian airline attendant who was erroneously recorded as the first known HIV patient, as "the Columbus of AIDS" (Howard, 2016). Other cases include The New York Times which reported about a child who was nicknamed 'the poison emperor' in China; a twenty-six-year-old Singaporean flight attendant, who infected several people, killing her parents and pastor, "turning her into a national scapegoat" when Singapore's minister of health accused her of infecting "all of us".

Western researchers and journalists seem to have a tendency of dismissing claims of white people as vectors, especially their compatriots and attributing such claims to black people and developing countries. Howard (2016) reports that a study found that Duga did not spread HIV and Campbell traces the disease to a Scandinavian who contracted it in Kinshasha, the DRC (2018). Campbell appears to mention DRC by name because it is an African country but conveniently fails to do the same with the Scandinavian country. In addition, Campbell describes Swine Flu as one of "infectious diseases of African origin, such as Ebola and HIV/AIDS". The outbreak narrative is also palpable in "Central Africa, seemed to sire new diseases with nightmarish regularity. Earlier that year, not far from Abumombazi, in a village along the Ebola River on the Zaire-Sudan border, a virulent outbreak of a horrifying new disease had demonstrated the dangers of primitive medicine and new viruses" (Shilts, 2007, p.3).

METHODS

Deploying Critical Discourse Analysis (CDA) as the methodology, this paper sought to conduct a thoroughgoing exegesis of two speeches that were made by Oppah Muchinguri between the 14th of March 2020 and 16th of January 2021. The two speeches were purposively selected because they threatened Zimbabwe's relations with its 'all weather friend' China and attracted global interest. In addition, Muchinguri-Kashiri's multiple roles as a Zimbabwean, grand(mother), friend, minister, decorated liberation fighter and veteran politician facilitates analysis of perceptions towards COVID-19 from a nexus of identities. Muchinguri-Kashiri is "considered as (former information minister, Monica) Mutsvangwa's senior in government circles" (Munhende, 2021). Studio 7 was chosen for analysis because it is popular among Zimbabweans across the globe and since its headquarters are in the US, it is free from intimidation and censorship which is common in Zimbabwe. The news report under study features representatives from the Zimbabwean government, the opposition MDC Alliance (now Citizens Coalition for Change, CCC), women and the audience. This provides balance to the reportage of stories. Simba Chikanza is a colourful figure in online journalism. He stirs controversy and makes important contributions, so he deserved academic scrutiny to establish the extent to which he balances the two. His novel way of gathering and reporting news has generated a lot of content and questions regarding ethics.

CRITICAL DISCOURSE ANALYSIS

CDA greatly influences framing in focusing on statements and their implications. Discourse refers to talk, text, speech, narratives, conversations, "stretching the meaning of discourse from a genre to a register and to a code and language" (Wodak & Meyer, 2009, p.3). CDA is multidisciplinary; it straddles fields such as psychology, linguistics, sociolinguistics among others. Michel Foucault has contributed immensely to the discourse of CDA. Foucauldian Discourse Analysis (FDA) regards discourse as a site of contestation between people who are in power and their subordinates. Power is reflected through names and titles ascribed to people according to their stations in society. Discourse affects both parties because as authorities seek to maintain their stranglehold, their subjects conform or resist. Names and terms which each group uses in reference to the other reflects their attitude.

Like Foucault's concept, Jurgen Habermas' Theory of Communicative Action (1981) recognizes the influence of power in relations. However, according to the Habermasian Discourse Analysis (HAD), human beings have a moral obligation to respect and tolerate each other for them to prosper. To Habermas, communicative action is a reflection of rationality in which the better argument wins which contrasts with Foucault's conceptualization of force influencing the outcome (Bernd-Carsten, 2004, p.4331). Nonetheless, Foucault concedes that there are instances that rationality may fall short hence he identifies an "ideal speech situation" in which few conditions must be met: discourse should be inclusive, everyone should have an opportunity to express themselves and participants should "mean what they say" (Habermas, 1998, p.282). Though it is almost impossible to achieve the ideal speech situation, it enables communicants to imagine its possibility which drives their interaction. However, as alluded to earlier, this paper adopts FDA though there will be instances in which elements of HDA are involved.

DISCUSSION AND FINDINGS

Muchinguri's celebration of rising COVID-19 cases in the United States promotes toxicity because it suspend humane, cultural values which encourage sympathy among people.. The suffix '-ka' in her use of the word 'masanctionska' (COVID-19 is a form of sanctions) has a similar function as saying '(you) see!' Ironically, as, apart from being the initial epicentre of COVID-19, China, Zimbabwe's 'all weather friend' had one of the biggest number of cases and the classification of the virus as a global pandemic on the 11th of March 2020 meant that it posed a threat everywhere. She also expresses satisfaction at the intensity with which as she claims, God has exacted a heavy punishment "Mwari abva ati zhii". The ideophone 'zhii' underlines the intensity with which God has descended on some countries in the form of COVID-19. Muchinguri's 'authoritative' claims that COVID-19 is a form of punishment are dubious because her portfolios as a minister of defence and identity as a war veteran hardly qualify her to interpret spiritual based issues. In addition, she demonstrates bias when she takes delight in the suffering of people in western countries which apparently reduces her reference to God as namedropping. Muchinguri's vindictiveness threatens the goodwill of western countries which regularly donate to Zimbabwe.

STUDIO 7 REPORTING

Reportage of Studio 7 blends several techniques to maximize the impact of the message in the limited time that is allocated to the bulletin. Ray Choto, the station's US based newsreader kickstarts the bulletin by introducing Muchinguri-Kashiri as the chairperson of ZANU PF as well as the minister responsible for the welfare of war veterans. Her portfolios do not suggest that Muchinguri-Kashiri has expert knowledge about health issues or COVID-19 which probably explains why Choto mentions them from the outset. Choto passes the baton to Nunurai Jena who is on the ground in Zimbabwe, to provide more context as well as implications of Muchinguri-Kashiri's comments. The Studio 7 duo of staffers indicate that Muchinguri-Kashiri surprised all and sundry "vakachamadza vanhu" when she described COVID-19 as God's way of exacting punishment to countries which imposed sanctions on Zimbabwe. Jena's commentary is more quantitative as he insinuates that Muchinguri-Kashiri shocked many people, "vanhu vakawanda". Though Muchinguri-Kashiri clearly revels in the misery of western countries' high Covid-19 carnage, it appears as if Choto and Jena distort her comments when they say respectively say "vachiti vanofarira" and "pavati vanofarira" which translates to 'when she said she is happy'. This creates the impression that those were the minister's words, yet the recorded clip proves otherwise though she said words to that effect. Jena subtly indicates that Muchinguri-Kashiri's comments are frivolous when he states that COVID-19 is ravaging the entire world, killing people indiscriminately yet she appropriates such a calamity to suit her narrative, that it is God's way of punishing countries which she accuses of imposing sanctions on Zimbabwe.

Furthermore, Choto metaphorically paraphrases Muchinguri-Kashiri's statement by saying she the minister described COVID-19 as a whip though she did not say so explicitly. Jena, however, uses a prosaic expression, "vachiti Mwari ari kutsiva" (she said God is avenging). It appears as though Muchinguri-Kashiri and by extension, ZANU PF and the government are paranoid because whenever things go wrong, they blame everyone except themselves. In addition, Choto and Jena's cynical attitude towards Muchinguri-Kashiri's statements is more palpable when they suggest that Muchinguri's comments are assumptious. The duo utters similar comments whose only difference is that Choto starts with the subject, western countries whilst Jena begins with the object. Choto says, 'nyika dzavati dzakatemera zim zvirango" (Countries which she said, placed Zimbabwe under sanctions and Jena says, "Zvirango zvavati zvakatemerwa Zimbabwe nenyika dzakaita seAmerica (sanctions which she said were imposed on Zimbabwe by countries like America). The root of the Shona word 'zvirango' for sanctions, 'ranga' denotes the act of punishing which explains why Muchinguri-Kashiri believes that COVID-19 is God's way of exacting penalty. Despite differing with the minister Choto and Jena maintain respect for her by calling her "Amai Muchinguri-Kashiri": 'Amai' literary translates to 'mother' and is an honorific form which is a form of address to a woman similar to "Ms".

NO ONE BENEFITS FROM THE ZERO-SUM POLITICS OF VINDICTIVENESS

Muchinguri-Kashiri comes across as vindictive when she states that COVID-19 is retribution for western countries which imposed sanctions on Zimbabwe, "Coronavirus iyi yauya iyi masanctionska aya. Masanctions auya kunyika dzinotiisira masanctions". Appearance of the plural noun "masanctions" three times serves two purposes. Firstly, it emphasizes that the virus' destruction is as big as sanctions on Zimbabwe's economy. Secondly, it shows the gleefulness with which Muchinguri-Kashiri responds to the calamity that has befallen western countries; it also creates an impression that she speaks authoritatively. In addition, Muchinguri-Kashiri celebrates restriction of citizens of people in western countries to staying indoors so their economies are 'screaming' just as they have suppressed the Zimbabwean economy, "economy yavo yaakuchema handiti yedu iri kuchemawo vari kutichemedza". Muchinguri-Kashiri seems to tie herself in knots because she admonishes then United States president Donald Trump from acting as if he is God but giggles and rhetorically asks Zimbabwe's imaginary enemies "murikuda kuti tisvinwe tiendepi chimbosvinwaio necoronavirus munzwe kurwadza kwazvinoita (where do you want us to go after we get squeezed? Get squeezed by Coronavirus so that you can understand how it feels).

MORE VOICES, MORE IDEAS, AND SOLUTIONS

Voice of America also provided opportunities to different people to respond to Muchinguri-Kashiri's claims of COVID-19 being a form of punishment. Choto paraphrases what Justin Munyaradzi, a Chinhoyi resident said Muchinguri-Kashiri's comments indicate that government officials are out of touch with what is happening in the world, that no one is immune to COVID-19. Though Munyaradzi's occupation is not provided, he contributes a well thought out, erudite analysis. For Munyaradzi, the minister's failure to comprehend that, as human beings, we ought to be guided by morals, is symptomatic ('chiratidzo') of Zimbabwe's leadership crisis. Words such as "mutungamiri" (leader) "hutungamiri (leadership) kutungamiririra (infitive term for 'presiding over'), 'gwara' (direction)X2 "tinofamba sei" (how we can navigate challenges) indicate that Muchinguri is expected to be a role model. As a leader, the minister should protect people in her society by preparing for the arrival of a crisis (in this case, the COVID-19 pandemic). So acute is the COVID-19 crisis that Munyaradzi does not mention its name, referring to it somewhat euphemistically as "njodzi" (calamity) two times, accompanied by words like "kungotiwira" (can befall us), kutiwira (to befall us) stressing possibilities of the virus spreading to Zimbabwe. To repel the devastating effects of the virus, The minister of defence whose ministry entails protection of the country's citizens, "kuchengetedzwa kwenyika" carries people's expectations, "watiri kutarsra". As such, Muchinguri ought to demonstrate a good sense of discretion, "ruzivo".

However, descriptions that are in the negative like "hutungamiri hwedu hausi kuziva" (our leadership is inept), "hauna gwara" (lacks vision) emphasize the glaring shortfalls of Muchinguri, the ministry of defence which she leads and the entire government which she is part of.

Though MDC-Alliance spokesperson at the time, Daniel Molokele was not available to comment, his predecessor, Jacob Mafume concurred with Munyaradzi that laughing at other countries was ill-advised. Mafume modifies a Shona saying, "chawana hama hachisekwe" (one should not make fun of the misfortune of one's kin) to "chawana mumwe hachisekwe" (one should not make fun of another person's misfortune). Shona language is so rich in ancient wisdom that, these few words have a similar impact to Munyaradzi's longer comments. Just as Munyaradzi expresses dissatisfaction at Muchinguri's enjoyment of other countries' COVID-19 challenges and expresses dismay at the government's failure to provide solutions, Mafume exposes the futility of such actions. Mafume suggests that the government should look for treatment methods and protection because a viral disease is like rain which reaches all corners of the earth. This pervasiveness is stressed in the repetition of the word "kwese" which means 'everywhere'.

SOUND EFFECTS

Music takes on a life of its own as acts as a soundtrack to the news. A jazz instrumental which accompanies all Voice of Africa bulletins has a nostalgic ring to it which resonates with many Zimbabweans around the world who listen to the news. Another track which can also be described as a signature tune of Studio 7 is an instrumental of Thomas Mapfumo, Chimurenga (folk Zimbabwean music)'s version of the folk song, "chave chemutengure vhiri rengoro" which loosely translates to 'the situation is now like the turning of a wagon's wheel. The song gained popularity during the colonial era when Zimbabweans bemoaned suppression of their freedom. In addition, Muchinguri-Kashiri's audience's singing provides a subtext. With lyrics of a hymn which say in part, "Amai vedu ava takavapiwa nashe (this mother of ours is heaven sent), in reporter, Nunurai Jena's background suggest Muchinguri-Kashiri's popularity.

In the same vein, the audience react in what one can describe as a call and response technique as they clap hands for the minister and share in her laughter.

SIMBA CHIKANZA'S CONVERSATION WITH MUCHINGURI-KASHIRI AS A JOURNALISM TECHNIQUE

Studio 7's coverage of Muchinguri-Kashiri's remarks about COVID-19 in a news report, the other text is a telephone conversation between Zim Eye journalist Simba Chikanza and Muchinguri Kashiri who he called masquerading as her acquaintance on the 15th of January 2021, hours after the death of minister of state and devolution Ellen Gwaradzimba. Chikanza pretends to sob and surreptiously records the conversation that he has with Muchinguri-Kashiri, Gwaradzimba's friend and colleague. As alluded to earlier, the Studio 7 text which is set in Chinhoyi on the 14th of March 2021 when the minister addressed war collaborators, is punctuated by the assumption that COVID-19 only targets Zimbabwe's enemies. On the other hand, hand, in the Zim Eye recording Muchinguri-Kashiri switches from her tonal arrogance to a sad tone.

Muchinguri's brokenheartedness is evident in the Zim Eye recording which is replete with emotive sentiments such as "COVID yatisorera" (COVID-19 has brought misery to us) and "COVID yatishurira" (COVID-19 has brought untold suffering to us). Muchinguri-Kashiri discloses that the virus once left all members within the Gwaradzimba household incapacitated though they later recovered; ZANU PF Secretary for Finance and Economic Development, Patrick Chinamasa and Joseph Chinotimba, an MP were fortunate to recover whilst a Mutare-based clerk, like Gwaradzimba succumbed to the lethal ailment. To put the devastation caused by the disease into perspective, Muchinguri-Kashiri seemingly realizes that she cannot identify all people who have been infected hence she refers anonymously to others as "ana aniko" (many different people). Despite acknowledging the enormous potency of the pandemic, Muchinguri-Kashiri remains adamant that she is fine: "Inini handis kurwaraba"(I'm not ill). To prove her fitness, the minister not only reiterates that she is fine, "nditori right" but adds that "ndri kuto batsra vamwe" (I am helping others to cope with COVID-19).

MINISTERS AS HUMAN BEINGS

COVID-19 gave Muchinguri-Kashiri a reality check to her assumptions. To her credit, she took everything in her stride; stoically spending sleepless nights nursing Gwaradzimba who she affectively refers to as her daughter and taking Gwaradzimba's widowed children with her to Manicaland where she sourced medication for them. Even when Chikanza entreats her to stay indoors as a precaution, Muchinguri-Kashiri, in a typical motherly manner, says she cannot neglect Gwaradzimba's children. Her reference to Gwaradzimba by her first name, "Ellen" consolidates the idea that the two were close friends. As early as halfway into the conversation after she exhorts Chikanza to remain strong when he 'cries', to show how caring she is, Muchinguri-Kashiri demonstrates her selflessness and sense of responsibility when she asks to be excused so that she can attend to Gwaradzimba's children as well as speak to her superiors.

In a further demonstration of her shift from feeling immune to COVID-19, she tells Chikanza after he pleads again with her to stay safe, that she is practicing social distancing, wearing a protective screen, four masks, steaming, drinking herbal concoctions which include zinc, garlic onion, honey. Muchinguri-

Kashiri concedes that she 'respects' this regimen because it enhances protection from infection, "ndozvatinorespecta manhingi zvekumaker sure kuti tiri protected".

Notwithstanding Chikanza's provocative questioning, the minister responds pragmatically when he asks what can be done to prevent the virus from decimating the country. Shei neither allays Chikanza's fears nor offers possible solutions. In fact, she seems to confirm Chikanza's fears when she agrees that the pandemic is a threat to the country's population and adds resignedly, "Zvakaoma" (it's not easy), "akomana zvakaoma haa yakaoma" haa chrwere chacho ichi chakaoma chinouraya chaizvo hachisi kumbotamba (it's not easy to deal with COVID-19). Chikanza moves on with his line of questioning, "toita sei mama toita sei" (what can we do mother? What can we do?) and Muchinguri-Kashiri's response is as honest as it is pragmatic, "zviri serious chaizvo, zviri serious" (it's very serious, really serious). Though she indicates that she is following a routine to protect herself from the pandemic, the minister concedes that "pachine rwendo" (there is still a lot of work to be done) to control the high mortality rate.

OLD HABITS DIE HARD: THE REEMERGENCE OF THE BLAME GAME

Towards the end of the conversation, Muchinguri-Kashiri eventually relents to Chikanza's lead questions. When the journalist claims to be worried that the president (Emmerson Mnangagwa)'s bodyguards may compromise his safety, the minister answers in the affirmative: "Ehe vanokanganiswa nekuti vanhu vacho ava vavengi vedu variktoshandsa vanhu vane zvrwere izvozvo kupa mashefu" (yes, the president's health may be compromised because these people are using infected people to infect senior officials). Buoyed by this sensational response, Chikanza asks why the Chinese are not assisting Zimbabwe to fight COVID-19. Again, he elicits a shocking response. Considering close ties which Zimbabwe shares with China, Muchinguri-Kashiri's comments that COVID-19 emerged after Chinese scientists lost control of experiments which they carried out in their laboratories. When she says, "vatinoti shamwari dzedu idzi honai kwavatisvitsa" (look at where our so-called friends have taken us), it seems as if she has always been cynical of the Zimbabwean leadership's friendship with its Chinese counterpart.

Interestingly, even the state broadcaster, the Zimbabwe Broadcasting Corporation (ZBC) which is regarded by many Zimbabweans as a government mouthpiece is not spared from suspicion. When Chikanza suggests that the state broadcaster increases its coverage of COVID-19-related issues, Muchinguri-Kashiri alleges that executives are only concerned about their interests.

FUTURE RESEARCH DIRECTIONS

There is need for more studies on the interface between leadership of women during a challenge such as the COVID-19 pandemic, their interactions with the media and implications on society. Mixed methods analyses involving people from a more representative sample drawn from diverse groups such as people from marginalized communities should be leveraged. A further examination of Oppah Muchinguri-Kashiri's responses to challenges facing the country, her current perceptions towards COVID-19 considering her previous controversial comments will a bring holistic analysis.

CONCLUSION

This study made the following findings: Opinion leaders have a huge influence on society, The power of information and Ethics as an indispensable part of humanity.

OPINION LEADERS HAVE A HUGE INFLUENCE ON SOCIETY

Leaders from areas such as religion, politics, science and society have a huge influence on people who look up to them. Therefore, they should behave in an exemplary way which means taking caution before speaking. They should also provide direction on how best to behave especially during times of a crisis or pandemic such as COVID-19. The media have a fundamental role of facilitating the flow of true information using different creative techniques though they should do so ethically.The tone-deaf behaviour of leaders like Muchinguri-Kashiri possibly contributed to the increases in COVID-19 cases. It took the arrival of COVID-19 in Zimbabwe, infection and deaths especially personal bereavement like the death Oppah Muchinguri-Kashiri's friend, Ellenn Gwaradzimba that the Zimbabwean government which she is a part of, to take the virus seriously. To her credit, Muchinguri representing the intersection of identities, such as mother, minister, friend realized her mistakes and assisted other people to take the necessary precautions.

THE POWER OF INFORMATION

Though COVID-19 is a lethal disease, knowledge of the disease, causes, prescriptions and proscriptions help in dealing with it. In the same vein, ignorance, myths impede progress in fighting the virus. Lack of access to information or coordination of efforts by key stakeholders nurtures misinformation, disinformation which all contribute towards increased infections. Experts should be allowed to do their work without restrictions that are based on untested claims. Citizens and journalists like Chikanza should be given access to information that they require. On their part, the experts should act responsibly.

ETHICS AS AN INDISPENSABLE PART OF HUMANITY

Ethics is an important aspect of human civilization which provides guidelines on what is morally good or wrong. As a product of culture and history, journalism, like any other profession, is guided by principles such as seeking consent, avoidance of harm and abiding by the truth. Opinion leaders like government officials should be diplomatic so that they avoid generalizations and spreading fallacies as truth because of their influence on others.

EXPECTED CONTRIBUTION TO RESEARCH AND RECOMMENDATIONS

It is hoped that this paper will stimulate interest among researchers in studying how different identities influence perceptions of COVID-19. The paper also aims to encourage public figures to ensure that they verify information before sharing because they have a huge influence on society. They must also unify instead of dividing people at all levels from community level to international level (country to country relations. On their part, journalists must always consider the greater good of society in their gathering and reportage of news. Containment of diseases requires unity of purpose among all people so governments, regional and international representatives should continue to encourage adherence to precautions though COVID-19 case have decreased.

REFERENCES

BBC. (2021a). Coronavirus in Zimbabwe: Nick Mangwana apologises for 'medical assassins' slur. https://www.bbc.com/news/world-africa-55797903

BBC. (2021b). Tanzania President confronts anti-Covid vaccine MP. http://www.channelafrica.co.za/sabc/home/channelafrica/news/details?id=ffe1c60b-0b22-426d-b567-fe6f5e9bd118&title=Tanzania%20President%20confronts%20anti-Covid%20vaccine%20MP

Bernd-Carsten, S. (2004). Whose Discourse? A Comparison of the Foucauldian and Habermasian Concepts of Discourse in Critical IS Research. AMCIS 2004 Proceedings. 538.https://aisel.aisnet.org/amcis2004/53

Brown, S., & Rosier, M. (2023). COVID-19 Vaccine Apartheid and the Failure of Global Cooperation. *British Journal of Politics and International Relations*, *25*(3), 535–554. doi:10.1177/13691481231178248 PMID:38602976

Bwire. (2021). As Tanzania Changes Tack on Covid-19, Leaders Have a Role to Play in Pushing Accurate Information. Africa Check. https://africacheck.org/fact-checks/blog/analysis-tanzania-changes-tack-covid-19-leaders-have-role-play-pushing-accurate

Cacciatore, M. A., Scheufele, D. A., & Iyengar, S. (2016). The End of Framing as We Know It… and the Future of Media Effects. *Mass Communication & Society*, *19*(1), 7–23. doi:10.1080/15205436.2015.1068811

Campbell, J. (2018). Outbreak of African Swine Flu in China is One of Many. https://www.cfr.org/blog/outbreak-african-swine-flu-china-one-many

Cassese, E. C., Farhart, C. E., & Miller, J. M. (2020). Gender Differences in COVID-19 Conspiracy Theory Beliefs. *Politics & Gender*, *16*(4), 1–10. doi:10.1017/S1743923X20000409

CBS. (2022). Conspiracy theorists claim bird flu is fake news: "It's just COVID for chickens". https://www.cbsnews.com/news/bird-flu-outbreak-2022-conspiracy-theories/

Chikowore. (2021). Zimbabwean Journalist Hopewell Chin'ono Still Fighting for Bail. Daily Maverick. https://www.dailymaverick.co.za/article/2021-01-14-zimbabwean-journalist-hopewell-chinono-still-fighting-for-bail/

Chingono, N. (2020). Zimbabwe Health Minister Facing Coronavirus Corruption Charge Sacked. The Guardian. https://www.theguardian.com/global-development/2020/jul/09/zimbabwe-health-minister-facing-coronavirus-corruption-charge-sacked

Cohen, B. C. (1963). *The Press and Foreign Policy*. Princeton University Press.

Coscieme, L., & Skodowska-Curie, M. (2020). Countries With Female Leaders Suffer Six Times Fewer COVID-19 Deaths. https://www.tcd.ie/news_events/articles/countries-with-female-leaders-suffer-six-times-fewer-covid-19-deaths/

Crandell, E. (2013). Framing in the Chinese Media: Who Framed Bo Xilai and How? American University Honors Thesis. Capstone.

Cuadrado, D. C. (2022). Corruption During Covid-19 Trends, Drivers, And Lessons Learned For Reducing Corruption In Health Emergencies. Chr. *Michelsen Institute*, *U4*(CMI), 16.

Davies, S. E., & Wenham, C. (2020). Why the COVID-19 response needs International Relations. *International Affairs*, *96*(5), 1227–1251. doi:10.1093/ia/iiaa135 PMID:34191916

Dludla, N. (2020). South Africa's chief justice unrepentant for linking vaccines to Satanism. https://www.reuters.com/article/health-coronavirus-safrica-vaccine-idUSL8N2IR2VW

Entman, R. M. (1993). Framing: Towards Clarification of A Fractured Paradigm. *Journal of Communication*, *43*(4), 51–58. doi:10.1111/j.1460-2466.1993.tb01304.x

Entmann, R. M. (2003). Cascading Activation: Contesting the White House's Frame After 9/11. *Political Communication*, *20*(4), 415–432. doi:10.1080/10584600390244176

Entmann, R.M. (2007). Framing Bias: Media in the Distribution of Power. Academic Press.

EWN. (2021). Madagascan Leader in Covid Vaccine U-Turn. https://ewn.co.za/2021/03/26/madagascan-leader-in-covid-vaccine-u-turn

Filio Marineli, F., Tsoucalas, G., Karamanou, M., & Androutsos, G. (2013). Mary Mallon (1869-1938) and the History of Typhoid Fever. Hellenic Society of Gastroenterology. *Annals of Gastroenterology*, *26*(2), 132–134. PMID:24714738

Foss, K. A. (2020). #TyphoidMary – Now a Hashtag – Was a Maligned Immigrant Who Got a Bum Rap. https://theconversation.com/typhoidmary-now-a-hashtag-was-a-maligned-immigrant-who-got-a-bum-rap-136571

France, S. (2020). Drogba Slam Medical Professors Over 'Racist' Remarks Coronavirus Vaccine Tests Should be Conducted in Africa. https://www.goal.com/en/news/etoo-drogba-medical-professors-racist-coronavirus-vaccine-tests-conducted-africa/1wuqs7zifvehm19gl6fq36yqgo

Furlong, A. (2023). WHO COVID Origins Investigation is 'Stymied'. https://www.politico.eu/article/who-abandon-covid-origin-investigation-china-data/

Gamson, W. A., & Modigliani, A. (1989). Media Discourse and Public Opinion on Nuclear Power: A Constructionist Approach. *American Journal of Sociology*, *95*(1), 1–37. doi:10.1086/229213

Global Compact Media, U. N. 2020. COVID-19: What makes a good leader during a crisis. https://unglobalcompact.org/take-action/20th-anniversary-campaign/covid-19-what-makes-a-good-leader-during-a-crisis

Goffman, E. (1956). *The Presentation of Self in Everyday Life*. Doubleday.

Goodrich, S. (2021). *Transparency International (TI). Track and Trace.: Identifying Corruption Risks in UK Public Procurement for the COVID-19 Pandemic*. Transparency International.

Habermas, H. (1998). *The Inclusion of the Other: Studies in Political Theory*. MIT Press.

Hawthorn, A. (2021). Apocalypse Then. Germ Warfare: Weaponizing an Illness Is Older Than You Might Think. https://www.cbc.ca/news/canada/newfoundland-labrador/apocalypse-then-germ-warfare-1.6052178

Henley, J. (2020. Female-led Countries Handled Coronavirus Better, Study Suggests. The Guardian. https://www.theguardian.com/world/2020/aug/18/female-led-countries-handled-coronavirus-better-study-jacinda-ardern-angela-merkel

Hotez, P. J. (2023). *The Deadly Rise of Anti-science: A Scientist's Warning*. JHU Press. doi:10.56021/9781421447223

Howard, J. (2016). The Truth About 'Patient Zero' and HIV's Origins. CNN. https://edition.cnn.com/2016/10/27/health/hiv-gaetan-dugas-patient-zero/index.html

Human Rights Watch. (2020). China: Covid-19 Discrimination Against Africans. https://www.hrw.org/news/2020/05/05/china-covid-19-discrimination-against-africans

Ivan Krastev & Mark Leonard. (2021). Every major crisis of the past decade has divided Europe. COVID is no different.Euronews. https://www.euronews.com/2021/09/08/every-major-crisis-of-the-past-decade-has-divided-europe-covid-is-no-different-view

Iyengar, S. (1991). *Is anyone responsible? How television frames political issues*. University of Chicago Press. doi:10.7208/chicago/9780226388533.001.0001

Iyengar, S. (1992). How Television News Affects Voters: From Setting Agendas to Defining Standards, 6 Notre Dame J.L. *Ethics & Public Policy,* 33.

Iyengar, S., & Kinder, D. R. (1987). *News that Matters: Television and American opinion*. University of Chicago Press.

Jacob, C., Hausemer, P., Zagoni-Bogsch, A., & Diers-Lawson, A. (2023). Policy Department for Economic, Scientific and Quality of Life Policies Directorate-General for Internal Policies. https://www.medicalbrief.co.za/as-tanzania-changes-tack-on-covid-19-leaders-have-a-role-to-play-in-pushing-accurate-information/

Kelly, A & Johnson, T. (2020). Research and Data Section. UN Women.

Koon, A. D., Hawkins, B., & Mayhew, S. H. (2016). Framing and the health policy process: A scoping review. *Health Policy and Planning, 31*(6), 801–816. doi:10.1093/heapol/czv128 PMID:26873903

Krishnatray, P & Shrivastava, S. (2021). Asia Pacific Media Educator. Coronavirus Pandemic: How National Leaders Framed Their Speeches to Fellow Citizen. University of Wollongong. doi. doi:10.1177/1326365X211048589journals.sagepub.com/home/ame

Kudzayi. (2020). Zimbabwe: Covid-19 Drugs Scandal Lays Bare the Rot in The System. https://www.theafricareport.com/30676/zimbabwe-covid-19-drugs-scandal-lays-bare-the-rot-in-the-system/

Lee, C. T., Kanji, R., Wang, A. H., Mamuji, A., Rozdilsky, J., & Chu, T. (2021). Cultural Contexts During a Pandemic: A Qualitative Description of Cultural Factors that Shape Protective Behaviours In The Chinese Canadian Community. *BMC Public Health*, *21*(1), 1897. doi:10.1186/s12889-021-11928-w PMID:34666726

Leopold Munhende. (2021). Ministers Clash Over Covid Jabs. https://www.newzimbabwe.com/ministers-clash-over-covid-jabs/

Liu, J., & McLeod, D. M. (2019). Counter-Framing Effects of User Comments. *International Journal of Communication*, 13.

Lucas, S. (2000). The River: A journey back to the source of HIV and AIDS. *BMJ (Clinical Research Ed.)*, *320*(7247), 1481A. PMID:10827067

Machaya, P. (2021). Zimbabwe Plays Vaccine Politics, Rejects Western Vaccines. https://www.zimlive.com/zimbabwe-plays-vaccine-politics-rejects-western-vaccines/

Makinana, A. (2020). Stella Ndabeni-Abrahams Pays R1,000 & Gets A Criminal Record for Lockdown Lunch. https://www.timeslive.co.za/politics/2020-04-22-stella-ndabeni-abrahams-pays-r1000-fine-after-covid-19-lunch-in-lockdown/

Makoni, M. (2021). Tanzania Refuses COVID-19 Vaccines. *Lancet*, *397*(10274), 566. doi:10.1016/S0140-6736(21)00362-7 PMID:33581810

Mavuso, S. (2020). Ramaphosa Backs Dlamini-Zuma in Cigarette Ban War. https://www.iol.co.za/news/politics/ramaphosa-backs-dlamini-zuma-in-cigarette-ban-war-47507125

McCombs, M., & Ghanem, S. I. (2001). The Convergence Of Agenda Setting and Framing. In S. D. Reese, O. H. Gandy, & A. E. Grant (Eds.), Framing public life. Academic Press.

McCoy, S. (2020). Africa's Elite Build VIP Hospitals for Themselves, Leaving Workers to Die. https://www.wsws.org/en/articles/2020/04/08/elit-a08.html

McGuire, K. (2021, March). COVID-19, Contagion, and Vaccine Optimism. *The Journal of Medical Humanities*, *42*(1), 51–62. doi:10.1007/s10912-021-09677-3 PMID:33587203

Moore, A., & MacKenzie, M. K. (2020, October 26). Policy making during crises: How diversity and disagreement can help manage the politics of expert advice. *BMJ (Clinical Research Ed.)*, *371*, m4039. doi:10.1136/bmj.m4039 PMID:33106231

Murhula, P. B. B., & Singh, S. B. (2022). The Impact of COVID-19 Vaccine Nationalism on Global Health and Human Rights to Health Standards. *The Oriental Anthropologist*, *22*(1), 93–101. doi:10.1177/0972558X221096263

Murrrey., R. (2015). Merit vs Equality? The argument that gender quotas violate meritocracy is based on fallacies. Academic Press.

Mutingwende. (2023). Religious sects shun health services as cholera spreads in Zvimba. Spiked Media. https://spikedmedia.co.zw/religious-sects-shun-health-services-as-cholera-spreads-in-zvimba/

Nagler, R. H., Vogel, R. I., Gollust, S. E., Rothman, A. J., Fowler, E. F., & Yzer, M. C. (2020). Public Perceptions of Conflicting Information Surrounding COVID-19: Results from a Nationally Representative Survey of U.S. Adults. *PLoS One*, *15*(10), e0240776. doi:10.1371/journal.pone.0240776 PMID:33085719

NewZWire. (2020). 'Open for all': Outrage as Sakunda Steps in to Revive Two Idle Hospitals For Coronavirus. https://newzwire.live/open-for-all-outrage-as-sakunda-steps-in-to-revive-two-idle-hospitals-for-coronavirus

Ogone, J. O. (2020). Mobile Phones in Africa: The Politics of Cultural And Material Integration into Local Economies. *International Journal of Cultural Studies*, *23*(4), 531–546. doi:10.1177/1367877920903739

Pieri, E. (2019). Media Framing and the Threat of Global Pandemics: The Ebola Crisis in UK Media and Policy *Response. Sociological Research Online*, *24*(1), 73–92. doi:10.1177/1360780418811966 PMID:34285639

Pindula. (2020). Zambia's Opposition Leader Says Sacking Health Minister Came ' a Little Too Late'. https://www.pindula.co.zw/2021/01/11/zambias-opposition-leader-says-sacking-health-minister-came-a-little-too-late/

Piscopo, J. M. (2021). Working Paper Effective, Decisive, and Inclusive: Women's Leadership In Covid-19 Response And Recovery. Leadership And Governance Section UN Women.

Reese, S.D. (2007). The Framing Project: A Bridging Model for Media Research Revisited. Academic Press.

Riebling, J.R., & von der Wense, I. (2019). Framing The Mass Media: Exploring 'Fake News' As a Frame Embedded In Political Discourse. *Journal of Alternative and Community*, 4.

Ritschel, C. (2020). Hulk Hogan Sparks Backlash For Suggesting Coronavirus Is Punishment From God: 'Maybe We Don't Need A Vaccine'. https://www.independent.co.uk/news/world/americas/hulk-hogan-coronavirus-vaccine-god-punishment-plagues-instagram-wwe-wrestling-a9452851.html

Rota, P. A., Oberste, M. S., Monroe, S. S., Nix, W. A., Campagnoli, R., Icenogle, J. P., Peñaranda, S., Bankamp, B., Maher, K., Chen, M., Tong, S., Tamin, A., Lowe, L., Frace, M., DeRisi, J. L., Chen, Q., Wang, D., Erdman, D. D., Peret, T. C. T., ... Bellini, W. J. (2003). Characterization of a Novel Coronavirus Associated with Severe Acute Respiratory Syndrome. *Science*, *300*(5624), 1394–1399. doi:10.1126/science.1085952 PMID:12730500

Rusike, T. (2023). My Mission is to Save Lives. https://www.sundaynews.co.zw/my-mission-is-to-save-lives/

Samad, A., Al Jerjawi, K., & Dadich, A. (2023). A. Crisis Leadership: Political Leadership during the COVID-19 Pandemic. *Sustainability (Basel)*, *15*(1), 266. doi:10.3390/su15010266

Scheufele, D. (1999). Framing as a Theory of Media Effects. *Journal of Communication*, *49*(1), 103–122. doi:10.1111/j.1460-2466.1999.tb02784.x

Scheufele, D. (2004). Framing-effects Approach: A Theoretical and Methodological Critique. doi:10.1515/comm.2004.29.4.401

Scheufele, D. A., & Iyengar, S. (2012). The State of Framing Research: A Call for New Directions. In The Oxford Handbook of Political Communication Theories. Oxford University Press.

Schmidt, T., Cloete, A., Davids, A., Makola, L., Zondi, N., & Jantjies, M. (2020). Myths, Misconceptions, Othering and Stigmatizing Responses to Covid-19 in South Africa: A Rapid Qualitative Assessment. *PLoS One*, *15*(12), e0244420. doi:10.1371/journal.pone.0244420 PMID:33351852

Shilts, R. (2007). *And the Band Played On* (20th ed.). St Martin Press.

Solvoll, M., & Høiby, M. (2023). Framing the Covid-19 Pandemic. *Mediekultur*, *73*(73), 6–27. doi:10.7146/mk.v38i73.131934

Tandwa, L. (2020). Cigarette Sales Ban: DA Labels Nkosazana Dlamini-Zuma A 'Liar', Says Ramaphosa Should 'Fire' Her. https://www.news24.com/news24/southafrica/news/cigarette-sales-ban-da-labels-nkosazana-dlamini-zuma-a-liar-says-ramaphosa-should-fire-her-20200529

Taruvinga, M. (2020). Mahomva's Reassignment Raises Stink. newzimbabwe.com.

Teicher A. (2023). Super-spreaders: A Historical Review. *Lancet Infect Dis.* . doi:10.1016/S1473-3099(23)00183-4

The Chanzo Reporter. (2021). Is This the End of Gwajima's Campaign Against COVID-19 Vaccines? The Chanzo. https://thechanzo.com/2021/08/17/is-this-the-end-of-gwajimas-campaign-against-covid-19-vaccines/

The Standard. (2020). Makandiwa, Bill Gates, vaccines and microchips. https://www.newsday.co.zw/thestandard/2020/04/12/makandiwa-bill-gates-vaccines-microchips

The Zimbabwe Mail. (2021). Outrage as Makandiwa blames vaccines for poverty in Africa https://www.thezimbabwemail.com/religion/outrage-as-makandiwa-blames-vaccines-for-poverty-in-africa/

Transparency International. (2021). Transparency International UK 2020-21. Impact report. file:///C:/Users/roya.witness/Downloads/Transparency%20International%20UK%20Annual%20Imapct%20Report%20and%20Accounts%20ye%2031%20March%202021.pdf

Türkili, C. (2022). Role of media framing on the formation of opinion. Master of Science Media and Cultural Studies Thesis. Çankaya Ankara: Middle East Technical University.

UNNews. (2020). None of us is safe until we all are, says UN chief at EU push to end COVID-19 pandemic. https://news.un.org/en/story/2020/05/1063132

Van Damme, W., Dahake, R., Delamou, A., Ingelbeen, B., Wouters, E., Vanham, G., van de Pas, R., Dossou, J.-P., Ir, P., Abimbola, S., Van der Borght, S., Narayanan, D., Bloom, G., Van Engelgem, I., Ag Ahmed, M. A., Kiendrébéogo, J. A., Verdonck, K., De Brouwere, V., Bello, K., ... Assefa, Y. (2020). The COVID-19 pandemic: Diverse contexts; different epidemics—how and why? *BMJ Global Health*, *5*(7), e003098. doi:10.1136/bmjgh-2020-003098 PMID:32718950

Voice of America. (2020). Panic Grips Faithful After Cameroon COVID Pastor Dies. https://www.voanews.com/a/covid-19-pandemic_panic-grips-faithful-after-cameroon-covid-pastor-dies/6189445.html

Wald, P. (2008). Contagious Cultures, Carriers, and the Outbreak Narrative WHO. Supporting Madagascar's COVID-19 vaccine uptake at 78. https://www.afro.who.int/countries/madagascar/news/supporting-madagascars-covid-19-vaccine-uptake-78

Willingham, E. (n.d.). COVID Vaccines Show No Signs of Harming Fertility or Sexual Function. Scientific American. https://www.scientificamerican.com/article/covid-vaccines-show-no-signs-of-harming-fertility-or-sexual-function/

Wingfield, M. (2021). Faith leaders are key to reaching herd immunity in U.S., researchers say. Baptist News Global. https://baptistnews.com/article/faith-leaders-are-key-to-reaching-herd-immunity-in-u-s-researchers-say/#.YxVUWuzMKNY

Wodak, R. & Meyer. (2009). Methods for Critical Discourse Analysis (2nd ed.). London: Sage.

Women, U. N. (2020) COVID-19 and Women's Leadership: From an Effective Response to Building Back Better. Policy Brief (18). https://www.unwomen.org/en/digital-library/publications/2020/06/policy-brief-covid-19-and-womens-leadership

Wood, M. L., Stoltz, D. S., Van Ness, J., & Taylor, M. A. (2018). Schemas and frames. *Sociological Theory*, *36*(3), 244–261. doi:10.1177/0735275118794981

Worobey, M., Watts, T.D., McKay, R.A., Suchard, M.A., Granade, T., Teuwen, D.E., Koblin, B.A., Heneine, W., Lemey, P., & Jaffe, H.W. (2016). 1970s and 'Patient 0' HIV-1 genomes illuminate early HIV/AIDS history in North America. *Nature*. 539(7627), 98–101. doi:10.1038/nature19827

KEY TERMS AND DEFINITIONS

Agenda Setting: A theory which acknowledges the influence of the media in determining issues that are considered topical in society.

COVID-19: A portmanteau of 'Coronavirus', the virus which cause it, 'disease' and '2019', the year it broke out in China, COVID-19 is a respiratory disease whose symptoms include shortness of breath and loss of appetite. It was declared a pandemic by the World Health Organization (WHO) on the 11th of March 2020.

Disinformation: Information that is deliberately spread with the aim of achieving certain ends.

Ethics: Is a subpart of philosophy which guides human behaviour, a sense of right and wrong

Framing: A theory and method which presupposes bias in the way information is presented with the aim of getting certain responses from recipients.

Misinformation: The unwitting spreading of wrong information.

Pandemic: When an epidemic spreads to more than one country.

Public Interest: What is considered as the greater good for society as opposed to individual preferences.

ENDNOTES

1 When SARS emerged in 2003, it was a rare phenomenon which was described by scientists as 'novel coronavirus' (Rota, et al.,2003, p. 1394).

2 The term super-spreader was coined in 1972, in relation to computer simulations of influenza epidemics (Teicher, 2023) but gained massive popularity after COVID-19 was declared a global pandemic by the World Health Organization to denote activities which promote the spread of the virus to many people.

3 In the 1980s, white gay men were stereotyped as vectors of HIV/AIDS (Schmidt, Cloete, Davids, Makola, Zindi et al., 2020).

4 McCombs notes that Lippman, who he calls the 'the intellectual father of agenda setting' (2018, p.2) regards the media as "the primary bridge between the vast array of events in the external world and the truncated views of these events in our minds" which means what people are exposed to conditions their minds to respond within that framework.

Chapter 15
Navigating Borders:
Communication and Language Experiences of African Migrants in South African Public Health Facilities

Ignatius Khan Ticha
Cape Peninsula University of Technology, South Africa

ABSTRACT

This chapter examines the communication and language experiences of African migrants in Cape Town public health facilities in South Africa, exploring strategies they employ to navigate language and communication challenges they may encounter in the healthcare system. About 2.9 million migrants, predominantly Africans, live in South Africa, and their movement to South Africa has brought linguistic diversity and linguistic and cultural complexity, creating unique communication dynamics in health-care settings. This mainly qualitative research draws on the responses of African migrants from various African countries purposively selected and surveyed to explore their lived experiences and perspectives. The study explores how African migrants experienced language use and communication, considering differences between migrant experiences in South African health institutions and their home countries and offering recommendations to improve communication in health facilities and, consequently, enhance the experiences of African migrants in South African health institutions.

INTRODUCTION

It has been estimated that South Africa is home to 2.9 million immigrants, which would account for about 5% of the overall population. 68% of African migrants come from the 16-country Southern African Development Community (SADC), with Zimbabwe alone accounting for about 24% of all immigrants. Besides the SADC region, South Africa hosts migrants from countries in other zones of the continent, such as Somalia, Congo, Cameroon, Nigeria, Ethiopia, and, in fact, from most countries on the continent. South Africa attracts many immigrants from Europe, North America and other world regions (United Nations Office for the Coordination of Humanitarian Affairs – OCHA, 2021). Still, the focus of this

DOI: 10.4018/979-8-3693-0624-6.ch015

chapter is African migrants. African migrants have received positive and negative responses from the South African public and institutions. They have been reported to impact society both positively and negatively, and their condition and experiences in South African society have also been portrayed in both a positive and negative light, depending sometimes on who is portraying them. African migrants have reported positive and negative experiences when accessing and using different institutions in South Africa. The rationale for this study is that healthcare is the most essential need of all members of society, local or migrant, and the material conditions of most African migrants only allow them access to the public health sector, where there seems to be a mismatch between the language competencies and language needs of African migrants and the language reality they encounter in the facilities, resulting in communication challenges that determine levels of service dis/satisfaction. These are critical issues that demand exploration.

Based on the background above, this chapter has as its primary objective to investigate the communication and language experiences of African migrants in South African public health facilities, considering how they navigate the language boundaries and create opportunities for communication. The study deals with the question, *how do African migrants experience communication and language use in public health facilities, and how do language challenges or opportunities respectively hinder or promote access to effective and efficient health care?* The study explores aspects such as how African migrants experienced language use and communication at South African health institutions, languages that they commonly used or are expected to use in communicating with health practitioners at the institutions, challenges that they have faced in communicating with health practitioners, whether cultural differences and expectations affect communication and interaction with healthcare practitioners, strategies that African migrants have employed to overcome communication challenges, the possible exposure of African migrants to discrimination, cultural insensitivity or bias in public health facilities, possible similarities and differences between migrant experiences in South African health facilities and experiences in their home countries and critically, recommendations from African migrants' perspectives on how language use and communication can be improved to enhance their experiences in South African public health facilities.

The implications of this research could be far-reaching. The findings can inform the development of policies, interventions, and training programs to improve communication, enhance cultural sensitivity, and reduce healthcare disparities for African migrants based on language and communication challenges. By understanding the language and communication challenges that African Migrants may encounter in public healthcare facilities and by engaging with suggestions (from the migrant perspective) on how to deal with the challenges, this research strives to suggest ways to create more inclusive and patient-centred healthcare environments for African migrants in public health facilities in Cape Town and South Africa broadly – through effective communication practices.

THEORETICAL/CONCEPTUAL FRAMEWORK AND LITERATURE REVIEW

The study is grounded in Communication Accommodation Theory (CAT), which emerged in the 1970s as a valuable framework for predicting and explaining the many adjustments individuals make to create, maintain, and decrease social distance in social interaction. CAT offers scope for critical engagement with interpersonal communication and communication in larger contexts of intergroup encounters such as the two intergroups in this study – African migrants on the one hand and healthcare practitioners on the other. Applied to this study, the theory allows space to explore what drives communication between migrants and healthcare workers. It has been suggested that CAT has some basic principles, which will be considered in framing the discussion in this chapter. These are: 1) Communication is influenced not only by the features of the immediate situation and participants' initial orientation to it but also by the social-historical context in which the interaction is embedded. 2) Communication is not only a matter of merely exchanging information about facts, ideas, and emotions; salient social category memberships are often negotiated during an interaction through communication. 3) Interactions have expectations regarding optimal levels of accommodation. These expectations are based on stereotypes about the outgroup members and the prevailing social situational norms, and many stereotypes are revealed on both sides in the study. 4) Interactions use specific communication strategies to signal their attitudes towards each other and their social groups, a key element in this study (Giles & Ogay, 2009).

Relegation of Communication Amid Other Pressing Imperatives of the Healthcare Sector

It has been suggested that communication across language and cultural barriers in the healthcare sector has received much interest in settings such as the U.S. However, in low- and middle-income settings such as South Africa, health communication tends to have low priority relative to other pressing issues in the health system (Hunter-Adams & Rother, 2017, p. 2). There is likely even less attention placed on migrant communication experiences in the health sector in settings such as South Africa. While Hunter-Adams & Rother (2017) focus on the importance of communication among women seeking maternal care, which, of course, is an essential area of healthcare, this study considers the communication experiences of migrants in all domains of public healthcare.

Recognising that both migrants and South Africans face a complex slew of challenges in accessing health services (e.g., long wait times and medication shortages), Hunter-Adams & Rother (2017, p2) argue that language is a crucial obstacle to adequate medical care. Issues that are highlighted in their study include the view of migrants that nurses refuse to speak English to them even where they can, and this is the standard language for both groups. Second, migrant women seeking antenatal care were forced to receive medical interventions that they did not consent, partly due to the lack of linguistic competence by some of the women, which placed a "burden" on their English-speaking (mainly) Congolese and Somali husbands to take time off work to act as ad-hoc interpreters (Hunter-Adams & Rother, 2017). Though described as a burden, these are the kinds of strategies migrants draw on to mitigate the impact of language challenges that this chapter explores. It is essential to acknowledge that the public health sector in South Africa faces many challenges that relegate matters such as effective communication and, particularly, effective, and inclusive communication with African migrants to the rear of attention-deserving matters. This is understandable, considering the enormity of the other challenges, but deserving of attention considering that the implications of in/accessibility to healthcare are enormous, justifying the relevance of this study.

Migrant Experiences of Health Communication in Other Contexts: Denmark and Thailand

In other contexts (beyond South Africa), migrants have been described as an underserved group, particularly during health crises like the recent COVID-19 pandemic. This makes them vulnerable to getting left behind in pandemic communication (Brønholt et al., 2021). During the COVID-19 pandemic, health and risk communication were critical to prevent the virus's spread and ensure awareness of the vaccine's effectiveness. This, as suggested by Brønholt et al. (2021, p. 1), is valuable as it is only when individuals have an accurate understanding of their risk of getting infected by or dying from the coronavirus disease that they can take responsibility and engage with the range of prevention practices and technologies available, something that Brønholt et al., (2021) report could not be done effectively by migrants in the Danish context due to communication challenges or deficiencies. In fact, despite the importance of health risk information during the pandemic, it is reported that fewer than half of European countries had online COVID-19 advice in at least one primary migrant language, with Denmark, the focus of the study by Brønholt et al. only publishing information in English (a language understood by many of the migrants) on how to avoid infection and information on testing only at the end of March 2020, approximately two weeks after the first national lockdown. There was, therefore, a communication gap at a crucial stage of the pandemic in Denmark and the world. In cases where language use excluded migrants, the implications were enormous, including leaving migrants vulnerable and at risk of infection. In the case of Belgium and as may have been the case elsewhere, including in South Africa, migrants resorted to social media and news from their home countries of origin to keep themselves informed and possibly safe. The complexity and challenge of communicating effectively with migrants in the health sector is not a uniquely South African challenge. Other countries face this challenge with severe implications during health challenges such as the COVID-19 pandemic. To have a holistic global picture, it is important to also engage with the challenges of communicating with migrants in the health sector in the East – Thailand.

Considering the case of Thailand, with a population of Sub-Saharan African migrants coming predominantly from Nigeria, Kenya, South Africa, Ghana, Mali, Zimbabwe, and Tanzania, Gonah et al. (2016) argue that these migrants from Sub-Saharan African countries and from elsewhere in the world face challenges in accessing healthcare services in Bangkok and that they rely on specific coping strategies in dealing with those barriers. Among the many challenges faced by migrants in Thailand are language and communication, with some of the migrants being unable to communicate and describe symptoms; migrants sometimes misunderstand, misinterpret, and fail to read the forms written in the Thai language. Language and communication challenges also affect healthcare workers who sometimes fail to understand immigrants and give appropriate care. These language and communication challenges may, in some cases, obstruct migrants' ability to get to the health care facilities as they face challenges communicating destinations with taxi drivers (Gonah et al. 2016: 241).

Migrant-Aware Health System for South Africa

In a paper that engages comprehensively and holistically with the link between migration and health, (Veareyi et al., 2017 p. 90) argue that "in the absence of a migration-aware approach to health and health-systems planning, inequities will persist, and South Africa will struggle to meet its key health targets. They adopt an expanded conception of migration that includes internal migration, arguing that, "despite popular assumptions to the contrary, the largest population of migrants within South Africa are South African nationals who move within the country, often between provinces … challenging the popular notion that South Africa is 'overwhelmed' by immigrants from other countries and particularly, other African countries (Veareyi et al., 2017 p. 90). The authors outline a plethora of structural determinants of health inequity experienced by internal and cross-border migrants in South Africa. Interestingly, communication and language are omitted from the list of determinants that the authors outline. The current study seeks to place communication and language at the fore of the conception and implementation of a migrant-aware health system, focusing on African migrants from across the South African border as this group of migrants comes to the health care system with a lot more vulnerabilities and may attract higher levels of bias, prejudice and scapegoating though they are in reality accused by locals and even government officials in unsavoury terms of congesting the health care system. However, as suggested by Veareyi et al. (2017), this is not to the extent that is often projected in the media and public discourse.

Medical Xenophobia in South Africa

Crush and Tawodzera (2011), in an interesting report titled Medical Xenophobia, argue that healthcare workers are part of the many professionals who bring xenophobia into their jobs when working with and assisting African migrants and, more specifically, Zimbabweans. I view the dynamics between migrants and South Africa(ns) and state institutions as too complex to be qualified (in all instances) simplistically as xenophobic when there is perceived unfavourable treatment of African migrants. When marginalisation, discrimination, exclusion, and bias occur in some cases, it may be xenophobic, but in other instances, the occurrences are more complex than just xenophobia. Unfortunately, the simplistic attribution of xenophobia is the easy explanation often provided. However, xenophobia exists in some instances and the report by Crush and Tawodzera (2011) highlights some interesting and significant ways in which these xenophobic tendencies are exercised against African migrants, one of which is that "communication difficulties arise when health staff refuse to communicate with patients in a common language [English] or allow the use of translators" (Crush and Tawodzera, 2011: 2). This, as indicated in the report affects predominantly African migrants and particularly, Zimbabweans who were the main subject of the study. Communication remains one of the significant factors affecting access to adequate health care for African migrants in South Africa, and this study will describe migrant experiences of communication challenges and the strategies they adopt to deal with communication challenges and mitigate its impact on their ability to access health care in public health facilities in Cape Town, South Africa.

METHODOLOGY

The study is mainly qualitative. The qualitative approach allowed for the collection of rich and detailed data that should help to reveal the nuances and subtleties of the language and communication experiences of African migrants in South African public health facilities. Attitudes towards African migrants and their experiences in public health facilities in South Africa have been a contentious subject. The qualitative data collection approach is well suited to offer a deep understanding from their viewpoint of "how" they experience these facilities and "why" they feel the way they do, with a focus on language and communication. The study sample included eleven African migrants selected using purposive sampling to ensure diversity in terms of country of origin, language spoken, gender, and length of stay in South Africa, Cape Town in particular. The population sample generated comprehensive, rich meaningful data, aligned with the research objectives, leading to in-depth insights. The research participants completed an online qualitative questionnaire, which allowed for the collection of open-ended, textual data to gain in-depth insights into their experiences, opinions, beliefs, and perspectives on African migrant language and communication experiences in public healthcare facilities in South Africa. Some of the respondents did not hold the language and technical competence to complete the online questionnaire, so they were assisted in achieving it, ensuring that the research process took the form of face-to-face interviews with the interviewer recording the responses provided as accurately as the respondent expressed them in a Google Form that had been shared with the respondents. The research participants who live mainly in the Northern Suburbs of Cape Town – particularly Parow and Bellville come from the following African countries – Zimbabwe, Cameroon, Democratic Republic of Congo, Lesotho, and Somalia. 54.5% were female, and 45.5 were female. 40% described themselves as self-employed, 40% as unemployed, 10 percent as employed and 10% as students. The participants identified themselves as first-language speakers of English 36%, French 9%, Pinyin 10%, Sesotho 9%, Shona 9%, and Somali 27%.

FINDINGS AND DISCUSSIONS

Overall Impression of Communication and Language Experiences

Although the study was mainly qualitative, a few quantitative items were embedded in the data collection. One of these was intended to gauge the overall impression of African migrants on how they have experienced communication and language use at public health facilities in South Africa. 81% of respondents described their experiences as good, 9% as unsure and 9% as bad. Overall, respondents in this study hold a positive impression of communication and language use at public health facilities. It is, however, essential to drill down into some of the perspectives they share to complement this statistical indicator or the expressed positive experience.

Some of the views that accompanied the overall impressions indicated above included the following:

- *Staff friendly, no language barrier*
- *Good, at the health facility they use mostly the international language which is English*
- *Assisted me in English*
- *I don't ubdrstsnt English well*

So, for African migrants, a marker of inclusive communication is the use of the English language to communicate with them. It is, in fact, for this reason that the respondents who for this item shared an unfavourable experience did so because they "don't ubdrstsnt English well". They seem to *own the challenge,* as seen in the possessive "I", rather than ascribing the blame for the challenge `to anyone else or the system. Considering the prescripts of the South African constitution and other language policy frameworks, promoting multilingualism, particularly the use of indigenous African languages in public health facilities, is vital. However, the language selected to communicate with African migrants at every instance should be congruent with the language repertoire of patients as it would defeat the purpose of communication if health personnel spoke an indigenous African language with all patients, including those who do not. For example, a previous study focussing on the experiences of Zimbabwean migrants in Cape Town "interpreted the language barrier as an unnecessary imposition," arguing that "nurses could speak English but tended to communicate in IsiXhosa, despite the fact that Zimbabweans could not understand this South African language" (Hunter-Adams & Rother, 2017 p. 4). Switching between the indigenous African languages and English is vital to ensure linguistic inclusivity and linguistically congruent practices, depending on the patient's or client's language competence and repertoire.

Balanced Attribution of Responsibility for Communication Challenge

Different respondents described their experiences of communicating with healthcare workers variously as "good / easy to communicate / easy and understandable", further explaining that "communication goes smoothly because, I can understand the Healthcare provider whereas the health care provider also understands me". These respondents' positive impression can be attributed partly to what they see as the "caring" temperament of the health professionals, claiming that the "Staff always ego to check if everything is alright, helpful". There is a clear link between caring qualities and effective communication in the health sector. However, there are challenges, as seen in the respondent who describes their experience of communicating with the health worker as "Xenophobic", implying that they experienced linguistic xenophobia. Therefore, as Crush and Tawodzera (2011) explain, this participant experiences xenophobia in how communication takes place but, as I cautioned earlier in this chapter, xenophobia should not be applied unquestioningly and simplistically to all situations where African migrants are made to feel discomfort or even exclusion. It is essential to consider other more nuanced but also complex explanations.

It is significant to note that the respondents are balanced in their perspectives. While some point to what they see as the "xenophobic" tendencies of the staff, others are fully aware of their culpability in the communication barriers that ensue in their engagements with healthcare workers. This is the case with the respondent who describes their experience of communicating with healthcare workers as "bad" on the basis that they "understand some words but not talk nicely", implying that for their experience to be entirely positive, they should understand and "talk nicely" in English which in their admission, they do not do. Adequate healthcare provision can only happen when communication challenges are identified and attended to.

The Good and the Bad: Balanced Migrant Perspective on Challenges

There is an even split between respondents who describe communication with healthcare workers as effective and those who do not. Suggesting that no challenges were experienced in communicating with healthcare workers, a respondent indicated, "I don't really have any challenges because I am fluent in English". Here, it is seen that the patient's fluency in English, which depends on the healthcare worker's openness to communicate in English, is a critical ingredient to effective communication with African migrants in the public health sector and, of course, a ticket to accessing adequate healthcare. The other respondents, reacting to the question whether they experienced any communication challenges, responded categorically, "Not at all. / No, Communication is good", and one would assume that, like the previously quoted respondent, "good communication" here is attributed to the possibility that both the patient and the healthcare worker are fluent in and open to using the English language.

African migrant communication experiences in public health facilities are not entirely without challenges, as seen in the comments that "some don't listen at all, but some do Can't answer well. Understand doctor but can not give well". Here, the respondent assumes some responsibility for the communication challenges experienced. They understand the doctor but cannot communicate effectively. Still, there is also a view that some healthcare workers "don't listen at all", which may imply that they do not listen effectively and do not communicate properly but it seems more likely that what is intended here is that the healthcare workers do not listen with compassion, care and patience but also do not communicate "answer" with compassion, care, and patience. The responses illustrate that English language proficiency is essential to effective communication but care and compassion are also highlighted by respondents as essential elements of effective communication. In other studies, this is a common finding where "good communication meant good care and enhanced satisfaction" (Sokhela et al., 2013, p.5).

Good-Intentioned With Unintended Outcomes: Specified Instances of Communication Barriers

Participants identified some specific instances of barriers to communication, including that "at times, most health officials like to speak their local language other than English, especially when they see a black person". This experience speaks to the point that Hunter-Adams & Rother (2017) make about healthcare workers avoiding using English to communicate with African migrants. It seems that when healthcare workers speak "their local language … other than English", this may not be with some malicious intention to disadvantage African migrants. It seems this is instead to ensure linguistic inclusivity or achieve effective communication, based on the claim that "especially when they see a black person". They assume that the patient speaks an indigenous African language because they are "a black" person". This shows that language dynamics are complex, and some good intentions, as in this case, may generate unintended results. In another instance, a respondent mentions a specific health institution, claiming that "doctors in …. [name omitted] they sigh and don't help because people is not same". When doctors in this health institution, and one that attracts many African migrants, exhibit the attitude described by the respondent, it may be assumed that this expression of frustration "sighing" by the doctors is possibly a result of difficult struggles to communicate with African migrants and possible, the lack of systems to assist them with the communication challenges. It is essential to consider ways to mitigate the impact of these communication barriers on access to healthcare.

A triad relationship of patient-interpreter-provider is highlighted as a way of dealing with communication challenges between healthcare workers and migrants but a respondent associates this with "wast of time because the Healthcare provider need to look for interpreter to translate the French speakers world into English before he or she will be able to identify the presenting problem and treat acoundlely". Identifying the use of interpreters as a viable solution to communication challenges, the respondent points to the fact that this would be time-consuming and delay the process to "identify" and "treat". Additionally, the respondent highlights the possibility that, by using the interpreter, "Communication will be very poor, they will Leads to poor diagnosis", identifying one instance involving an interpreter where, as they indicate, "I couldn't explain my problem clearly" and was "unable to ask follow up questions". This defeats the purpose of the whole process with disastrous consequences, and this is not an isolated challenge experienced when using interpreters. In another context, (Fatahi, 2010, p.5) found that despite the value they add to the communication process, "interpreters experienced a number of difficulties, including "problems of diverse health beliefs … shortage of time and lack of specific knowledge … factors that obstructed the communication process". On their part, Shamsi, et al., (2020) argue that interpreter services contribute indirectly to increased costs and the length of treatment visits. Therefore, interpreters should be used with an awareness of the value but also, shortcomings of using them in healthcare provision.

Impact of Cultural Differences or Expectations on Interaction With Healthcare Providers

Commenting on whether cultural differences impact their interactions with healthcare providers, a respondent states "No, I am a Christian most of the health care provider are Christians with only few Muslims", suggesting in a tone that is discriminatory that religion, as an element of culture is a factor in how they relate with healthcare providers. Yet another respondent indicates that "When doctor fo not understand it is because of culture. Because the people I'd dark inside. White propel always try to understand". The most significant element of this point is that the respondent feels that the people other than White doctors are "dark inside" while white people "always try to understand". This is possible prejudice and stereotyping and demanding further interrogation but it suggests that African migrants hold the view, rightly or wrongly that doctors of White background try to understand them a lot more than doctors of other racial groups whom they describe as "dark inside". An additional aspect highlighted by a respondent is that "Can't pronounce surnames correctly..some do make a morkery of it". It is taken that this refers to mispronouncing the surnames of patients and making a mockery of it, which could add hurt to the already hurt or ill. While the respondent holds a positive experience of communication and the nature of health care received from healthcare personnel of another racial group, Eshiett & Parry (p. 229) who acknowledge that "a recent migrant to the UK may feel culturally isolated during illness" and they identify a different racial dynamic in the UK health context where "the behaviour of healthcare professionals towards those of a different race can lead to feelings of discrimination and lack of sympathy, so that a gulf can be allowed to develop", impacting negatively on healthcare.

It should be noted that, while the respondent quoted earlier attaches race to discrimination and cultural insensitivity and bias, like in the UK case, some (45.5% of respondents) in this study reported experiencing instances of discrimination, cultural insensitivity, and bias in their interactions with health care workers while a majority, 54.5 did not. In a specific instance, a respondent claimed that they "Had to be taken into a interrogation though my papers were legit". In another instance, a respondent reported that they were discriminated against "Because of broken English", suggesting that weak mastery of English becomes a mechanism that shapes the attitude of healthcare workers towards them. In what is a balance to these negative experiences, another respondent states that "I have never experienced discrimination", additing that "at the health facility everyone is treated acounding to their problem and it fast come fast serve" which points to the fairness of the system. Clearly, migrant experiences of communication at health care facilities is varied and diverse but it can be noted that fewer participants felt discriminated against on the basis of cultural bias and language capability and repertoire.

Communication in South African Public Health Facilities Compared to Other Countries

The intention here was to use data provided by African migrants who had lived in a country other than their country of origin besides or before migrating to South Africa. However, none of the respondents identified themselves as having lived in a transit country and so could not compare South Africa to a transit host country. It is believed that a respondent who has experienced both South Africa and another country as a migrant would provide a more objective comparative perspective than when comparing their experiences of communication in the country of origin with South Africa. However, the comparison of South Africa with their countries of origin still offers valuable insights. A respondent who identifies themself as Cameroonian states that "health care [in their country of origin] is for all, Nigerians etc are not discriminate upon". While one would see this as an attempt to portray the healthcare sector in Cameroon as being inclusive and non-discriminatory, the claim would hold more sway if it was made by someone who identified themselves as having lived as a migrant in Cameroon such as the "Nigerians" referenced here. Yet another respondent expresses the view that their experiences were more positive in "Somalia because is talking same language", valuing monolingual communication in Somali health facilities but here again, this may not represent the whole reality as such monolingualism would exclude any non-Somali patient who may not master the language. In another reflection that suggests that the language and communication challenges reported by respondents in this study are not unique to South Africa, the respondent declares, "Cameroon in term of Communication, me at Anglophone site we only speak English in facilities why the French side mostly speak French". This demonstrates an even more complex language situation where even citizens are excluded from effective healthcare by language. Cameroon practices sectional bilingualism, where one section of the country speaks French and the other English. In this instance, it would be difficult not just for migrants who do not speak these languages but also for citizens from the other section to access healthcare effectively in the language of the other section that they may not master. Finally, comparing their country of origin to South Africa, a respondent declares, "Health care providers in South communicate more clearly". These comparative reflections suggest that the language and communication challenges experienced in public health institutions are not a uniquely South African phenomenon. Other countries struggle with similar challenges, the key among which is language barriers. The universality of language barriers in healthcare is demonstrated in a survey study that included 14 studies conducted in various developed and developing countries, covering a total of 300 918 participants. In the study, Shamsi, et al., (2020) found that "language barriers in healthcare lead to miscommunication between the medical professional and patient, reducing both parties' satisfaction and decreasing the quality of healthcare delivery and patient safety. Dynamics may be different in different countries, but this chapter deals with a universal problem, and, in some cases, the problem may not only affect international but also, local migrants.

Strategies to Overcome Language Barriers

Respondents highlighted several strategies adopted to mitigate language and communication challenges. In response to the concern that healthcare workers speak to them in South African indigenous languages, regardless of whether they understand the languages, a respondent's strategy is to "speak first to them in English" with the intention to influence the language used. Commenting on the same issue, a respondent indicates that "Often health care providers switch to local language when interacting with me, but I am assertive to redirect the language", and assertiveness here is a valuable strategy that this respondent, like the one who speaks English first uses to direct and influence the language of choice in the conversation. Faced with a similar challenge (being spoken to in indigenous South African languages they do not understand), another respondent reports "I will simply asked the health care provider to repeat in English". One sees a rich variety of strategies that African migrants adopt in response to their limited proficiency in indigenous South African languages, but healthcare practitioners are also shown to play a valuable role in overcoming language barriers. A respondent reports, "Doctor always understand what I say because doctor know Somalian people, doctor now understand Somalian broken". While this can be attributed to experience gained over a long period of time working with African migrants and mastering the skills to understand "Somalian broken" English, it is partly because of a strategy where the respondent reports

"Doctor use google yo translate somalian". Nonverbal communication is also highlighted as a useful strategy where a respondent reports that "Sometimes I use hand and sometimes", but when this does not work, there is a switch to using members of the patient community as interpreters whereby "the doctor call another Somalian come help your sister". Both parties are aware that the use of interpreters is useful, as another respondent reports that" I cope by finding an interpreter". Despite the challenges associated with the use of interpreters in healthcare, Shamsi, et al., (2020) posit that "the use of interpreter services contributes to increased patient satisfaction and improved patient care among patients with language barriers. Interpreter services have a significant association with increased physician visits, prescription drugs by physicians, and receipt of preventative services among patients". Through the strategies adopted by both African migrants and healthcare personnel, there is some indication that communication, though far from perfect, enables improved healthcare provision and satisfaction.

Respondent Recommendations to Improve Communication

Drawing on their experiences, respondents made useful suggestions for improving communication between African migrants and healthcare workers in public health facilities. Most respondents called for English medium communication, with one respondent declaring that "migrants should be recognised and English be made mandatory", another made a call "To make English a primary language" and another to "Promote English speaking all the time" and yet another, "English language should be used as a medium of communication". The repetitive quoting of these responses is intended to show the unmistakable appeal of migrants to adopt English medium communication as a solution to communication challenges between African migrants and healthcare workers. While there are calls for English medium communication, it should be noted that some of the migrants do not also master the English language well enough to communicate with healthcare workers, which is the reason for the response by one of the participants that "I must be teach English", highlighting the need to teach English proficiency to African migrants as a recommendation. Some of the respondents take a more linguistically inclusive position in what seems to be a call to migrants to embrace "South African official languages [which] should be used", and yet another proposes "Knowing at least some words of another one's language" and another, "They [I assume African migrants] should speak national South African languages". In making recommendations on how to deal with the language challenge, migrants' perspectives are balanced between calling for homogenic English language monolingual practices and inclusive multilingualism that places what I see as a fair responsibility on African migrants living in South Africa to gain some conversational competence in indigenous African languages or at least, those of the regions in which they live – isiXhosa and Afrikaans for the Western Cape.

In addition to the suggestions on language medium to be adopted are other useful ones which include the call by migrants for "sensitivity training", in my estimation, on the part of the health care worker in particular but also, the African migrants, in other words, a call "To treat people equal with respect and dignity" to "Try to accommodate everyone..." for Patients [to] be treated with love and compassion", by "having workshops with health care providers, "No racist approach", "By promoting English speaking and let African, in general, be one" and finally a call for "proper listening". These are very valuable suggestions that should improve the quality of communication and by extension, healthcare provided to African migrants. It should however be noted that these suggestions, if implemented would not benefit just African migrants but also, local patients. In what I see as stereotyping but include for the sake of reporting objectively and fully on the finding, is the view that "I would like to always communication white pepople b cause give me respect, not sick inside and try to listen to me". As suggested earlier, this is a very contentious, troubling, and possibly prejudicial viewpoint but it deserves to be explored further not just in the public health sector but in other spheres of South African society. These are very valuable elements that should ensure effective and improved communication between African migrants and healthcare workers in public facilities. The issue of communication and language barriers in the healthcare sector stands out but it is complex and there is no single solution. Considering this complexity in the South African context, Hussey (2012: 192 -193) suggests that "the ideal is for the health service to employ health professionals who are already culturally and linguistically capable. Health professionals who would be proficient in the language of their patients should be identified and recruited", further explaining that "If mother-tongue speakers are not available, health professionals must learn to speak the language of the majority of their patients". This proposal can be applied as a feasible response to language barriers between local patients and healthcare workers but would not assist African migrants who come with a variety of languages that healthcare workers may not be proficient in and would require a very sustained period to learn. Considering that this and some of the other suggestions may not apply to African migrants, the ideal solution may be for English to be adopted in communication with African migrants, and for African migrants to acquire conversational competence in English and the regional South African languages.

CONCLUSION

This chapter studied the perspectives and views of African migrants on how they have experienced language and communication in public health facilities in Cape Town, South Africa. The study explored perspectives shared by eleven African migrants from five different African countries speaking six languages, including English, French and indigenous African languages spoken in different countries on the continent. Overall, respondents hold a positive impression of their communication and language experiences in public health facilities but also identify challenges such as healthcare professionals communicating with them in indigenous South African languages regardless of whether they understood and spoke those languages. They also identify experiences of bias and insensitivity of some healthcare workers and point to their (African migrants') low proficiency in the English language as a major challenge. African migrants amplify these and make them evocative by enunciating specific instances of these challenges that they experience, explaining how they attempt to mitigate these by adopting strategies that include using interpreters, using assertiveness to control language use but also relying on the strategies that healthcare workers have adopted to function under the challenging communication contexts. A comparative perspective on patient-healthcare worker communication in South Africa and in their home countries demonstrates that language and communication challenges in the health sector are a universal phenomenon that requires carefully thought out but dynamic and contextual solutions. Drawing on the findings of this study and the recommendations of respondents and considering that this is a very complex but neglected healthcare imperative, it is recommended that: 1) Health-communication strategies and policies should give effect to the legislative framework that emphasises inclusivity and, in the process, expand inclusivity to include African migrants. 2) while multilingualism is encouraged in the healthcare sector, the study's findings lead me to recommend that when dealing with African migrants, English should be adopted as a language of inclusion, but migrants also need to be equipped with conversational skills to function in English but also, conversational skills in the indigenous languages of their host society – South Africa. The language and communication experiences of African migrants in the healthcare sector are varied and sometimes dependent on the language repertoires that they bring with them and on the background and personality of the healthcare worker assisting them, requiring that strategies to mitigate the challenges and the impact on healthcare be varied, dynamic and contextual.

ACKNOWLEDGEMENT

I would like to acknowledge the contribution of Ms Ziphora Ramaila for the initial conceptualisation of the study.

REFERENCES

Brønholt, R. L., Langer Primdahl, N., Jensen, A. M. B., Verelst, A., Derluyn, I., & Skovdal, M. (2021). Challenges and Tactics Adopted by Migrants in Denmark When Accessing Health Risk Information about COVID-19. *International Journal of Environmental Research and Public Health, 18*(17), 8932. Advance online publication. doi:10.3390/ijerph18178932 PMID:34501520

Crush, J., & Tawodzera, G. (2011). *Medical Xenophobia: Zimbabwean access to health services in South Africa.* Idasa.

Eshiett, M., & Parry, E. (2003). Migrants and health: A cultural dilemma. *Clinical Medicine, 3*(3), 229–231. doi:10.7861/clinmedicine.3-3-229 PMID:12848255

Fatahi, N. (2010). *Cross-cultural encounters through interpreter: experiences of patients, interpreters and healthcare professionals.* Geson Hylte Tryck.

Giles, H., & Ogay, T. (2009). Communication accommodation theory. Explaining Communication: Contemporary theories and examples. Lawrence Erlbaum Associates.

Gonah, L., Corwin, A., January, J., Shamu, S., Jokomo, Z. N., & Putten, M. (2016). Barriers to Healthcare Access and Coping Mechanisms among Sub-Saharan African Migrants living in Bangkok, Thailand: A Qualitative Study. *Medical Journal of Zambia, 43*(4), 238–246. doi:10.55320/mjz.43.4.315

Hunter-Adams, J., & Rother, H. A. (2017). A Qualitative study of language barriers between South African health care providers and cross-border migrants. *BMC Health Services Research, 17*(97), 97. Advance online publication. doi:10.1186/s12913-017-2042-5 PMID:28143514

Hussey, N. (2012). The Language Barrier: The overlooked challenge to equitable health care. *SAHR*, 13, 189 – 195. https://journals.co.za/doi/pdf/10.10520/EJC133688

Office for the Coordination of Humanitarian Affairs – OCHA. (2021). South Africa Reckons with Its Status as a Top Immigration Destination, Apartheid History, and Economic Challenges. https://reliefweb.int/report/south-africa/south-africa-reckons-its-status-top-immigration-destination-apartheid-history

Shamsi, H. A. (2020). Implications of Language Barriers for Healthcare: A Systematic Review. *Oman Medical Journal, 35*(2), e122. Advance online publication. doi:10.5001/omj.2020.40 PMID:32411417

Sokhela, D. G., Makhanya, N. J., Sibiya, N. M., & Nokes, K. M. (2013). Experiences of Fast Queue health care users in primary health care facilities in eThekwini district, South Africa. *Curationis*, *36*(1). Advance online publication. doi:10.4102/curationis.v36i1.60 PMID:23902165

Veareyi, J. (2017). Towards a migration-aware health system in South Africa: a strategic opportunity to address health inequity. SAHR. https://www.hst.org.za/publications/South%20African%20Health%20Reviews/9_Towards%20a%20migration%20aware%20health%20system%20in%20South%20Africa_a%20strategic%20opportunity%20to%20address%20health%20inequity.pdf

KEY TERMS AND DEFINITIONS

African Migrants: Are individuals who have moved from their countries of origin within the African continent to settle in a different African country or, in some cases, to other parts of the world.

Communication and Language Experiences: Refer to impressions left by interactions and encounters of African migrants when it comes to using and navigating languages and communication in public health facilities. This includes the various ways in which language and communication impact their experiences when seeking healthcare services.

Communication Barriers: Refer to the various factors, circumstances, or obstacles that hinder effective and meaningful communication between individuals or groups. These barriers may be linguistic, cultural, psychological, or physical, and can impede the exchange of information, ideas, and emotions.

Healthcare Workers: Also known as healthcare professionals or healthcare providers, are individuals who are trained and employed to deliver medical and healthcare services to patients.

Language Barriers: Refer to the obstacles or limitations arising due to differences in language proficiency and level of language mastery between individuals or groups who need to communicate.

Patients: Are individuals who seek or receive medical care, treatment, or attention from healthcare providers or institutions. Patients of all ages and backgrounds may require healthcare services for a wide range of reasons, including illness, injury, preventive care, chronic conditions, routine check-ups, and more.

Public Healthcare Facilities: Are institutions or centres that provide a range of healthcare services and medical care to the general population, typically under government or public ownership and operation.

Chapter 16
About Time:
The Justification for Publishing Media Literacy and Fact Checks in African Indigenous Languages

Ganiyat Tijani-Adenle
North-West University, South Africa

Israel Ayinla Fadipe
https://orcid.org/0000-0003-0862-6377
Ajayi Crowther University, Nigeria

Abiodun Salawu
https://orcid.org/0000-0002-1687-4621
North-West University, South Africa

ABSTRACT

Fact-checking and media literacy promoting organisations are now more committed than ever to combatting misinformation in Africa. The challenge, however, is that they have been publishing the bulk of their contents in colonial legacy languages of the African countries, thereby losing the opportunity to enlighten a significant part of the population that are not on the internet nor conversant with those global languages, particularly as it relates to misinformation about public health. Interestingly, a few Nigerian fact-checking organisations have commenced publishing contents in the three major indigenous Nigerian languages. This chapter reviews the efforts of three purposively selected Nigerian fact-checking organisations in reaching media publics who are not likely to be English-literate nor on the internet. Key findings are that indigenous speaking publics prefer audio-visual contents to texts, and the efforts of the media literacy organisations in reaching indigenous publics is significantly impacted by funds.

DOI: 10.4018/979-8-3693-0624-6.ch016

INTRODUCTION

The need to beam searchlight on language exclusion and development implications usually becomes paramount when it concerns people's well-being. It is the reality of the world we live in now considering the plight of numerous people in African nations. Information disorder worldwide and the critical impact of information communication technologies with social networking platforms have further heightened this concern. With the emergence of information glut comes infodemic that necessitates the need for media literacy for people that are being infected psychologically to discern this pervasive infodemic and fight its hold on them in a practical manner. The capacity of information disorder syndrome gives no regard to people's level of education; it exerts direct and indirect effects on all and sundry, causing mild to virulent effects capable of altering human life forever. The intrusive nature of information and communication technology use by the people enables information disorder prevalence. Information disorder is a complex network of human activities that have been categorised into three: misinformation, disinformation and malinformation (Wardle, 2019; Wardle and Derakhshan, 2017) depending on their level of harm. Whichever of these categories befalls society still poses a certain level of threat that needs to be tackled before information disorder destroys the world. At this juncture, efforts that have been geared towards eradicating this menace have further exposed the problem of language exclusion that has often negatively impacted human developments, especially of the African continent whose indigenous languages and cultural realities usually are not reckoned with, with regards to solutions being propounded to combat information disorder. Despite the special status accorded to colonial languages to the detriment of several African languages, many Africans who still reason, think and speak these major indigenous languages can never access many media literacy skills and fact-checking solutions. Thus, it is argued that to fully combat information disorder no human or society should be deliberately or unintentionally left behind because of language barrier. Unfortunately, many studies with regards to information disorder, media literacy and fact-checking have failed to explore the significance of indigenous languages in fighting and proffering solutions to information disorder. African indigenous language-based media literacy skills and fact-checking solutions can further positively change conversation surrounding information disorder effects in our society if consideration is given to people-oriented advocacy and solutions. Mass communication institutions' role is significant in actualising this kind of objective, especially if the mass media activities are integrated and complemented with indigenous language media. The social responsibility of all media organisations, non-governmental organisations and media practitioners is to represent the voiceless and the excluded in human communities everywhere. Therefore, this study seeks to investigate if those responsible for inclusion of indigenous language speakers in media and information literacy programmes against information disorder have done the job, and to determine challenges encountered in the process and solutions they have applied.

LITERATURE

This section foregrounds the concepts relevant to this study, empirical studies that are pertinent to this study and the theory that underpins this study.

CONCEPTUAL FRAMEWORK

This sub-section briefly discusses the concepts relevant to this study. *Misinformation* Misinformation is one of the three members of information disorder of the Internet age (Wardle, 2019), and infodemic in the news media industry has bred mistrust from which lens people currently view the industry (Forum for Information & Democracy, 2021). According to Wardle and Derakhshan (2017), misinformation happens when false connection or misleading content is shared by people unintentionally to form identity. It is driven by psychological factors. In the long run, it is believed that this gradually leads to disinformation which gives room for false content, imposter content, manipulated content and fabricated content. The third part of information disorder is mal-information that appear as hate speech, leaks and harassment which are also intended to cause harm. Moreover, Horowitz and Lowe (2020:175) foreground the impact of misinformation on humanity thus: Viral false information, siloed information habits, and growing distrust in the media are amongst today's most alarming challenges to digital media markets. These phenomena impact trust in media at all societal levels – global, regional, national, and local.

The prevalence of misinformation that has significantly impacted world citizens has been enabled by economic, socio-cultural and technological transformations that have equally destabilised media industry. Cunliffe-Jones et al. (2021) found that false and misleading information in sub-Saharan Africa has caused a wide range of harms from vigilante violence and civil unrest in Ethiopia and Nigeria, the use of wrong medical treatments for Ebola, malaria or Covid-19, and harms to mental health, politics and businesses. No wonder, Wardle (2019) acknowledges the complexity of information disorder like click-bait headlines, sloppy captions and satire that is highly deceptive as low-level information pollution in society. De la Piscina et al. (2016) surveyed European media professionals' and the internet users' opinions with regards to social networks impact, digital media quality, citizens' willingness to pay for content, degree of interactivity in the digital and future of journalism. Professionals were more critical of news quality evaluation, and thus recommended critical analysis, promotion of quality over quantity and niche specialization to combat information disorder. Equating fake news to misinformation and disinformation on social networking sites, Aïmeur et al. (2023) categorised fake news into two: intent-based and content-based. While intent-based fake news encompasses clickbait, hoax, rumour, satire, framing, propaganda, and conspiracy theories, content-based fake news consists of text (headline, hyperlinks, source and body) and multimedia (image, video, audio and animation). Although they identified artificial intelligence-based detection mechanism of fake news or misinformation such as crowdsourcing, fact-checking, block-chain methods and hybrid methods, they conclude that misinformation identification on social media platforms is still a challenge. This challenge is further highlighted by Baptista and Grandim (2020) that misinformation is made attractive in the title and language used to convey it such that people continue to share and consume it which is the main objective of perpetrators in the first place. Thus, tackling misinformation has been an engaging challenge that advocates need to deploy more, people-oriented and practicable resources to make any meaningful impact.

Fact-Checking Benefits

Considering appalling level of information disorder in human societies worldwide, fact-checking becomes significant to media practitioners due to the war against traditional media institutions and the unbridled licence the Internet has bestowed social media platforms' users to disseminate unverified information (Posetti, 2018). Fact-checking revolves around truth-telling, impartiality, verification and clarity of presentation (Wasserman and Madrid-Morales, 2022) which is anti-information disorder practice. Surveying Pakistani journalists' perceptions about the benefits of fact-checking in the news room in the age of information disorder, Ghani and Khan (2020) note that majority of the journalists reasoned that applying fact-checking in work is significant for discountenancing the narrative the media spread about misinformation which has resulted in public mistrust in them. However, even though the journalists were aware of fact-checking, they could hardly differentiate between misinformation, mal-information and disinformation. Similarly, with regards to fact-checking, Abu-Fadili (2018) advocates inculcation of news literacy that endows listening audience the understanding of the language and the conventions of news as a genre through which they can recognise how these features can be exploited with malicious intent. Its benefits to people include media knowledge, criticism, perceived realism, influence, behavioural beliefs, attitudes, self-efficacy and behaviour (Cunliffe-Jones et al., 2021). Al Zou'bi (2022) also found that media and information literacy (MIL) has a significant impact on Jordanian students' acquisition of skill needed to detect fake news. Shawcross equally (2016) posits that fact-checking has increasingly become a popular way of fighting back against the deluge of disinformation in the world today. Thus, he proposes that fact-checking advocates need to mainstream fact-checking in the media, understand and penetrate echo chambers, export fact-checking technology, encourage education and regulation, and establish a Transparency International for disinformation. The benefits of fact-checking in checkmating misinformation or fake news in news industry are dependent on adequate funding in AI, not only in sub-fields of machine learning, computer vision and planning, scheduling and optimization, but also in other sub-fields (de-Lima-Santos and Ceron, 2022). Focusing on integrating indigenous African languages into journalism education using AI, Iyinolakan (2023) also highlights improvement of journalism quality and equipping journalists with necessary skills to succeed in a digital age. Yet, he laments sluggish attitude integrating indigenous language journalism beyond entry level. As before, he canvasses for funding to train veteran and budding journalists with regards to fact-checking application in their duties.

Empirical Review

The reality about fact-checking in African languages may have been foretold by the submission of Tshabangu and Salawu (2021) with regards to the dearth of research in indigenous African language media by scholars who have long favoured colonial language media research. Fact-checking in African languages by news media may be non-existent. Highlighting the significance of African languages to news media, Salawu (2006) notes that African language pedagogy should transcend classroom learning to include the media of mass communication. Since, then there has been a considerable but not sufficient attention given to African language learning in news media as a form of mass communication. Even with the proliferation of fake news and the need to curb it through fact-checking and media literacy in news media, using indigenous language news, Onyenankeya (2022) laments insufficient funding and dwindling patronage of indigenous media as banes of the news industry. Moreover, Cheruiyot and Conie-Ferrel (2018:971) argued that 'fact-checking carries both journalistic and epistemic discourses that go beyond the figure of the journalist, and that when adopted by extra-journalistic actors, expand data-driven practices by shaping fact-checking within news organisations, but also by bypassing news media and reaching citizens directly.' Fact-checking here is seen as serving both news media organisations and media audience, which is how it can prove effective against incidence of fake news. Using three African fact-checking organisations: Code for Africa, Open Up and Africa Check, the authors state that they gather and corroborate data to verify depending on data source, and serve as watchdog to hold accountable government institutions and media organisations. Similarly, Gagnon et al. (2023) explored how platforms, news publishers, and fact-checkers described gains they made in partnerships to counter misinformation. Findings reveal that their partnerships relied on resources and news values, contributing knowledge about fighting misinformation and misinformation types that matter to the public. The authors however, recognized lack of coordination and cooperation as problems facing anti-misinformation advocacy. For Himma-Kadakas and Ojamets (2022), they reasoned that Estonian journalists employed traditional fact-checking skills in specific combinations. Moreover, they observed when the journalists were under duress, they trusted their professional experience to publish unchecked information, when the information appeared official or derived from official social media platforms or personal social media page. However, when presented with video manipulation and decontextualized photo presentation, the journalists found it difficult to fact-check the information. Markowitz et al. (2023) investigated US fact-checkers' agreement' (The Washington Post and PolitiFact) with regards to President Trump's false and misleading statements. They submit that fact-checking is a difficult business, considering variability between the fact-checkers and selection and scaling account for apparent discrepancies among fact-checkers.

Theoretical Framework

The advent of the internet and social networking sites evidently has created information disorder syndrome that makes it difficult for people using computer and phones to control themselves at times. Kandel (2020) says information disorder syndrome is the sharing or developing false information with or without the intent of harming. It involves sharing misinformation, disinformation and malinformation on digital media. She believes people engage in information for sharing sake, money and political gains, and harm. Consequently, many solutions ranging from psycho-counselling to multiliteracies model involving analytical skills that can help to thoughtfully questioning and ethically engaging civic dialogues have been proffered (Damasceno, 2021). With regards to Nigerian context, Tijani-Adenle (2021) describes information disorder as an intent to compromise the integrity of published information, act of which has affected Nigerians' trust in the news media and led to the politicians' continuous campaign to gag the media generally. Mare et al (2019) equally adduce to the fact that understanding the nature of information disorder theory in an African context goes beyond applying Western gaze. They submit that reckoning with the African contexts of news production and consumption with regards to resource-constrained newsrooms, an ever-shifting communication ecology, realignment of the relationship between producers and consumers of content, digitization of political communication, media repression, digital literacy and competencies and competing regimes of truth and non-truth will give a better understanding and appreciation information disorder nature.

METHODS

This section details the data gathering and analysis approach used for this study, which includes the research methods used in gathering data and the method of data analysis used in making sense of the gathered data.

This study is based entirely on a qualitative research approach. Qualitative research designs are research procedures focused on understanding individuals and institutions' experiences, perspectives and/or procedures without the use of numerical data (Merriam & Tisdell, 2015). Qualitative research procedures, therefore, privilege small samples with deep insights compared to quantitative procedures that utilise larger number of samples (research subjects/objects) but with minimal insights into the investigated subject (Stratford & Bradshaw, 2016). We decided on a qualitative approach because we wanted to assess, in a detailed manner, three sampled organisations' perspectives and publications as they relate to publishing fact checks and media literacy information in indigenous languages. We therefore utilised two qualitative methods (interviews and textual analysis) to appreciate Nigerian fact check and media literacy organisations' policies on the use of indigenous languages in reaching media audiences. The study also investigated the various ways in which the sampled organisations actualised these principles and their implications for media literacy awareness and indigenous language use in Nigeria.

Our study population are 12 fact checking organisations in Nigeria and those are the entire members of the Nigeria Fact-checkers' Coalition [NFC] (Egwu, 2023; Anjorin, 2023). But not all the 12 members of this coalition are full-time fact-checking and media literacy organisations. Some are mainstream news organisations while others are media-development civil society organisations. For this study, only the three members of the coalition who are recognised by the International Fact-Checking Network [IFCN]; (Dubawa, Fact Check Hub and Africa Check) are sampled for the study. The International Fact-Checking Network (IFCN) at Poynter Institute is the global association of fact-checking organisations committed to promoting truth and combatting information disorder in the world. The network empowers its members using trainings, publications, grants, conferences, and collaborations. It has strict membership rules and Code of Principles for members committed to promoting excellence and integrity in global fact-checking and the fight against information disorder. Purposively selecting these three organisations for the study ensured that the organisations sampled have the requisite experience, and they utilise best practices in their operations as they have been reviewed by the International Fact-Checking Network [IFCN] for professionalism, ethics, and integrity.

We used textual analysis and semi-structured interviews in investigating the sampled organisations' publications of fact checks and media literacy information in indigenous languages. Textual analysis involves reviewing pre-existing secondary data to obtain information that are required to answer research questions (Kuckartz, 2019). Archival materials and/or secondary data can be in several forms like text, audio, video or in any form that permits the storing and retrieving of information (Garderen, 2007). For the purposes of this study, the archival materials reviewed were the publications that could be accessed on the websites of the three Nigerian fact-checking organisations sampled (Dubawa, FactCheck Hub and Africa Check). The authors accessed the websites of the three sampled organisations for information that would aid the understanding of the organisations, as well as for fact checks and media literacy information published in indigenous languages (by the organisations). We examined the sampled organisation's websites for indigenous language fact-checks and media literacy publications, as well as audios, videos and/or podcasts. We coded for available indigenous language publications and the variety of publications' formats, as well as any information that could help us to understand the indigenous language publication/promotion praxis of the sampled fact checking and media literacy organisations.

For the interviews, we applied the semi-structured interview format. Semi-structured interviews are interview formats used in gaining information for a study by combining a pre-determined set of questions with emerging or follow-up questions that the researcher deems appropriate while conducting the interviews Naz, Gulab & Aslam (2022). This means that the researchers have predetermined set of questions that all participants in the study will/should be asked, but they vary the questions or ask additional questions not in the interview guide based on the flow of thoughts or comments of the interviewer/interviewee while the data is being gathered (Dolczewski, 2022). This format was favoured for this study because while the three sampled fact check and media literacy organisations perform similar tasks, their organisational structures, operations, and philosophies are different, and the researchers took this into account in conducting the interviews.

We were only able to interview the professionals working in two of the sampled organisations; Dubawa and FactCheck Hub. Africa Check did not respond to requests for interview. The interviews were conducted in October 2023. Two individuals were interviewed in Dubawa [the Editor and a Researcher/ Fact-Checker] while the Editor of FactCheck Hub was interviewed for the medium. We asked questions about their motivations for publishing in indigenous languages, the reception of those publications, the manpower and technical resources used, the financial implications of the venture, how they promote the publications so that Nigerians are aware of such publications and general questions about how they planned to sustain the practice. The interviews were done via chat messaging on WhatsApp and WhatsApp calls which the first author recorded and transcribed. The shortest verbal WhatsApp interview was 13 minutes while the longest was 48 minutes. Interviews of the Editors of both Dubawa and FactCheck Hub involved verbal interviews and WhatsApp chats (more than once, and on different days) while the interview with the Dubawa Researcher and FactChecker was completely via WhatsApp chats.

We utilised thematic analysis in examining and presenting the findings obtained from the use of the two research methods. Thematic analysis is a method of data analysis that presents similar findings from different methods or instruments together in a form that aids understanding and perspective (Terry, Hayfield, Clarke & Braun, 2017). We derived four broad themes from the interviews and textual analysis used in gathering data. The four broad themes are: motives, technology and workforce, reception, and funding. These themes are discussed in the findings and discussion section in detail below.

FINDINGS AND DISCUSSION

We present the findings from the data gathered based on the four themes we identified from the textual analysis and interviews conducted: motives, technology and workforce, reception, and funding. Each broad finding (based on the themes) is noted, and their implications are discussed before moving to the next.

Motive

The sampled fact checking organisations are all non-profit media organisations committed to curbing information disorder, holding public office holders accountable, and preventing the spread of information likely to harm individuals and societies in Nigeria and/or Africa. These motives are true for the three sampled organisations.

The main objectives of the sampled organisations are relatively the same: curbing information disorder and promoting media literacy. The organisations also have more detailed objectives like empowering journalists, researchers and newsrooms with the education and skills that they require to fact-check information and create more factual contents, as well as holding public officials and opinion leaders accountable for their comments.

None of the three sampled organisations specifically note their reasons for publishing contents in Nigerian/African languages in their mission, vision and/or objectives, as well as on their websites, but the two organisations interviewed (out of the three sampled) mentioned that they started publishing in

Table 1. The motives of fact checking organisations

Organisation	Motive for Publishing About Information Disorder and Media Literacy
Africa Check	"We seek to reduce the spread and impact of misinformation and promote accurate, evidence-based understanding in the public, governments and media. This will ultimately strengthen democracy, foster engaged citizenship and improve life outcomes across the continent" (Africa Check, 2023a)
Dubawa	"Through media literacy articles, fact-checks, explainers, fact sheets and online/offline engagement, encourage a more engaged and information-literate citizenry who are capable of making informed decisions a bout issues that affect their development" (Dubawa, 2023).
FactCheck Hub	"To promote and create awareness on public issues through the dissemination of balanced and evidence-based reports, while also combating rumours and misinformation" (FactCheckHub, 2023).

Source: (Africa Check, Dubawa & FactCheckHub, 2023)

indigenous languages with the intention to reach media audiences who understand and/or prefer/appreciate communication in their indigenous languages.

Our intention is to be able to reach almost all audience categories, including those conversant in indigenous languages and who will prefer to consume media contents in those languages (Kemi Busari, Editor, Dubawa).

I believe no one should be left-behind, regardless of their educational status. False information spreads so fast and when it gets to these 'uneducated people', just like every other person, they believe it, and if verified information is put out there, they don't have the privilege to read this, so as translators, I think we are doing a lot to get the information to the grassroots in a language they can easily understand. I still consistently engage in reading Yoruba literature to learn more (Elizabeth Ogunbamowo, Researcher, Dubawa).

We could not get Africa Check's policy on publishing in indigenous African languages since they were unavailable for interview, but we reviewed their websites for publications in indigenous Nigerian and/or African languages but none was found. We also searched the website for fact checks and information literacy publications (in major Nigerian languages) by searching for "Yoruba", "Hausa" and "Igbo" but no publications in these languages surfaced. What we got on the websites were fact checks about issues relating to these ethnic groups, but none of such contents was published in any Nigerian and/or other African countries' indigenous languages. All published contents were in English Language. As there was no evidence of their publishing in any indigenous language, we did not find any statement on why they were or were not publishing in Nigerian/African indigenous languages.

While the Dubawa team noted that their organisation prioritised publishing in indigenous languages because they wanted to be able to reach all media audiences by reducing the language barrier to understanding information disorder and improving media literacy, the Editor of FactCheckHub remarked that in addition to reaching all segments of the population, his organisation is also proud to help "in the revitalisation of major Nigerian indigenous languages" (Opeyemi Kehinde, personal communication, October 2023) through their consistent use in the public domain and for critical issues.

We do not think that the organisations interviewed (Dubawa and FactCheck Hub) are deficient by not specifically mentioning or highlighting their motives for publishing in indigenous languages, as they cannot highlight all policy decisions on their websites. Reaching indigenous language speaking populations fit into their broad aims of educating people about information disorder, promoting media literacy, publishing fact-checks, preventing the havocs that misinformation can cause and holding politicians, institutions, and prominent individuals accountable for their claims.

Technology and Workforce

Publishing in indigenous languages in developing economies is always a challenge because the received technologies are in the languages of the more technologically advanced nations. This reality does not discountenance the fact that some applications have options for users to choose from major indigenous languages (in their country/location) when accessing online contents. However, there is a major difference between accessing contents in indigenous languages and creating contents in indigenous languages. A major challenge with publishing contents in indigenous languages is that content creators are stuck with computer hardware and software that are not localised for their languages.

Africa Check's head office is at Johannesburg, South Africa. They also have offices in Nairobi (Kenya), Dakar (Senegal) and Lagos (Nigeria). The team (across the countries) is made up of 40 professionals (including 5 interns) but none of these team members was cited as overseeing indigenous languages or translation (Africa Check, 2023b). The organisation's website was also thoroughly reviewed but all content were published in English Language. We conclude that Africa Check does not currently publish fact checks and media literacy information in indigenous languages on their website (as at October 2023 when the data gathering was concluded). This conclusion is based solely on the review of the organisation's website, as we did not check the other platforms that they were using to publish their fact checks and information literacy content to their publics. The technology for translation question, therefore, does not apply to Africa Check.

We asked the representatives of the two organisations interviewed (Dubawa and FactCheck Hub) about the technologies that they use to publish text contents in indigenous languages, and they mentioned that they have hardware and software resources that allow their content creators to publish in the three major indigenous languages in Nigeria without compromising on the standards of those languages like the signs, vowels, and intonations.

Yes, I use G-board keyboard. It includes the ami Yoruba. Even those who translate for Igbo, Hausa, can use the keyboard for their translation (Elizabeth Ogunbamowo, Dubawa).

Our translators use the Google Yoruba keyboard, and they also have the keyboards compatible with the Hausa and Igbo languages which they use in writing and/or translating in the three prominent Nigerian languages which we publish in (Opeyemi Kehinde, FactCheck Hub).

We see this as a great development because previous studies have noted that publishing text contents in African indigenous languages was a challenge because of the absence of text creating hardware and software compatible with African indigenous languages. But we note that this opportunity may be limited to only the three main indigenous languages in Nigeria, and the hundreds of other minority indigenous languages in the country may not enjoy a similar benefit.

Regarding *workforce* and/or *manpower* for publishing in indigenous languages (particularly in text format), there is no uniformity in how the two organisations interviewed manage this aspect.

Dubawa utilises members of staff who are already part of the team for translation:

We have two in-house fact checkers who are very sound in Yoruba language. Our Editor, Prof. Ropo Sekoni is also very good in Yoruba language, and he helps reviews these contents before they are published. For the Hauwa language, we have an in-house consultant with numerous years of experience working with multinational news organisations like Deutsche Welle (Kemi Busari, Editor, Dubawa).

I am originally a researcher and fact-check officer. Apart from sourcing and fact-checking claims, I write explainers and media/information literacy articles. I believe that as journalists or media practitioners, it is our duty to put out factual information regarding events or concepts for people (Elizabeth Ogunbamowo).

FactCheckHub, on the other hand employed personnel specifically for the role of translating publications into the three prominent indigenous languages in Nigeria (Hausa, Igbo, Yoruba).

We have a team of 9 people specifically employed for the writing and translation of fact checks into the three prominent Nigerian indigenous languages. We have three for Hausa, three for Igbo and three for Yoruba (Opeyemi Kehinde).

This has greatly enhanced the organisation's ability to publish factchecks, as its website has numerous factchecks and media literacy contents in the three prominent Nigerian indigenous languages (Hausa, Igbo and Yoruba). However, it is one thing to publish contents in indigenous langauges, but ensuring the intended audience have access to the publications is another issue. The next theme addresses how these media literacy organisations ensure their publications get adequate exposure.

Reception

There are assumptions in indigenous language research that the citizens of former colonies feel deprived of the use of their indigenous languages and that they are excited to drop the use of colonial legacy languages and commence using their (indigenous) languages in all sectors, as well as in the private and public sphere. This assumption is not always correct as there are residents of former colonies who continuously prioritise communication in English, French or Spanish, because the legacy colonial languages are the languages of power, social influence, and wealth. At the same time, some others do not have adequate mastery of their indigenous languages, and so they are more comfortable and fluent in the use of the colonial legacy languages. The Nigerians who can listen to and speak in their indigenous languages are more than those who can read in and write well in the same indigenous languages. More media audiences therefore appreciate indigenous language communication better through audio-visuals, compared to text.

The elderly (which we categorise as being from 60 years and above) and those in their middle-ages (characterised in this study as from 30 – 59 years of age) are the targets of most indigenous language publications, particularly those in text formats because most young Nigerians (30 years and below) do not have adequate mastery (in text form) of the major indigenous languages in the country. This means that some cannot even speak nor understand, while those who can speak and understand have challenges writing and reading in those languages. Unfortunately, the people with phones connected to the internet (mostly android) would rather read media contents in English Language, while those who are unable to read in English are not likely to have internet enabled mobile phones. The implication of this is that the audience for media literacy contents published in indigenous languages (particularly in written form) are not mainly on the internet.

People don't read the factchecks published in Yoruba and Hausa languages like they read the ones published in English. I guess it is more difficult and not as convenient as the English publications that they find easy reading (Kemi Busari, Editor, Dubawa).

The views are low for indigenous fact checks and media literacy contents. The views of English publications are in thousands while indigenous language texts struggle to get 100 views (Elizabeth Ogunbamowo, Dubawa).

I must admit that the contents published in text format (using indigenous languages) do not get as many views/reads like the content published in English language. But that is only for text, but they watch the videos published in indigenous languages and share them on their social media groups. (Opeyemi Kehinde, FactCheckHub).

These findings support the literature on people having different capacities regarding indigenous languages. The media literacy organisations therefore ensure that they not only publish written contents in indigenous languages, but they also almost always publish those same contents in audio-visual formats (also in indigenous languages). The sampled organisations then share the videos on their social media handles and also share on social media groups that can ensure adequate exposure to the target population based on their languages. These formats ensure higher views of publications, and the organisations mentioned that it is tough to confirm the accurate number of views, as some people download them and then share, or share the links among their social networks.

People prefer what they can watch. We create media literacy information and share them via social media to Nigerian indigenous language speaking communities. People watch the indigenous language contents a lot and we find people sharing them on their personal pages on social media or in the groups that they belong to on different social messaging applications (Kemi Busari, Editor, Dubawa).

To ensure further engagements with their contents, the two sampled organisations partner with mainstream media organisations (particularly radio) to publish their fact checks and media literacy contents (on radio programmes or as spot advertisements – in indigenous languages) in order to enhance media literacy among their target audience.

We partner with Garkuwa FM in Sokoto and Passion FM in Uyo so as to get the fact-checking contents to the grassroots. We are currently publishing 13 episodes of podcasts on Radio Nigeria Network service. This is in English Language, but we plan to include indigenous languages if we see the success of this phase (Opeyemi Kehinde).

Every 6 months, we train newsrooms (on fact-checking and information disorder) and give journalists fellowships that fund their trainings, and also pay them to publish fact-checks and media literacy contents using their employers' media. This has resulted in the publishing of several contents on information disorder in the broadcast media, and this helps us reach many sectors that we may be unable to reach with text contents (Kemi Busari, Editor, Dubawa).

These confirm that Nigerians are more receptive to consuming fact-checks and media literacy contents (in indigenous languages) in audio-visual format compared to print. This means that there is a huge need for the improvement in the writing and reading skills of Nigerians in the major indigenous languages to protect the languages. In addition, the findings highlight the need for fact checking and media literacy organisations to create more audio-visual contents and publish such contents via social media and mainstream media in order to ensure that all sectors of the society get the adequate information that they require.

Funding

The findings from the *reception theme* above shows that factchecking and media literacy organisations fund the production of fact checks and media literacy contents, the translation of the publications into indigenous languages, the conversion of published texts into audio-visual formats, as well as the exposures of the publications on social media and mainstream media so that they can reach all publics. These are very expensive processes for not-for-profits to handle, and it is impacting their abilities to ensure that key fact checks and media literacy information reach all sections of the population.

The cost of engaging personnel that can create and/or translate contents into the three major Nigerian languages is huge. Dubawa is optimising the existing hands, and this has reduced their capacities to reach their targets. Dubawa currently operates in five English speaking West African countries (Nigeria, Ghana, Sierra Leone, Liberia, and The Gambia). The organisation also planned to start their publishing in indigenous languages with five major languages [Hausa, Igbo and Yoruba, Kanuri, and Krio], as well as in Twi in Ghana. However, they only currently publish in two indigenous languages (Hausa and Yoruba) even though they have sections of their websites ready for this role. Indeed, the organisation is known for professionalism and excellence, as well as in employing young and creative minds while helping them grow professionally. Funds is actually the only challenge standing in its way.

We do not current;y have any grants or endowments dedicated to publishing media literacy and fact check contents in indigenous languages (Kemi Busari, Editor, Dubawa).

On the other hand, FactCheckHub which started operations two years after Dubawa currently publishes in the three most prominent indigenous Nigerian languages, because, unlike Dubawa, the organisation currently has funding to do that.

We currently have funding to publish in indigenous languages and that is why we can afford to do all that we do and also employ staff dedicated to this (Opeyemi Kehinde).

The reality is that a one-off funding cycle will not be adequate for this huge task that the organisations are performing. They will require consistent support to be able to sustain their contributions to media literacy among indigenous populations.

We stopped the Hausa publications sometime in 2021 but we have commenced again (Opeyemi Kehinde).

We see an opportunity here, for an integrative funding approach, which can result in funders interested in combating misinformation, as well as those focused on protecting and reviving indigenous languages in Africa to come together and support credible organisations working against misinformation in Africa. That is the only way that the hard work involved in fact checking and promoting media literacy in Africa can be sustained.

RECOMMENDATIONS AND CONCLUSION

The efforts of fact check and media literacy organisations in Nigeria cannot be understated. They have consistently debunked misinformation and promoted media literacy for up to a decade (from 2014 when the oldest of the three sampled organisations was registered). However, their critical efforts may not amount to much if these publications are not published in the languages that their audiences understand and through the media platforms that they can be reached by. Fact checking organisations in Nigeria, while they have identified this gap, need to focus on how to optimally fill the gap.

We believe that Dubawa and FactCheckHub need to be commended for commencing and sustaining publications in indigenous languages even without full or partial funding. This confirms their dedication and determination to protect their publics and ensure that no section of the population is let behind. Exposing these through traditional media is also evidence of their commitment to reaching all stakeholders, particularly the minorities not adequately represented online. Notwithstanding, the organisations have to seek ways to ensure that this effort is consistent regardless of the fact that funding can sometimes be unpredictable. While this may pose a challenge, being inconsistent in their publications may make them lose their publics and this will not only affect their brands, but it will also make minorities and indigenous communities vulnerable to the havocs that misinformation can cause.

Dubawa and FactCheckHub may have to consider employing versatile hands who can be effective in creating contents in both English and any one or more of the major Nigerian indigenous languages. This will ensure consistency and serve as a stopgap when funds are slow in coming. The current style employed by Dubawa in publishing in Yoruba language, for instance, is a great sample of how this can work.

The use of indigenous languages breaks barriers and make minority and indigenous communities more open to fact checks and media literacy contents published in their languages. This will promote better health practices and imbue in them confidence to query misinformation. Promoting media literacy using indigenous languages is therefore a huge gap that media literacy and fact checking organisations have to consistently seek the fill.

This study reviewed Nigerian internationally recognised media literacy organisations' use of indigenous languages in publishing fact checks and media literacy content. While there was adequate information on the current efforts of Dubawa and FactCheckHub in reaching indigenous communities, we did not study how indigenous communities review the fact checks and media literacy information that they are exposed to. A future study on indigenous communities' reception of fact check and media literacy information will fill this gap.

REFERENCES

Abu-Fadili, M. (2018). Combatting Misinformation and Disinformation through Media and Information Lietracy (MIL). In C. Ireton & J. Posetti (Eds.), *Journalism, 'Fake News' and Disinformation: Handbook for Journalism Education and Training* (pp. 70–80). UNESCO.

Aïmeur, S., Amri, S., & Brassard, G. (2023). Fake News, Disinformation and Misinformation in Social Media: A Review. *Social Network Analysis and Mining*, *13*(1), 30. doi:10.1007/s13278-023-01028-5 PMID:36789378

Al Zou'biR. M. (2022). The Impact of Media and Information Literacy on Students' Acquisition of the Skills Needed to Detect Fake News. Journal of Media Literacy Education Pre-Prints. Retrieved from https://digitalcommons.uri.edu/jmle-preprints/28

Baptista, J. P., & Grandim, A. (2020). Understanding Fake News Consumption: A Review. *Social Sciences (Basel, Switzerland)*, *9*(10), 185. doi:10.3390/socsci9100185

Bradshaw, M. B., & Stratford, E. (2010). *Qualitative research design and rigour*. Oxford University Press.

Cheruiyot, D., & Conie-Ferrel, R. (2018). Fact-Checking Africa. *Digital Journalism (Abingdon, England)*, *6*(8), 964–975. doi:10.1080/21670811.2018.1493940

Cunliffe-Jones, P. (2021). The State of Media Literacy In Sub-Saharan Africa 2020 and a Theory of Misinformation Literacy. In Misinformation Policy In Sub-Saharan Africa: From Laws and Regulations to Media Literacy. London: University of Westminster Press. doi:10.16997/book53.a

Damasceno, C. S. (2021). Multiliteracies for Combating Information Disorder and Fostering Civic Dialogue. *Social Media + Society*, *7*(1), 1–10. doi:10.1177/2056305120984444

de-Lima-Santos, M.-F., & Ceron, W. (2022). Artificial Intelligence in News Media: Current Perceptions and Future Outlook. *Journalism and Media*, *3*(1), 13–26. doi:10.3390/journalmedia3010002

Dolczewski, M. (2022). Semi-structured interview for self-esteem regulation research. *Acta Psychologica*, *228*, 103642. doi:10.1016/j.actpsy.2022.103642 PMID:35716626

Forum on Information & Democracy. (2021). A New Deal for Journalism. https://informationdemocracy.org/working-groups/sustainability-of-journalism/

Gagnon, V. B., Larsen, R., Graves, L., & Westlund, O. (2023). Knowledge Work in Platform Fact-Checking Partnerships. *International Journal of Communication*, *17*, 1169–1189.

Ghani, A., & Khan, S. (2020). *Disorder in the Newsroom: The Media's Perceptions and Response to the Infodemic*. Media Matter for Democracy.

Himma-Kadakas, M., & Ojamets, I. (2022). Debunking False Information: Investigating Journalists' Fact-Checking Skills. *Digital Journalism (Abingdon, England)*, *10*(5), 866–887. doi:10.1080/21670811.2022.2043173

Horowitz, M. A., & Lowe, G. F. (2020). Public service media in the era of information disorder: Collaboration as a solu- tion for achieving universalism. In P. Savage, M. Medina, & G. F. Lowe (Eds.), *Universalism in public service media* (pp. 175–190). Nordicom, University of Gothenburg.

Iyinolakan, O. (2023). Exploring the Potential of Artificial Intelligence for Supporting Indigenous Language Journalism Pedagogy in Nigeria. Symposium on African Journalism Education in the Post-COVID-19 digital era, 1-8. 10.31730/osf.io/jak43

(2020). Kandel (2020). Information Disorder Syndrome and its Management. *JNMA; Journal of the Nepal Medical Association*, *58*(224), 280–285. PMID:32417871

Kuckartz, U. (2019). Qualitative text analysis: A systematic approach. *Compendium for early career researchers in mathematics education*, 181-197.

Mare, A., Mabweazara, H. M., & Moyo, D. (2019). "Fake News"and Cyber-Propaganda in Sub-Saharan Africa: Recentering the Research Agenda. African Journalism Studies, 40(4), 1–12. doi:10.1080/23743670.2020.1788295

Markowitz, D. M., Levine, T. R., Serota, K. B., & Moore, A. D. (2023). Cross-checking journalistic fact- checkers: The role of sampling and scaling in interpreting false and misleading statements. *PLoS One*, *18*(7), e0289004. doi:10.1371/journal.pone.0289004 PMID:37490489

Naz, N., Gulab, F., & Aslam, M. (2022). Development of qualitative semi-structured interview guide for case study research. *Competitive Social Science Research Journal*, *3*(2), 42–52.

Onyenankeya, K. (2022). Indigenous language newspapers and the digital media conundrum in Africa. *Information Development*, *38*(1), 83–96. doi:10.1177/0266666920983403

Patrick. (2023). "We can't do this alone": Nigerian fact-checkers teamed up to debunk politicians' false claims at this year's election. https://reutersinstitute.politics.ox.ac.uk/news/we-cant-do-alone-nigerian-fact-checkers-teamed-debunk-politicians-false-claims-years-election

Peter van Garderen. (2007). Archival Materials: A practical Definition. Van Garderen, P. (2007). Archival materials: a practical definition. *Blog. Archivemati. Ca*. https://vangarderen.net/posts/archival-materials-a-practical-definition.html

Posetti, J. (2018). News Industry Transformation: Digital Technology, Social Platforms and the Spread of Misinformation and Disinformation. In C. Ireton & J. Posetti (Eds.), *Journalism, 'Fake News' and Disinformation: Handbook for Journalism Education and Training* (pp. 55–69). UNESCO.

Ramirez de la Piscina, T., Zabalondo, B., Aiestaran, A., & Agirre, A. (2016). The Future of Journalism—Who to Believe? *Journalism Practice*, *10*(1), 71–92. doi:10.1080/17512786.2015.1006932

Salawu, A. (2006). Indigenous Language Media: A Veritable Tool for African Language Learning. *Journal of Multicultural Discourses*, *1*(1), 86–95. doi:10.1080/10382040608668533

Shawcross, A. (2016). *Facts We Can Believe in: How to Make Fact-Checking Better*. Beyond Propaganda Series. Legatum Institute.

Terry, G., Hayfield, N., Clarke, V., & Braun, V. (2017). Thematic analysis. The SAGE handbook of qualitative research in psychology, 2, 17-37.

The Nigeria Fact-Checkers' Coalition showed how collaborative journalism can work in West Africa. (n.d.). https://www.niemanlab.org/2023/10/the-nigeria-fact-checkers-coalition-showed-how-collaborative-journalism-can-work-in-west-africa/

Tijani-Adenle, G. (2021). *Information Disorder and Future of Journalism in Nigeria*. Centre for Journalism Innovation and Development.

Tshabangu, T., & Salawu, A. (2021). Indigenous-language Media Research in Africa: Gains, Losses, Towards a New Research Agenda, African. *Journalism Studies*. Advance online publication. doi:10.1080/23743670.2021.1998787

Wardle, C. (2019). Understanding Information Disorder. First Draft. https://creativecommons.org/licenses/by-nc-nd/4.0/

Wardle, C., & Derakhshan, H. (2017). *Information Disorder: Towards an Interdisciplinary Framework for Research and Policymaking*. Council of Europe.

Wasserman, H., & Madrid-Morales, D. (2022). *An Assessment of Media Literacy and Fact-Checking Training Needs of South African Schools and Universities. African Check.*

Chapter 17
Participatory Intervention in Eliminating Harmful Traditional Practices:
A Review of Female Genital Mutilation Practices in Nigeria and South Africa

Didunloluwa O. Tella
KolaDaisi University, Ibadan, Nigeria

ABSTRACT

Concerning female genital mutilation practice in Africa, much of the abolition approach has focused on mass-mediated approaches: heavy reliance on mass campaigns and enlightenment programs in the affected communities. However, little or no attention has been given to the cultural adherents/perpetrators of this practice. Thus, in order to achieve a pragmatic and sustainable outcome regarding this practice, this chapter intends to broaden the theoretical discourse (democratic participant theory), seeking to highlight participatory interventions to put an end to this harmful traditional practice in selected African countries (Nigeria and South Africa). Primarily, it intends to explore the concept of participation and dialogue by incorporating the concerted effort of all stakeholders, particularly that of the cultural adherents/perpetrators of this practice. Thus, in order to achieve a colossal decline in female genital mutilation in Africa, active participation/involvement of cultural adherents is pertinent.

INTRODUCTION

Female genital mutilation (FGM), otherwise known as female cutting or female circumcision is defined by the World Health Organization (WHO) as "all procedures which intentionally alter or damage the external female genitalia organs for non-medical reasons and which have no benefit for the health of young girls and women"(World Health Organisation, 1998, Toubia & Sharief, 2003). It is mainly classified into 4 types; Type I: partial or total removal of the clitoris and/or the prepuce (clitoridectomy),

DOI: 10.4018/979-8-3693-0624-6.ch017

Type II: partial or total removal of the clitoris and the labia minora, with or without excision of the labia majora (excision), Type III: narrowing of the vaginal orifice with covering by cutting and appositioning the labia minora and/or the labia majora, with or without excision of the clitoris (infibulation) and Type IV: all other harmful procedures to the female genitalia organs for non-therapeutic purposes, such as pricking, piercing, incision, scarification, and cauterization. It has also been defined as a cultural practice done to girls/young women to uphold a cultural practice of a rite of passage to womanhood and to curb sexuality" (World Health Organisation, 1998, Toubia & Sharief, 2003). Female genital mutilation is mostly carried out on girls between the ages of 0 and 15 years. However, occasionally, adult and married women are also subjected to the procedure. The age at which female genital mutilation is performed varies with local traditions and circumstances, but is decreasing in some countries. Therefore, social and cultural claims cannot be evoked to justify female genital mutilation (International Covenant on Civil and Political Rights, Article 18.3; UNESCO, 2001, Article 4 & UNICEF, 2005).Statistically, more than 200 million women and girls have undergone this practice and another 2million are estimated to experience it every year (World Health Organisation, 2023; Toubia & Sharief, 2003).

In other words, it (FGM) is any procedure that causes injury to the female genitals without medical indication (Epundu et al, 2018). This practice dates back to uncertain origin. Recent evidence suggests it pre-dates Christianity and Islam (Lane & Rubinstein, 1996). It was first practiced in African and European continents in countries such as Egypt, Ethiopia and Greece. Likewise, twentieth-century obstetricians in America were also reported to have performed FGM as treatment for clitoral enlargement, hysteria, lesbianism and erotomania.

In Africa, the practice of female genital mutilation (FGM) is prevalent and can be traced in 28 African nations. This is despite the fact that the use of nationality as a predictor is less significant as compared to the traditional culture. Statistics have it that each year, not less than three million women are circumcised, and more hundred million females have already been circumcised (Alhassan et al, 2021).

In Nigeria, recent statistics indicate that the practice is particularly prevalent, and still persists in Southern geopolitical zones of the country, among the Yoruba and Igbo ethnic groups (NPC, 2014; NBS, 2017; UNICEF, 2017). Although the commonest types practiced in Nigeria are types I and II, the other types of FGM (types III and IV) are also carried out, particularly in the northern parts of the country (Johnson & Mandara, 2004; 2012). While FGM is not considered to be wide-spread in South Africa; it is practiced in some parts of the Eastern Cape and Kwazulu-Natal (Immigration and Refugee Board of Canada, 2003). This is as reiterated by (Kitui, 2012) who stated that FGM remains one of the cultural practices embedded amongst the Venda community of North-East, South Africa. She explained that eight weeks or less after childbirth, Venda women undergo a traditional ceremony called '*muthuso*'. *Muthuso* is a process of cutting the vaginal flesh of the mother by a traditional healer. The flesh is mixed with black powder and oil and applied on the child's head to prevent *goni*. *Goni* has been described as a swelling on the back of a child's head. The Venda people believe that *goni* can only be cured using the vaginal flesh of the child's mother. Women who experienced FGM stated that they bleed excessively after the ceremony. Moreover, the women stated that there is no postnatal care in Venda. Consequently, the women use traditional medicine and sometimes this leads to death because of sub-standard treatment. Thus, there exists FGM in both countries.

In an effort, the World Health Organisation (WHO) together with other international bodies are aggressively making sure that this practice is eliminated or at best reduced to its barest minimum by collaborating with all stakeholders in the endemic area-this includes the perpetrators and cultural adherents of this practice (El-Defrawi, et al, 2001).

Female genital mutilation (FGM) persists despite a growing body of knowledge about its health and psychological harm. Presently, it is practiced in some 28 African countries and affects some 125 million females in the world. More than 80 million females worldwide are estimated to have been damaged by the practice. Like male circumcision, FGM is thought to have evolved independently in Africa, Australia, and America (WHO, 1998; Eke, et al, 1999).

REVIEW OF RELEVANT LITERATURES

While there are existing interventions and activities aimed at eradicating the practice, there are little or no scholarly work focusing on the cultural perpetrators and adherents of the practice. Hence, the knowledge gap. Other existing literatures have approached this practice from the perspective of women's attitude towards FGM and its association with selected socio-demographic factors. The study adopted survey method, with questionnaire being used as instrument for data collection. Findings reveal that respondents who had undergone circumcision were more likely to have their daughters circumcised and almost all of the circumcisions were performed by traditional practitioners. Results indicate that in Nigeria, FGM remains a widely prevalent phenomenon with an increasing number of women experiencing this practice. Important regional and socioeconomic disparities were used as indices, which has negatively contributed to the prevalence of the practice.

In South Africa however, FGM is a cultural practice done in certain provinces in South Africa. This is despite the fact that FGM in South Africa is officially considered to be non-existent and non-endemic. As a result, most information obtained on FGM in South Africa is based on research by individuals or international organisations (Kitui, 2012).Thus, in a way, more research must be done on FGM in South Africa to know and fully understand the extent of the problem.

Going further, another study by Kandala et al (2009) examined the Spatial Distribution of Female Genital Mutilation in Nigeria. The study leveraged on the 2003 Nigeria Demographic and Health Survey data to determine the spatial distribution of the prevalence of FGM and associated risk factors. Data were available for 7,620 women; 1,673 (22.0%) interviewed had had FGM and 2,168 women had living children, of whom 485 (22.4%) daughters had undergone FGM. The study adopted survey research design while questionnaire was used as the instrument of data collection. The population of the study comprised 7,620 women with ages between 15 and 49 years. Findings reveal that unmarried women were more likely to report a lower prevalence of FGM. Modernization (education and high socioeconomic status) had minimal impact on the likelihood of FGM, thus education plays an important role in the mother's decision not to circumcise her daughter. Summarily, the study revealed that community factors have a large effect on FGM, with individual factors having little effect on the distribution of FGM. The study recommended that individual factors such as education and community such as area and state of residence, which are strongly associated with FGM, are important in considering the economic implications of FGM in policy designs in Nigeria.

Further studies by (Whitethorn et al, 2002) indicates that female genital mutilation (FGM) is widely practiced in several regions of the world and often associated with physical, psychological, sexual and social problems. However, its continued perpetuation is dependent on the interplay of culture, lack of awareness and acceptance in some societies. Thus, health professionals must be aware of these issues in their interventions, without being judgmental. Thus, from a bigger picture, this requires the concerted effort of all stakeholders (the international, non-governmental, human rights and national organizations) on the deleterious effects of female circumcision.

Other studies by Orji and Babalola (2006) investigate the correlates of female genital mutilation and its impact on safe motherhood among 500 women aged 15-45 years in Southwest Nigeria. Survey method was used; while data was collected using a structured questionnaire from five hundred consenting subjects. Vulva examination was carried out by the investigators to confirm the presence or absence of female genital mutilation using the WHO classification. Further findings revealed that the incidence of female genital mutilation is 85%. Out of this, 86.8% had type I mutilation, while 13.2% had type II mutilation. There were no type III or IV mutilation. The lowest trend in female genital mutilation was found in the age of 15-19 years. Culture/tradition was the strongest reason for the practice. Female genital mutilation decreased with increasing level of education. Only 11.7% of those with type I mutilation compared to 48.2% of those with type II mutilation had long term complications. The mode of delivery was spontaneous vaginal delivery in majority of them with no major complications. The result of the study revealed that most of the married respondents supported the practice unlike the single respondents. This may be because a higher percentage of the married were of lower educational class coupled with pressure from in-laws. The apparent lack of support by the singles could be connected with their educational level. The practice of FGM was significantly lower among daughters of uncircumcised mothers (7.8%) compared to those in circumcised mothers (61.2%). These findings have implications when considering strategies for the elimination of this harmful tradition.

While the above reviews constitute the different aspects in which scholars have approached the phenomenon, there is scarcity of literatures on studies focusing on cultural adherents/perpetrators of the practice. The few existing ones only talk about the cultural adherents in passing. Thus, in an attempt to find sustainable, lasting solution to this practice, the effort is to evolve best communicative strategies to engage with the cultural adherents/perpetrators of this practice. These efforts should be such that information, messages, and activities can be tailored to them (cultural adherents/perpetrators) accordingly (Orji and Babalola, 2006).

Going further, Orji and Babalola (2006) assert that it is not enough to fight the practice; rather efforts must be made to include the perpetrators/adherents of the practice. As such, dialogue must be incorporated in order to put an end to this practice. It is important to state that these cultural adherents/perpetrators are traditional men and women who are deeply ingrained and /knowledgeable in their respective cultural beliefs/traditions. Hence, a local communicative approach is most suitable.

Furthermore, some factors that have enabled the practice of FGM in Nigeria and in some other climes includes: environmental, health, biologic, lifestyle, globalization, gender, religion and politics (Kolawole & Anke 2010). While all the above-listed factors remain valid, the role and impact of cultural adherents/ perpetrators of FGM practice have been neglected and remains under-researched- hence this study.

Therefore, and in order to evolve a pragmatic as well as a sustainable solution to this practice, the democratic participant theory postulated by Dennis Quail (1987) was used to interpret and give meaning to the subject matter. This theory was considered suitable because it highlights the essence of individual/ grassroot participation towards governance. In this case, it is towards the eradication of FGM practice in Nigeria. Thus, and according to this theory, can active dialogue/participation with the cultural adherents adequately put an end to the practice? In addition, what kinds of structures are in place to ensure effective participation? This is needed in order to evolve an approach which would enable participation and dialogue of the cultural adherent/perpetrators.

Going further, the lack of agency to interpret culture, evaluate options and make genuine choices on the part of the adherents is one of the reasons attributed to the continued and unabated practice of FGM (Shell-Duncan et al, 2018). In other words, the inability of the adherents to make relevant and informed decisions has served as a barrier in eliminating this practice. Thus, for them, culture holds sway and is usually presented as a justification for the continued perpetration of this practice.

Furthermore, the Democratic Participant theory proposes that participation in societal decision making and involvement in communication activities should not be the exclusive preserve of the rich but of all citizens. Summarily therefore, and in the words of Baran and Davis (2012:149-150) "democratic-participant theory advocates media support for cultural pluralism at grassroots level.

Drawing on the democratic participant theory above which serves as the theoretical base of this article, the theory states that all individuals (cultural adherents/perpetrators) are eligible to have equal access to public governance. Thus, public participation and plurality remains the core theme of the theory. The next rational question to then ask is: how can they (cultural adherents) be made to participate in the campaign to end female genital mutilation in the selected countries- Nigeria and South Africa?

In a multi-ethnic and heterogeneous country like Nigeria and South Africa; what structures/mechanisms are in place to make these adherents participate? Do they (cultural adherents) consider FGM a harmful and dangerous practice? It is expedient to state that many of these cultural adherents are masked under pseudo title of traditional birth health attendants, women leaders, and local medicine men/women. Hence, they are 'human factors' that cannot be downplayed in the fight against FGM.

Another reason this practice is prevalent and thrives in Africa -particularly Nigeria is because FGM serves as a means of livelihood for these traditional circumcisers who are often regarded as Traditional Birth Attendants (TBA). Thus, and in order to preserve the legacy of this practice, the occupation is transferred down the generations (Dare et al, 2004; Walker and Parmar, 1996). While most of the practice of FGM is perpetuated by traditionalists (circumcisers, barbers, birth attendants), licensed medical professionals are not left out as they have been found complicit to the crime. In 2011, 17% of all FGM in Nigeria was carried out by medical personnel, especially nurses /midwives. The perception of FGM as being harmless, 'good' or less risky when performed by professionals have been put forward as reasons for the practice of medical FGM and Medical FGM has come under severe criticism by the WHO.

Summarily therefore, and as stated above, the effect of FGM is a violation of the human rights of the women and girl child. FGM categorically violates the right to health, security and physical integrity, freedom from torture and cruelty, inhuman or degrading treatment and the right to life when the procedure results in death. It constitutes an extreme form of violation, intimidation and discrimination. Despite its numerous complications, this harmful practice has continued unabated, notwithstanding the VAPP Act and the resolutions that the government of Nigeria has entered into. This includes the Maputo Protocols and the sponsored resolution at the 46th World Health Assembly calling for the eradication of female genital mutilation in all nations (Klouman et al., 2005; ACHPR, 2003; Idowu, 2008). Thus, in view of all these, what needs to be done to ensure that FGM is permanently eradicated -particularly with the cultural adherents/ perpetrators?

FACTORS RESPONSIBLE FOR FEMALE GENITAL MUTILATION IN AFRICA

Existing literatures highlighted many factors aiding female genital mutilation in Africa. However, all of these factors have been grouped into five main factors namely: socio-cultural, health, biological, lifestyle, globalization, gender, religion and politics (Kolawole & Anke, 2010). It should be noted that these factors are also applicable in other countries involved in the practice.

Furthermore, and in the context of this study, the socio-cultural factor ranks high and it is one factor that has allowed for the continued existence of the practice of FGM. While this is not to underscore the relevance of other factor(s), FGM continues to thrive because it is perceived as part of the socio-cultural norms handed down by mothers and grandmothers. Thus, any attempt to discontinue the practice is met with societal pressure and risk of isolation (Babatunde, 1998, Rahman & Toubia, 2000). According to Maria Gabriella De Vita of UNICEF cited in Kelly (2006) "Female genital mutilation or cutting may be considered a social convention which is ensured through non-written system of rewards and punishments". Asides the socio-cultural reason, it has also been argued that get-rich-quick syndrome of some people is also one of the factors responsible for Female Genital Mutilation in Nigeria. (Kandala et al, 2009) submit that the socio-cultural factors are often given as reasons for the practice of FGM more than the economic reasons. However, there are instances in which those who perform the cutting get paid in cash and that the cut parts are either buried or sold.

Thus, in view of all these, what is the way out and how can such socio-cultural norms/ beliefs be eradicated or abandoned?

Participation of Cultural Adherents as a Means to End Female Genital Mutilation in Africa

There are little or no scholarly literatures on the participation of cultural adherents in the quest to end female genital mutilation in Africa as well as the countries in focus (Nigeria and South Africa). The few existing ones are sketchy and only talk about cultural adherents in passing. Hence, the knowledge gap. The reason for the absence of relevant literatures could possibly be as a result of the lack of proper structures/agency that are meant to trace and identify the perpetrators of this practice especially in remote rural places in Africa. Thus, it is as a result of lack of enforcement of the law criminalizing the practice (VAPP Act) as well as the lack of awareness of this Act in Nigeria (Nnamdi, 2019). Furthermore, and in view of the above mentioned thoughts, the next question to then ask is: what are the efforts of the government in desensitizing the (cultural adherents) and ensuring their participation in the campaign against FGM in Africa?

In 1994, Nigeria joined other members of the 47th World Health Assembly to resolve to eliminate FGM (resolution 47.10). Further steps taken include; establishing a multi-sectoral Technical Working Group on Harmful Traditional Practices (HTPs), conducting various studies and national surveys on HTPs, launching a Regional Plan of Action, and formulating a national policy and plan of action, which was approved by the Federal Executive Council for the elimination of FGM in Nigeria (Nnorom, 2000).

In South Africa, Sections 30 and 31 of the 1996 South African Constitution provide for the right to culture which must be done in compliance with the Bill of Rights. Section 211 of the Constitution recognizes the existence of cultural institutions which must comply with the Constitution. Furthermore, there are other subsidiary and regional legislations to address FGM in South Africa. These includes: (i) The Promotion of Equality and Prevention of Unfair Discrimination Act (Equality Act) which outlaw discrimination of any person on grounds of gender and culture, including FGM and,(ii) Section 12(2)(a), the Children's Act explicitly prohibits genital mutilation or circumcision of female children.

Despite all these legislations however, it is obvious the practice still persists as there are lack of structures/ laws to enforce it. Summarily, and just as UNICEF (2013:106) puts it:

Nigeria still has many customary laws in place that provide institutional support for practices such as FGM, child marriage, and dis-inheritance that limits women's right to equality. Even where laws exist to outlaw these practices, evidence shows that the enforcement level is negligible.

Thus, in view of all these, there is the need to educate and re-orientate the (cultural adherents). As stated above, there is no doubt that the bulk of the efforts/ strategies adopted by the government and other well-meaning international organizations have been done via mass-mediated platforms such as TV, radio, billboards, etc. Despite this however, the practice has continued unabated as there are currently over 20 million women and girls that have been mutilated in Nigeria (Nnamdi, 2019). In South Africa, there are increasing reports of North-East African migrant women arriving in South African hospitals showing signs of genital mutilation (Smillie, 2022). This is despite the fact that FGM in South Africa is officially regarded as non-existent.

Thus, and in order to engender participation of the adherents in a bid to end the practice, there is need to tailor the messages according to the demographics of these cultural adherents. By demographic, there is need to take into consideration the level of education, language, and other factors while passing across the message. Hence, it is not just about educating; the effort is to ensure the message is well received and acted upon.

Educating the Cultural Adherents: A Way to End Female Genital Mutilation (FGM) in Africa

Many scholars have suggested education as one of the principal ways to tackle FGM in Africa (Agboli, 2021; Okeke et al, 2012; Titilayo et al, 2015). In addition, the prevalence of FGM in many countries (especially Nigeria) suggests that FGM can only be effectively eliminated when its practitioners are presented with a safe alternative that preserves their culture and, at the same time, protects the health and well-being of women (Jones et al, 2004). Recognizing that there is no simple solution to the problem; Jones et al, (2004) further states that such interventions for preventing FGM should be non-directive, culture-specific and multi-faceted to be of practical relevance. According to the authors, such interventions should not only motivate change, but should also help communities to establish practical means by which that change can occur. As such, prevention interventions should be targeted at local practitioners of FGM, parents, at-risk adolescents, health and social workers, governments, religious authorities, the civil society, and communities are presented.

Focusing on the local practitioners, and in view of the fact that FGM is predominantly done by 'traditional female excisors" (WHO, 1999). Jones et al, (2004) argues that since FGM is considered a skill, and women who perform it are being paid for it; it would only be fair on the part of these women to be offered the opportunity to be re-trained in alternative skill. The authors further suggest that without offering to re-train and pay these circumcisers, the women would have no way to support themselves and it would be unlikely that they would stop practicing their trade. Thus, while re-training efforts would vary slightly depending on the local infrastructure and needs, these women could be re-trained as village health workers or birth attendants. The re-trained women could then begin to work toward solving the most pressing problems facing their communities, such as communicable diseases and malnutrition. In addition to providing skilled workers to combat growing health problems many of which are of greater immediate concern than FGM, re-training traditional circumcisers would allow these women to retain their place of importance and respect in society without continuing the practice of FGM (WHO, 1999).

Furthermore, and having established the fact that education remains valid in the fight against FGM, there is need to be familiar with the demographics of the recipient of the message. Furthermore, information about FGM/C must be tailored to fit the needs of the target populations, as this increases the acceptability of the program and leads to quicker dissemination of information among communities (Waigwa et al, 2018). This is needed in order to channel the intended message to the recipient (cultural adherent). This is to avoid misinterpretation and ambiguity of the message.

As such, consideration of the target population's characteristics must be present in order to contextualize educational interventions that use a rights-based approach. Thus, contextualizing involves the full inclusion of the communities in planning the programs, by involving community members as facilitators or research assistants. Religious and other key leaders must be empowered by helping promote the interventions (Asekun-Olarinmoye and Amusan, 2008).

The recipients of the message here are (cultural adherents) are usually grassroot people. Thus, the message and the medium of dissemination should be simple, clear, and unambiguous.

Usually, education of this sort takes the form of health talks/seminars, health campaigns, and other health interventions towards the eradication of FGM. However, very little results have been achieved (Awolola & Ilupeju, 2019).

Some other measures targeted towards the circumcisers includes the provision of alternative sources of income for the circumcisers, legislation, awareness campaigns, community leaders' participation in the abandonment, education of the girls, and the efforts of the non-governmental organizations and professional bodies (Titilayo et al, 2015).

However, all of these measures yielded poorly mainly because they were not well implemented/ enforced or not the best approach to eliminating FGM. Thus, while community-based educational initiatives are critical and have become a key component of campaigns worldwide. Government action is necessary to create a political and legal environment that deters people from practicing FGM/C, but it is ultimately the women, their families, and their communities who must be convinced to abandon the practice (Mohammed et al, 2016).

AN ENABLING ENVIRONMENT: A WAY TO ELIMINATE FEMALE GENITAL MUTILATION IN AFRICA

The Law and Female Genital Mutilation in Nigeria

Legislation is an important tool for eradicating FGM/C, as it can challenge the traditional status quo by providing legitimacy to new behaviors—but unless it is accompanied by measures aimed at influencing cultural traditions and expectations, it tends to be ineffective (UNICEF, 2013). In Nigeria and shortly before the introduction of the VAPP (Violence Against Person Prohibition) Act in 2015. There were no specific legislations outlawing female genital mutilation practice. Hence, most lawyers, non-governmental organizations (NGOs) and anti-FGM campaigners in Nigeria relied solely on the Nigerian Constitution and the Child Rights Act (CRA) to help speak out against FGM/C in the country. In addition, thirteen (13) out of 36 states in Nigeria have their own individual state laws expressly prohibiting FGM/C. These states are Lagos, Osun, Ondo, Ekiti, Bayelsa, Ogun, Delta, Ebonyi, Oyo, Imo, Edo, Cross-River and Rivers. Thus, there are no generally articulate laws criminalizing FGM in Nigeria. This, in a way created a gap towards outlawing and criminalizing the practice. Despite these however, human rights activists and lawyers continued to make use of the provisions in both Acts (The Nigeria Constitution and the Child Rights Acts) which are as follows:

The 1999 Constitution of the Federal Republic of Nigeria (CFRN) Section 34, states that *"no person shall be subjected to any form of torture, inhuman or degrading treatment or punishment"*. FGM/C falls under the above categories and thus can be punishable under this section. Furthermore, the Child Rights Act (CRA), which was passed in 2003 in Nigeria, also has some provisions that outlaw this practice. *Section 11(B) of this Act states that "no child shall be subjected to any form of torture, inhuman or degrading treatment or punishment".*

While these two legislations appear to deem FGM/C illegal, they don't specifically mention the practice. As a result, lawyers, NGOs and anti-FGM campaigners in Nigeria came together and started to advocate for a law which would specifically mention FGM/C as a criminal offence. Consequently, in the year 2015, the VAPP (Violence Against Persons Prohibition) Act was passed into law. This particular legislation explicitly mentions FGM/C as a criminal act. It also makes FGM/C and other forms of gender-based violence such as rape, spousal battery, and forceful ejection from home and harmful widowhood practices punishable offenses in Nigeria. The VAPP Act also arranges provisions for the maximum protection of victims and for the distribution of effective remedies to them.

In addition, the VAPP Act outlines a set of punishments for FGM. These punishments include:

1. Anybody who performs or engages another to perform FGM/C on any person is liable to a term of imprisonment not exceeding 4 years or to a fine not exceeding N200,000 or to both.
2. Anybody who attempts, aids, abets, or incites another to carry out FGM/C is liable to a term not exceeding 2 years' imprisonment or to a fine not exceeding N100, 000 or to both.

In most cases, the persons convicted under the law are liable to fine and imprisonment. However, enforcement of the law is not satisfactory and many believe this poor enforcement is the result of low fines and short duration of imprisonment (Kandala et al, 2009). Till date, there hasn't been any convictions/prosecutions regarding FGM/C in Nigeria. Another reason for the lack of enforcement is that the VAPP Act cannot apply in a particular state unless it is domesticated. This is because the VAPP Act is a federal law hence it cannot be enforced unless it is accepted and domesticated in that particular state. Currently, however, only three (3) out of the 36 states are actively enforcing VAPP Act. They are Anambra, Oyo, Ebonyi and the FCT. This current statistic shows that achieving an enabling environment for outlawing FGM is still a long walk in the park in Nigeria. Thus, there is need for consistent laws and enforcement across the country and efforts need to be intensified in the areas as well.

One other reason for the lack of enforcement is the lack of awareness of this Act in Nigeria. Many Nigerians do not know about the VAPP Act. Currently, it is estimated that 1 out of every 100 Nigerians knows about the existence of this law. It is also estimated that only 10 out of every 200 Nigerians really know what this Act says.

To further validate the point above, a study was recently conducted in the Nsukka Local Government Area (LGA) of Enugu, Nigeria. The purpose of this study was to determine the level of awareness among Enugu citizens of the VAPP Act in 2015.

A multi-staged sampling procedure was used and 210 women who accessed various health services in the 35 public primary health facilities in Nsukka were selected. The data was collected through self-developed questionnaires and was analyzed using figures and percentages to answer the research questions. 10 women out of the 210 participants had heard of the VAPP Act, meaning that 200 (95.2% of the pool) had not. After explaining the meaning of the Act to the women, they were then asked if they thought this law should be domesticated in Enugu. 190 women (90.47% of the pool) said that it should be. Those that were against its domestication said that FGM/C is part of their culture and that it helps to curb promiscuity among women.

THEORETICAL FRAMEWORK

As stated above, this study made use of the Democratic Participant Media Theory, proposed by Denis McQuail (1987). The theory emerged in recognition of new media developments and of increasing criticism of the dominance of the main media by private or public monopolies. The idea of Democratic Participant Theory was started by grass-root level media in 1960s. It emerged because of the dissatisfaction with other models such as libertarian theory, social responsibility theory, etc. The democratic-participant theory believes there is democratic and professional hegemony in the media today and the media is totally commercial. Thus, all these ill practices should be removed to enable the media to be democratic and be easily accessible or participatory. It considers there should not be monopolization (public/private), centralization of press and top down approach in the media. The press should be pluralistic, decentralized, bottom-up or horizontal and must have equality. The major concept is participation and full circular communication. The theory places greater importance to the receivers. The theory is otherwise known as Democratization Theory of the media. Another central theme that this theory emphasized is the need for equal and unhindered access regardless of their status, wealth, and position. Participation in societal decision making and involvement in communication activities should not be the exclusive preserve of the rich but of all citizens.Hence, all stakeholders (cultural adherents inclusive) have access and the right to freely participate in public and societal governance. In this case - eradicating FGM.

Baran and Davis (2012, pp.149-150) posits that "democratic-participant theory advocates media support for cultural pluralism at grassroots level. Thus, media should be used to stimulate and empower pluralistic groups. The media institutions created according to this theory should be more closely related to social life and should be under control of the audiences. This will afford them (the audience) opportunity to have access to the media and participate in information dissemination according to their own needs, rather than, the interest of the controllers of the media (Aleyomi, 2021).

METHODOLOGY

The kind of methodology used was a search strategy. This is as a result of the nature of the study and the focus of the subjects of the study (the cultural adherents). In view of the fact that it is nearly impossible to trace/track down a cultural adherent to be used as a primary source; the researcher decided to use a search strategy methodology. This is a kind of methodology done through the use of internet search engines, to search, collate and sift through relevant literatures/resources on the research topic.

Thus, the bulk of this methodology was done using secondary sources from relevant books and literatures through the search engines and database. Hence, the researchers searched and reviewed books and journal articles retrieved using the different database. Internet search was done using the PubMed, Google and Google Scholar Search engines. Data was also retrieved from the electronic archives of the World Health Organization websites (WHO), Social Science and Medicine websites and Nigeria Demographic and Health Survey (NDHS) of 2003.

CONCLUSION

There is no doubt that a socio-cultural challenge of this dimension requires the concerted effort of all stakeholders. Thus, the effort was to approach it from the cultural adherents' perspective, and to evolve ways to put an end to the practice of FGM in Africa. In view of the different names/appellations given to these set of people (cultural adherents, circumcisers, excisors, perpetrators, traditional birth attendants, etc.) which is largely dependent on the context/usage; their role and impact in the quest to eradicate FGM cannot be ignored. Thus, there is need to expand the extent of research on the cultural adherents as their role/impact cannot be undermined in the quest to end FGM in Africa-particularly in the selected African countries: Nigeria and South Africa.

Having established above that the participation of these adherents is required to completely eradicate FGM; there is also need to create an enabling environment by the Nigerian as well as the South African government in creating consistent laws to criminalize and outlaw the practice. Finally, in Nigeria; there is need for enforcement of the VAPP (Violence Against Persons Prohibition) Act and create more awareness to the public. Also at the policy-making level, there is an urgent need among concerned stakeholder to strengthen the national legal framework to publicize this law and enforce it into the Nigerian legal environment. In South Africa, there is need for government to continue partnering with civil societies to sensitize communities and encourage them to reflect on the implication of FGM and make a conscious decision to end the practice. In all, and as a means to end this harmful traditional practice in Nigeria and South Africa, a multi-faceted human rights approach should be instituted in order to prevent continuous practice.

REFERENCES

Abdul Rauf Alhassan, A.R., & Anyinzaam-Adolipore, J.N. (2021). Female Genital Mutilation in Ghana: Prevalent and Socioeconomic Predictors. *Journal of BioMed Research International.*

Agboli, A. (2021). Overcoming female genital mutilation and internalised social norms in the context of migration: turning points and explanatory mechanisms (Doctoral dissertation, UCL-Université Catholique de Louvain).

Aleyomi, T. P. (2021). *Democratic Participant Theory. A Postgraduate Seminar of the Department of Mass Communication.* Kaduna State University.

Asekun-Olarinmoye, E. O., & Amusan, O. A. (2008). The impact of health education on attitudes towards female genital mutilation (FGM) in a rural Nigerian community. *The European Journal of Contraception & Reproductive Health Care, 13*(3), 289–297. doi:10.1080/13625180802075174 PMID:18609348

Awolola, O.O., & Ilupeju, N.A., (2019) Female genital mutilation; culture, religion, and medicalization, where do we direct our searchlights for it eradication: Nigeria as a case study. Tzu Chi Medical Journal, 31(1), 1–4.

Babatunde, E. D. (1998). *Women's Rights versus Women's Rites: A study of circumcision among the Ketu Yoruba of South Western Nigeria*. Africa World Press, Inc.

Baran, S. J., & Davis, D. K. (2012). *Mass Communication Theory: Foundations, Ferment, and Future*. Wadsworth Cengage Learning.

Canada: Immigration and Refugee Board of Canada,14 March 2003, South Africa: Reports on female genital mutilation (FGM) and or female circumcision; where practised (urban and/or rural areas); the tribes, religions and cultures that practise it, whether it is legal or not; the government's position and availability of state protection. Available at: https://www.refworld.org/docid/3f7d4e3e2a.html

Centre for Reproductive Rights. (2006). Female Genital Mutilation, A Matter of Human Rights - An Advocate's Guide to Action. Author.

Daniyan, B., Ekwedigwe, K., Sunday-Adeoye, I., Yakubu, E., Uguru, S., & Dantani, D. (2018). Review of the Practice of Female Genital Mutilation in Nigeria. *Journal of Epidemiology*, *8*(4), 356.

Dare, F. O., Oboro, V. O., Fadiora, S. O., Orji, E. O., Sule-Odu, A. O., & Olabode, T. O. (2004). Female genital mutilation: An analysis of 522 cases in South-Western Nigeria. *Journal of Obstetrics & Gynaecology*, *24*(3), 281–283. doi:10.1080/01443610410001660850 PMID:15203627

Eke, N., & Nkanginieme, E. O. (1999). Female Genital Mutilation: A Global Bug That Should Not Cross the Millennium. *World Journal of Surgery*, *23*(10), 1082–1083. doi:10.1007/s002689900627 PMID:10512951

El-Defrawi, M. H., Lotfy, G., Dandash, K. F., Amany, H., Refaat, A. H., & Eyada, M. (2001). Female Genital Mutilation and its Psychosexual Impact. *Journal of Sex & Marital Therapy*, *27*(5), 465–473. doi:10.1080/713846810 PMID:11554208

Epundu, U. U., Emelumadu, O. F., Nwabueze, A., Nebue, C. C., & Ilika, A. (2018). The Epidemiology of Female Genital Mutilation in Nigeria-A Twelve Year Review. Afrimedic Journal, 6(1), 1-10.

Federal Ministry of Health. (2007). Elimination of Female Genital Circumcision in Nigeria. Author.

Idowu, A. A. (2008). Effects of female genital-mutilation on human rights of women and female children: The Nigerian situation. *Research Journal of International Studies*, *8*, 13–26.

International Covenant on Civil and Political Rights, adopted 16th December, 1966 (entry into force, 23 March 1976).

Johnson & Mandara. (2004). An Exploration of Attitudes Toward Female Genital Cutting in Nigeria. *Journal of Population Research and Policy Review*, 26(1).

Jones, S., Ehiri, J., & Anyanwu, E. (2004). Female Genital Mutilation in Developing Countries: An Agenda for Public Health Response. *European Journal of Obstetrics, Gynecology, and Reproductive Biology*, *116*(2), 144–151. doi:10.1016/j.ejogrb.2004.06.013 PMID:15358454

Kandala, N.B., Nwakeze, N., Spatial, Ngianga, S., & Kandala, I.I. (2009). Distribution of Female Genital Mutilation in Nigeria. *Journal of the American Society of Tropical Medicine and Hygiene*, *81*(5), 784–792.

Kitui, B. (2012) *Female Genital Mutilation in South Africa.* AfricLaw: Advancing the rule and role of law in Africa. https://africlaw.com/2012/06/07/female-genital-mutilation- in-south-africa/

Klouman, E., Manongi, R., & Klepp, K. I. (2005). Self-reported and observed female genital cutting in rural Tanzania: Associated demographic factors, HIV and sexually transmitted infections. *Tropical Medicine & International Health, 10*(1), 105–115. doi:10.1111/j.1365-3156.2004.01350.x PMID:15655020

Kolawole, A. O. D., & Anke, V. K. (2010). A review of determinants of female genital mutilation in Nigeria. *Journal of Medicine and Medical Sciences, 1*(11), 510–515.

Lane, D.S., & Rubinstein, R.A. (1996). Judging the Other: Responding to Traditional Female Genital Surgeries. doi:10.2307/3527930

Mandara, M. (2012). Family planning in Nigeria and Prospects for the Future. *International Journal of Gynaecology and Obstetrics: the Official Organ of the International Federation of Gynaecology and Obstetrics, 117*(1), 1–4. doi:10.1016/j.ijgo.2012.01.002 PMID:22342053

McQuail, D. (1987). *Mass communication theory: An introduction.* Sage Publications, Inc.

Mohamud, M., Kaba, M., & Tamire, M. (2016). Assessment of Barriers of Behavioural Change to Stop FGM Practice among Women of Kebribeyah District, Somali Regional State, Eastern Ethiopia. *Global Journals Inc,* 16(6).

National Bureau of Statistics, United Nations Children's Fund, and United Nations Population Fund (UNFPA). (2017). Nigeria Multiple Indicator Cluster Survey 2011. Abuja, Nigeria: NBS. Available at https://www.unicef.org/nigeria/media/1376/file

National Population Commission and ORC Macro. (2014). *Nigeria Demographic and Health Survey 2003.* National Population Commission and ORC Macro.

Nnamdi, S. U. (2019). FGM in Nigeria: Combative Legislation and the Issue's Impact on the Economic Growth of Women. https://impakter.com/female-genital-mutilation-in- nigeria-combative-legislation-and-the-issues-impact-on-the-economic-growth-of- women/

Nnorom, C. C. (2000). *Female Genital Mutilation Practice in Nigeria: Patterns.* Preference and Remedies.

Okeke, T. C., Anyaehie, U. S. B., & Ezenyeaku, C. C. K. (2012). An overview of female genital mutilation in Nigeria. *Annals of Medical and Health Sciences Research, 2*(1), 70–73. doi:10.4103/2141-9248.96942 PMID:23209995

Orji, E. O., & Babalola, A. (2006). Correlates of Female Genital Mutilation and Its Impact on Safe Motherhood. *Journal of the Turkish German Gynecological Association, 7*(4), 319–324.

Rahman, A., & Toubia, N. (Eds.). (2000). *Female genital mutilation: a guide to laws and policies worldwide.* Zed books.

Shell-Duncan, B., Moreau, A., Wander, K., & Smith, S. (2018). The role of older women in contesting norms associated with female genital mutilation/cutting in Senegambia: A factorial focus group analysis. *PLoS One, 13*(7), e0199217. doi:10.1371/journal.pone.0199217 PMID:30044770

Titilayo, A., Palamuleni, M. E., & Anuodo, O. O. (2015). Female Genital Mutilation/Cutting in Nigeria: Any Abandonment yet? *Ife Social Sciences Review*, *24*(2), 109–122.

Toubia & Sharief. (2003). Female Genital Mutilation (FGM). Have we Made Progress? International Journal of Gynecology and Obstetrics, September; 82(3), 251-261.

UNESCO. (2001). *UNESCO Universal Declaration on Cultural Diversity*. UNESCO.

UNICEF. (2005). *Female Genital Mutilation/Female Genital Cutting: A Statistical Report*. UNICEF.

UNICEF. (2013). Female Genital Mutilation/Cutting: A Statistical Overview and Exploration of the Dynamics of Change. UNICEF.

UNICEF. (2017) Approach to the Elimination of Female General Mutilation: A Decade of Action to Achieve Gender Equality. https://www.unicef.org/media/88751/file/FGM- Factsheet-2020.pdf

UNICEF. (2019). Statistical Profile on Female Genital Mutilation. https://www.unicef.org/

Union, A. (2003). *Protocol to the African Charter on Human and People's Rights on the Rights of Women in Africa*. African Union.

Waigwa, S., Doos, L., Bradbury-Jones, C., & Taylor, J. (2018). Effectiveness of health education as an intervention designed to prevent female genital mutilation/cutting (FGM/C): A systematic review. *Reproductive Health*, *15*(1), 1–14. doi:10.1186/s12978-018-0503-x PMID:29650025

Walker, A., & Parmar, P. (1996). *Warrior marks: Female genital mutilation and the sexual blinding of women*. Harvest Books.

Whitehorn, J., Ayorinde, O., & Samantha, M. (2002). Female Genital Mutilation: Cultural and Psychological Implications. *Sexual and Relationship Therapy*, *17*(2), 161–170. doi:10.1080/14681990220121275

World Health Organisation. (1998a). Gender and Health: Technical Paper. WHO.

World Health Organization. (1998b). Female Genital Mutilation: An Overview. WHO.

World Health Organization. (2008). *Sixty-First World Health Assembly: Resolutions and Decisions*. World Health Organization.

Yaya, S., & Ghose, B. (2018). Female genital mutilation in Nigeria: A persisting challenge for women's rights. *Social Sciences (Basel, Switzerland)*, *7*(12), 244. doi:10.3390/socsci7120244

Chapter 18
Impact of Town Criers Using Indigenous Yoruba Language in COVID-19 Awareness on Radio for Behavioral Change Among Rural Dwellers in Lagos

Akpan Unwana
https://orcid.org/0000-0003-0862-6377
University of Lagos, Nigeria

Maureen Samuel
Lagos State University Teaching Hospital, Nigeria

ABSTRACT

In 2020, a study was carried out to show the roles of the new fusion between the indigenous and traditional media (traditional town criers and radio) using indigenous Yoruba language in creating the awareness of COVID-19 among select rural dwellers in Lagos state, and which was published in 2023. This study revealed a novel scene where traditional town criers were brought into language radio stations to create awareness for COVID-19 using Yoruba language. However, this study did not investigate the impact these media fusions had on the minority rural dwellers in Lagos state; rather, it only revealed the roles these media played in creating awareness for COVID-19. Therefore, this chapter investigates the impact the fusion between the traditional town criers as an indigenous media and radio as a traditional media had on select minoritized rural dwellers in Lagos state during the pandemic. This study adopts the health belief model and framing theory, while the instrument for collecting data would be interviews.

DOI: 10.4018/979-8-3693-0624-6.ch018

INTRODUCTION

Numerous studies have revealed that health messages thrive and fulfill their purpose at targeted audiences based on some sociological factors that are culturally, traditionally, religiously, and sometimes economically induced (Pew Research Center, 2020; Gallotti, Valle, Castaldo, Sacco, De, 2020; Agley, Xiao, Thompson, Golzarri-Arroyo, 2021; Bloom, Cadarette, Ferranna, 2021; Scales, Gorman, Jamieson, 2021). Most African communities are culturally, traditionally and religiously hyper active to their environment. According to Akpan (2023, p. 136), "rural Africa has a long history of failure of health campaigns where the planners do not consider the basic elements underlying the traditional communication system such as the town crier in information dissemination. The town crier is still relevant today in many rural areas." During pandemics and epidemics, health workers rely heavily on sensitizing and creating awareness to the populace, and the rural dwellers who are sometimes the hard-to-reach and minority groups for precautionary purposes. In this article, we leverage and extend on Akpan's (2023) study on how language radio stations in Lagos state, Nigeria, made use of the traditional newsman, popularly called the town crier to create awareness of COVID-19 among the rural dwellers in the four rural local government areas (Epe, Ibeju-Lekki, Ikorodu and Badagry) of Lagos state. These rural dwellers in these four rural local government areas in Lagos state fall within the minoritized groups in Lagos state that this study seeks to study. Akpan had observed a new development in media channel fusion. According to him:

In Lagos during the pandemic In Lagos state, the two language stations (Bond FM and Radio Lagos) employed the services of the traditional newsman popularly known as the "town crier" during their programmes (Koko Iwe Iroin, Afobata, Kokoro, etc.) to use the local language in creating awareness of the ongoing pandemic on radio to prevent deaths in these rural areas. These rural dwellers were able to identify and adhere to the messages of the town criers because they are familiar with them. (Akpan, 2023, p. 135)

Akpan's (2023) study found out that first, the rural dwellers were fascinated and thrilled to hear their local town criers live on radio; and second, this fostered their believability because of the dual message channel (the town crier and radio) that are traditional to the majority of the rural dwellers in Africa. According to Akpan (202):

The author observed two radio stations in Lagos State (Bond FM and Radio Lagos) who used these town criers in their studio to create awareness of COVID-19. These town criers were brought from the rural areas of Ikorodu, Badagry, Ekpe and Ibeju-Lekki to use the airwaves in reaching the rural dwellers in these areas. The author also observed that these town criers were scheduled in the four major radio segments (morning, afternoon, evening and midnight) in order to reach out to these rural dwellers listening to various radio segments. Akpan (2023, p. 136).

First, let's seek to understand the impact of health awareness campaigns on the behaviorial pattern of people, why some health campaigns fail; and the influence of the application of a single (exact) message on dual media channels on people; as well as the attendant effect of the fusion of traditional media and indigenous media for the dissemination of a single message on people.

HEALTH AWARENESS

Nigeria being the most populous and one of the most populated countries in the world is as diverse as its cultural realities with over 250 ethnic groups and languages. These ethnic communities have very unique cultural and traditional methods of communication that is native to each of them. As a result, inadequate or ineffective channels of communication strategies, including the use of non-indigenous languages in health campaigns and a fusion of the mainstream media, can hinder the reach and impact of public health initiatives among minority communities. This also can impede behavioral health change. However, it is key to note that the effectiveness of health campaigns depends on how these various forms of indigenous communication and media can be harnessed for this common goal. Health awareness has been in existence for decades, and it is a method used by governments to combat pandemics and epidemics. It is a global phenomenon because governments around the world have understood the potent power and significant roles it plays in promoting individual and community well-being. Most often, health awareness combines the tools of sensitization, education and information dissemination about various health-threatening themes, and in so doing empower individuals to make informed decisions and take health decisions and actions to maintain and improve their wellbeing that is of importance to the community.

During health campaigns, individuals and communities are educated about best preventive health measures that could keep them alive, such as vaccinations, and disease prevention and control strategies. When using the various means of communication in raising awareness about the importance of health alertness, prevention and attitudinal change are guaranteed. Wild, Kunstler, Goodwin, Onyala, Zhang, Kufi M, et al. (2021) reveal that health awareness can go a long way in helping individuals and communities to take control of their own health behaviours and habits for healthy living. For instance, when governments furnish people with information about health attitudes, people can make informed choices and decisions, and adopt healthier lifestyles. This could promote community and individual self-care and reduce the risk of attendant preventable diseases. Nigeria engages in frequent awareness campaigns because of the health needs of her people; and these awareness campaigns targeted at health-related issues go beyond individual well-being to community health needs most times. During these campaigns, information dissemination about contagious diseases, pandemic, vaccination campaigns, sanitation practices, and safe behaviors are incorporated which assist in preventing the spread of diseases and promote a healthier environment for all community members, especially in minority communities.

Additionally, as World Health Organization (2020) posits, health awareness campaign initiatives can help in addressing health discrepancies and promoting health equality among minoritized groups of people in a community. When targeting minority communities in addressing roadblocks to healthcare accessibility and reach, health policy makers most often factor in the communication angle. Awareness campaigns most times are also aimed at reducing health inequalities of these minority groups and hard-to-reach groups and ensuring that every member of the community has an equal chance to access and achieve quality health provisions, and this can be achieved by the effective use of message design and plan. According to Ptil, Rao, Agarwal (2013), health awareness campaigns, especially among the rural dwellers, play a key role in advocating and recommending evidence-based policies and public health interventions in minoritized communities. The education of the public and policymakers about health challenges, pandemics, epidemics, risks, and effective interventions; awareness campaigns can influence health policy decisions, resource distribution, and the implementation of public health programmes and policies. That is why health awareness is important for promoting preventive measures, especially empowering individuals and communities, promoting behavioral change, managing diseases, ensuring community health, addressing health disparities among minoritized groups, and advocating for sound health policies. Governments by increasing the knowledge and understanding of health-based themes through health awareness, individuals and communities can make sound choices that could positively impact their well-being that could foster healthier societies.

REASONS FOR FAILED HEALTH MEDIA CAMPAIGNS

In the past, there have been cases of failed health campaigns in Africa largely because of language barriers and media sources used for such campaigns. A classical example of such a case was the Ebola outbreak response in West Africa in 2014-2016. According to reports, in some regions that were hit by it, methods of information dissemination were faulty because basically, information was disseminated through mainstream media outlets using western languages that were not widely spoken or understood by rural dwellers. This resulted in confusing messages, suspicion, mistrust, distrust and vaccine hesitancy and community resistance to the containment and awareness campaigns efforts. The total failure of the awareness campaigns in the rural areas during the Ebola outbreak due to non-inclusion of the media the local population were familiar with caused the health policy makers to go back to the drawing table; and realized the importance and the place of indigenous language and media for effective health campaigns. This explains Akpan's (2023) position that:

...any communication initiative geared towards health campaigns must consider the culture of the people and seek ways of incorporating it into the health message. Chances are that people will receive more messages that are in line with their cultural systems than the ones which are outside such culture. Therefore many communication campaigns do not see the light of the day on account of the audience (rural dwellers) resisting the messages because they contradict long-held beliefs, norms, habits and ingrained behaviours. (Akpan, 2023, p. 36).

This realization brought about the involvement of local contents (local language and media) in containing the outbreak and subsequent ones (Nutbeam, 2021; Seale, Harris-Roxas, Heywood, Abdi, Mahimbo, Chauhan, Woodland, 2022; Bennett, 2022; Seale, Harris-Roxas, Heywood, Abdi, Mahimbo, Chahan, Woodland, 2023).

SINGLE MESSAGE ON DUAL MEDIA CHANNELS/FORMATS

Placing a particular message on two different media formats that is targeted at different people or a particular set of people has been in existence for decades, and it is as old as the mainstream and indigenous media. Historically, in ancient African communities, such as soon west African rural communities where the village town crier was one of the credible and instituted sources of information dissemination, the village council used to pass information across to the people via the town crier, and as well as folklore and cultural groups who performed and entertained the community in the cool of the evening at the village square. Before such displays, the cultural troupes would first reiterate the message of the village council disseminated earlier by the town crier. This was a message strategy for message effectiveness. The idea was that, if anyone misses the message conveyed by the town crier, then the possibility is that they would not miss the same message that would be passed across by the village cultural dance troupe. In other words, the practice of placing the same message on dual media formats is not new to the rural Africans because it helps to strengthen the message and give it importance and high premium.

Similarly, we have seen in the contemporary times where corporate organizations and individuals place their message across different mainstream media formats (radio, television, newspaper, magazine, billboards); and lately they place the same message on social media. This practice is solely aimed at message effectiveness. On most occasions, these messages are placed on these channels based on the media preference of the audience. That is the reason health policy makers should be deliberate on the media channels or formats they should use in health awareness campaigns, if they really want results in the area of behavioral change. Just like every other study, Akpan's (2023) groundbreaking study of the role of town criers on radio for COVID-19 awareness in the rural areas in Lagos state had some gaps that needed to be studied further. One of them is the behavioral change in their exposure to the same message on dual media formats (the town crier and the radio) influenced during the pandemic.

MEDIA FUSION BETWEEN INDIGENOUS MEDIA AND MAINSTREAM MEDIA

Media fusion is not entirely a new phenomenon. For instance, the multiplatform media channels where one can watch or listen to a live broadcast of his/her favorite television/radio show on any of the social media platforms (Facebook, Twitter, Instagram, etc.). This is regarded as media fusion. During the pandemic, an unusual media fusion occurred in Lagos state, Nigeria, where the village town criers in the rural communities in Lagos state, were used on language radio stations in creating COVID-19 awareness. These town criers used the native Yoruba language, and a command display of local adages, proverbs and short didactic stories to warn the rural dwellers of the consequences of not adhering to the health safety measures that can help prevent the virus. Akpan's (2023) study dwelled indepthly on the roles of these two media channels in creating COVID-19 awareness, but failed to find out if it brought behavioral health changes to the targeted audiences, hence this study. According to Akpan (2023), the use of the traditional newsman, which is the town crier was strategic because the rural people in the community are familiar with the town crier as a credible source of information, and second, the rural dwellers are also familiar with the radio as a credible medium as well. Asides that, these villagers were thrilled to listen to their town criers go on air on radio. For them, it could be a thing of honor and prestige. Some studies have also asserted that the radio is an African medium (WHO, 2012; Dasgupta, 2019; Westoff & Bankole, 1997; Rogers, Vaughan, Swalehe, Rao, Svenkerud, Sood, 1999; Asiedu, 2012). This means, Africans rely more on radio due to its affordability and portability, than the television set. The combination of these two media channels that the rural dwellers in Africa are fascinated about, and have developed some high level of believability was the magic wand. The combination of these two powerful media channels to a great extent could have a powerful and influential effect on their health behavior during the pandemic.

THEORETICAL EXPLANATION

This study adopts a health belief model and framing as theoretical explanations. The Health Belief Model (HBM) is typically a psychological theory that seeks to give epistemological explanations and predictions about individualistic health-related behaviors. The model posits that people's cultural beliefs and perceptions about a specific health issue or behavior can have a great influence on their likelihood of taking preventive actions to curb or address that particular issue (Glanz and Oldenburg, 2001). According to Boston University School of Public Health (2022, para. 1):

The Health Belief Model (HBM) was developed in the early 1950s by social scientists in the U.S. Public Health Service in order to understand the failure of people to adopt disease prevention strategies or screening tests for the early detection of disease. Later uses of HBM were for patients' responses to symptoms and compliance with medical treatments. The HBM suggests that a person's belief in a personal threat of an illness or disease together with a person's belief in the effectiveness of the recommended health behavior or action will predict the likelihood the person will adopt the behavior. The HBM derives from psychological and behavioral theory with the foundation that the two components of health-related behavior.

This model is based on the notion that the likelihood of people engaging in health-related behaviors if they perceive themselves to be at risk of a particular health challenge, believe that the health issues have severe consequences, and feel that the recommended behavior change will effectively reduce the risk if applied. This is the case with using native town criers to influence behavioral change. The key components of the Health Belief Model include:

Perceived Susceptibility: The individual's belief system about the likelihood of developing a health problem if not checked, as done by the town criers on radio.

Perceived Severity: The individual's perception of the seriousness, intent and severity or impact of the health problem perceived.

Perceived Benefits: The individual's notion that taking action or adopting some specific health behaviors will minimize the risk or severity of the health problem being perceived.

Perceived Barriers: This has to do with an individual's assessment of the barriers, costs, or difficulties typical with adopting the recommended health behavior.

Cues to Action: This addresses external or internal elements of what is perceived as triggers that prompt the individual to take action, such as reminders, media campaigns, or personal experiences.

Self-Efficacy: This speaks to the individual's confidence in their ability and willingness to successfully perform the recommended health behavior.

According to Gochman (1997), it is believed that the Health Belief Model, individuals are more likely to support and engage in health-promoting behaviors that would promote health if they perceive a higher risk of health challenges, perceive the health related challenge as severe, have a firm belief that the recommended actions will be health effective, see fewer obstacles to taking action, and are inspired by cues to action (Kasl and Cobb, 1966; Noar and Zimmerman, 2005). Self-efficacy also plays a key role in determining whether individuals will take action or not. According to Smedley and Syme (2000), the Health Belief Model has been numerously applied in various health-related fields, such as public health campaigns, health education, health policies, and behavior change interventions as done by the town criers. This initiative inturn provides a functional framework for understanding and promoting healthier behaviors by targeting individuals' beliefs, perceptions, and motivations as seen in these local areas in Lagos, Nigeria.

On the other hand, framing theory is a concept from the field of communication and media studies, as well as sociology that looks at how the packaging, presentation and interpretation of information can influence the perception and understanding of an issue or event by individuals. Framing theory says that the way information is framed, packaged, or presented, can significantly shape the meaning people attribute to it and subsequently may impact individuals' opinions, attitudes, and behaviors and belief systems. This is the case of the indigenous town crier on the language radio stations in Lagos, using the native Yoruba language in creating COVID-19 awareness campaigns among the rural dwellers in Lagos state, Nigeria. According to framing theory, the media, policymakers, and other influential entities have the power to frame issues by emphasizing certain aspects while downplaying or omitting others. Here, the frame is the town crier on radio, because the rural dwellers are familiar with the town crier. The chosen frames can evoke specific interpretations, emotions, and responses from the audience. Framing involves selecting and highlighting certain aspects of a topic, such as its relevance, implications, causes, or solutions, to guide how people perceive and interpret it. Frames can be accomplished through various means, including word choices, metaphors, images, and emphasis on specific events or actors. Different frames can lead to contrasting understandings of the same issue. Framing theory suggests that frames can influence public opinion by shaping the context and meaning attributed to information. It also posits that individuals may be more receptive to frames that align with their existing beliefs, values, and worldviews, such as the town crier on radio.

METHODOLOGY

The study area was Lagos State, a cosmopolitan state with intercultural, inter-tribal, multilingual community. It was a community-based study whose study population were residents in rural local government areas (LGA) of Lagos State. These LGAs were Ikorodu, Badagry, Epe and Eti-osa LGAs. This study adopted a mixed method to obtain data. Qualitative and quantitative data were collected through interviews, first-hand observation and online questionnaires in two language radio stations in Lagos State, among the four rural local government areas in the state.

Observation and questioning came handy here as there are forms of first-hand experience that capitalize on watching the observed carry out actions that would help reveal further information to the observer in order to generate data (Kitzinger, 1995). This gave the participants room to express themselves, especially in the midst of the task they are doing. Observation and interview helped to investigate participants on subjects such as language as a form of identity, and a fusion of it can influence and impact behavioral patterns (Creese, and Kambere, 2003). The authors observed two radio stations in Lagos State (Bond FM, Radio and Radio Lagos) who used these town criers in their studio to create awareness of COVID-19; as well as some respondents in villages in the four rural communities in Lagos state. These town criers were brought from the rural areas of Ikorodu, Badagry, Epe and Ibeju-Lekki to use the airwaves in reaching the rural dwellers in these areas. The authors also observed that these town criers were scheduled in the four major radio segments (morning, afternoon, evening and midnight) in order to reach out to these rural dwellers listening to various radio segments. The list of these respondents and their villages are listed below. Please note that the names of the respondents are pseudo so as to protect their identity:

Table 1. Interview participants and related demographic data

Name	Local Government	Village	Age
Alake	Badagry	Abia	44
Azeez	"	Agonvi	33
Iya Sikira	"	Ajido	54
Alakija	"	Apa	64
Kemi	"	Dado	71
Taiwo	"	Iworo	43
Bola	Ibeju-Lekki	Eleko	65
Kehinde	"	Emu	59
Shola	"	Iba	52
Folashade	"	Eputu	64
Dele	"	Losoro	47
Segun	"	Lakowe	65
Ebun	"	Igando	38
Bisi	Ikorodu	Aga	45
Orekoya	"	Ajana	34
Iyioola	"	Aleke	53
Popoola	"	Elepete	38
Adepoju	"	Gbadi	42
Ajibade	"	Ewenla	65
Oketunde	Epe	Akata	41
Ajilore	"	Erese	54
Jimoh	"	Erepoto	43
Tope	"	Oko Egan	57

Study Area/Location: Epe, Badagry, Eti-osa and Ikorodu LGA

Study Population: Rural dwellers in these 4 LGA whose major means of communication is in Yoruba language.

Study Design: Cross-sectional, Mixed method study (Quantitative – questionnaire and Qualitative – In depth Interview

Sample Size Determination: A sample size of 230 was calculated and online questionnaires were distributed randomly to the respondents from four of the selected local government areas in Lagos state.

SAMPLING METHODOLOGY

Data Analysis: Data was analyzed with SPSS version 25. Descriptive statistics were collected and inferential statistics were calculated.

Ethical Consideration: Permission and consent were sought from the respondents before interviewing and questionnaire filling respectively.

DISCUSSION OF QUALITATIVE FINDINGS

The findings for the qualitative study are hereby presented. Following the in-depth qualitative interview conducted by the researchers on the rural dwellers in the four rural communities in Lagos state, the findings were revealing on the impact of their exposures to the town criers on radio during the COVID-19 awareness. Out of 22 respondents that were successfully interviewed, 20 of the respondents were in the affirmative that fusing the two modes of media channels impacted on them to take the warnings and the precautions of the pandemic seriously. These interviews were interpreted and transcribed. For Mr. Alakija in Ewenla village, Ikorodu:

"The day I heard our community town crier on radio, using our local dialect to talk to us about the pandemic, I knew it was real. In fact we believed it because we believe anything sad from the radio. In fact, my neighbor ran to me and notified me of the announcement, and that our Baba town crier is the one announcing it himself. That radio station, Radio Lagos is our station because they communicate in Yoruba language."

For Iya Sikira in Oko Egan village in Epe:

"After the pandemic, I took radio messages very seriously, because for our Bale and Oba to have allowed our town criers to get involved in creating the awareness, I meant it was not a child's play."

While in the neighboring Ibeju-Lekki, a certain Mr. Alake in Losoro narrated:

"Each time our town cider comes on air, most of us in the community would gather to listen to him, and it propelled us to adhere to the precautions on how to stay safe during the pandemic."

In Iworo community in Badagry, the impact was the same, as Mr. Azeez narrated:

"Most of us had to sit up and adhere to the safety measures that we heard from our town cider on radio during the pandemic. Immediately we heard our Alaga getting involved, we knew that it is not something to joke with. Bond FM tried by inviting our village Alaga. This honestly made us sit up, because the message was for our common good."

The other remaining 2 were just indifferent.

QUANTITATIVE RESULTS

A total of 230 respondents were sampled but 212 responses were eligible for analysis.

Table 1. Socio-demographic characteristics of respondents

Characteristics	Frequency N=212 n (%)
Age in years	
18-24	31 (14.6)
25-34	80 (37.7)
35-44	79 (37.3)
45-54	17 (8)
>54	5 (2.4)
Mean age	**35.21±8.9**
Gender	
Male	70 (33)
Female	142 (67)

Figure 1. A Chart showing the distribution of the respondents by gender

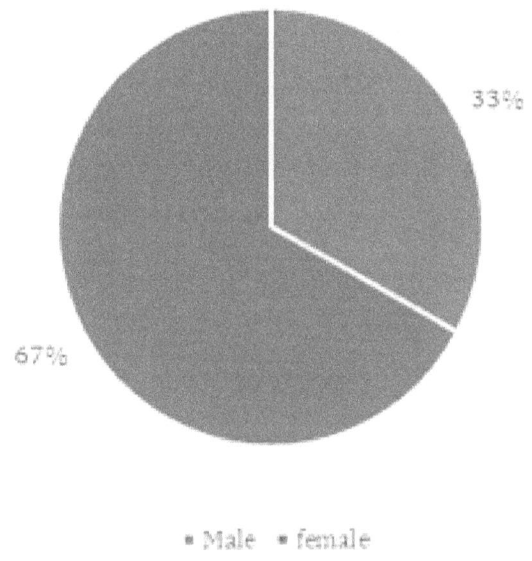

The table above describes the age and sex orientation of the respondents. The age distribution ranged between 21 years and 61 years, with a mean age of 35.2 ±8.9 years. There were more females than males across the age groups (67% for females and 33% for males).

The pie chart above indicates the gender distribution with female preponderance (67%).

Over 159 (75%) respondents were between the ages of 25-44 years. And nearly 15% of the respondents were aged 18-24 years.

The frequency of access to COVID-19 information was not statistically significant to their age or gender.

There is no statistically significant association of the respondents' improved understanding of the COVID-19 messages with their socio-demographic characteristics.

Figure 2. Distribution of respondents by age groups

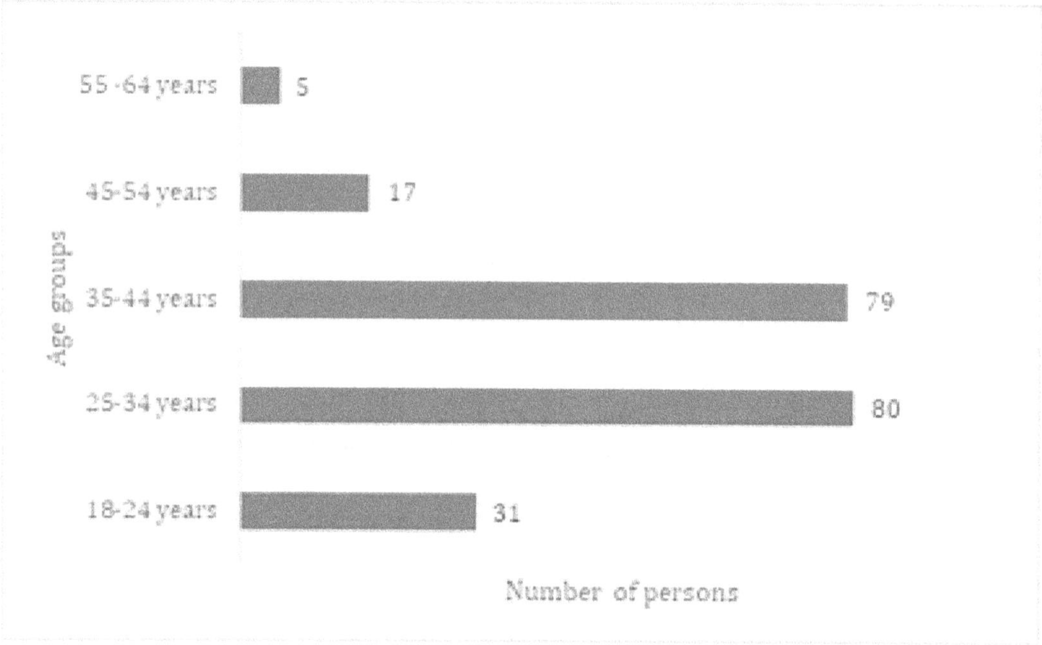

Table 2. Frequency of access to preventive information on COVID-19 by town-criers using radio settings

Sociodemographic Characteristics	Pearson Chi Square	P-Value
Age group in years **Gender** **Male** **Female**	 296 57.72	 0.00 0.00

Table 3. Improved understanding of COVID-19 messages by town-criers in radio houses

Sociodemographic Characteristics	Pearson Chi Square	P-Value
Age group in years **Gender** **Male** **Female**	 197.1 34.2	 0.00 0.00

A total of 41 respondents (78%) were aware that local town criers were being utilized to communicate important information related to COVID-19 prevention and health hygiene practices.

The above chart reveals that 62% of respondents had improved hygiene behavior while 16% felt there was no change. Also, almost half (55%) of the respondents had a good level of satisfaction with the use of local town criers in radio houses as a means of communication during the COVID-19 pandemic, while 45% of them were indifferent.

Table 4. Awareness and access to COVID-19 messages in radio houses by town criers

Responses	**Frequency N=212 n (%)**
Awareness of COVID-19 via Town criers in radio houses	
Aware	165 (78.0)
Not aware	47 (22.0)
Access to channels of COVID-19 messages via	49 (23.1)
Radio	15 (7.1)
Never	48 (22.6)
Rarely	53 (25.0)
A few times a week	47 (22.2)
Daily	
Multiple times a day	

Figure 3. Relationship between the respondents' level of satisfaction of listening to COVID-19 messages to their improved hygiene behaviour

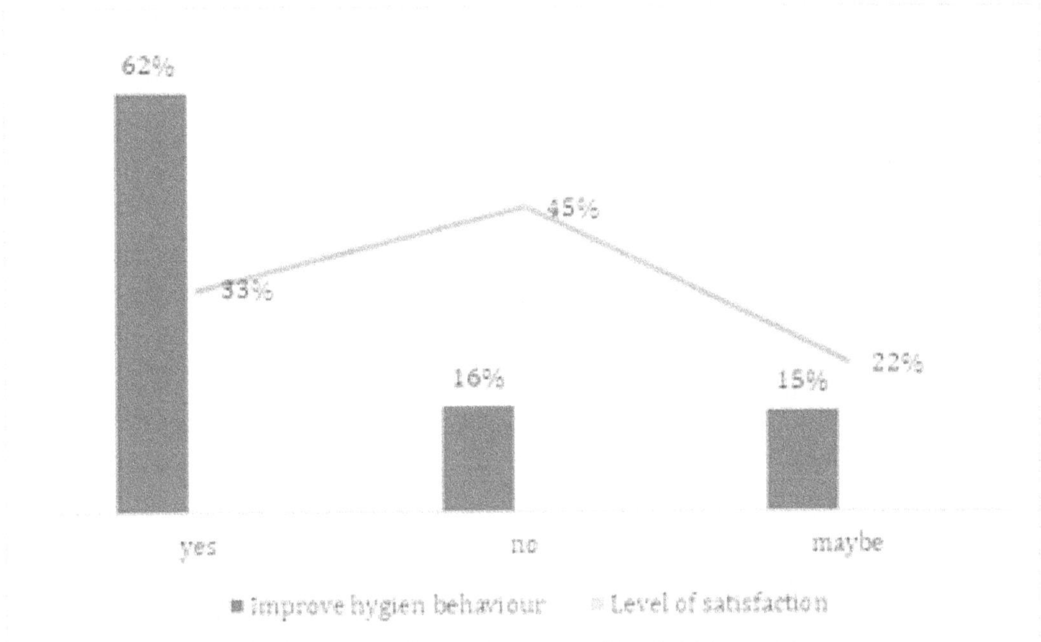

DISCUSSION OF QUANTITATIVE FINDINGS

Generally, the message reduced risk and spread hope though not statistically significant. Better understanding was achieved by the rural dwellers regarding mode of transmission and prevention of COVID-19. Over 55% of the respondents were satisfied with the information passed across by the rural town criers. In conclusion, behavioural change occurs when the medium used to deliver the message is familiar to the people in the community. Social integrity is therefore sustained as both the personalities as well as the media are conversant with the community.

CONCLUSION AND RECOMMENDATIONS

In addressing health behavioral change among the rural dwellers in Africa, it is important for health policy makers to prioritize culturally-all-embressing sensitive and traditionally-context-specific communication strategies, such as the fusion of the indigenous and the mainstream media in reaching out to the rural dwellers for message effectiveness and health behavioral change, as done in the rural areas of Lagos state, Nigeria. This should include engaging the town crier, cultural troupes, community leaders, indigenous, folklore specialists, local orators, local language media outlets, engaging community health workers who are natives of the community and are fluent in the indigenous languages spoken by the rural dwellers. Government should carry out a more comprehensive quantitative survey and involve other locations and spread in terms of more participants involvement. Government should also utilize culturally and traditionally friendly and appropriate messages that the people are at home with, and as well as channels of communication native to the people. These message strategies could help in bringing long lasting health behavioral change among the rural dwellers and assist in improving the effectiveness of health campaigns among rural African communities with minority groups during epidemics or pandemics.

REFERENCES

Agley, J., Xiao, Y., Thompson, E.E., & Golzarri-Arroyo, L. (2021). Factors associated with reported likelihood to get vaccinated for COVID-19 in a nationally representative US survey. *Public Health*. 196, 91–94. https://doi.org/.009 doi:10.1016/j.puhe.2021.05

Akpan, U. S. (2023). The role of traditional town criers using indigenous Yoruba language in COVID-19 awareness on radio for rural dwellers in Lagos. In P. Mpofu, I. A. Fadipe, & T. Tshabangu (Eds.), *African Language Media* (pp. 127–139). Routledge. doi:10.4324/9781003350194-13

Asiedu, C. (2012). Information communication technologies for gender and development in Africa: The case for radio and technological blending. *The International Communication Gazette*, *74*(3), 240–257. doi:10.1177/1748048511432606

Bennett C. (2022). Where did Victoria go so wrong with contact tracing, and have they fixed it? Melbourne: The conversation. theconversation.com/where-did-victoria-go-so-wrong-with-contact-tracing-and-have-they-fixed-it-147993

Bloom, D. E., Cadarette, D., & Ferranna, M. (2021). The societal value of vaccination in the age of COVID-19. *American Journal of Public Health*, *111*(6), 1049–1054. doi:10.2105/AJPH.2020.306114 PMID:33856880

Boston University School of Public Health. (2022). Behavioral change model: Health belief model. https://sphweb.bumc.bu.edu/otlt/MPH-Modules/SB/BehavioralChangeTheories/BehavioralChangeTheories2.html

Dasgupta, S. (2019). Impact of exposure to mass media on female empowerment: Evidence from India. *International Journal of Development Issues*, *18*(2), 243–258. doi:10.1108/IJDI-10-2018-0156

Gallotti, R., Valle, F., Castaldo, N., Sacco, P., & De Domenico, M. (2020). Assessing the risks of "infodemics" in response to COVID-19 epidemics. *Nature Human Behaviour*, *4*(12), 1285–1293. doi:10.1038/s41562-020-00994-6 PMID:33122812

Glanz, K., & Oldenburg, B. (2001). Utilizing theories and constructs across models of behavior change. In R. Patterson (Ed.), *Changing patient behavior: Improving outcomes in health and disease management*. Jossey-Bass.

Gochman, D. S. (1997). Health behavior research: Definitions and diversity. In D. S. Gochman (Ed.) Handbook of health behavior research, Vol. I. Personal and social determinants. Plenum Press.

Kasl, S. V., & Cobb, S. (1966). Health behavior, illness behavior, and sick-role behavior: Health and illness behavior. *Archives of Environmental Health*, *12*(2), 246–266. doi:10.1080/00039896.1966.10664365 PMID:5322534

Noar, S. M., & Zimmerman, R. S. (2005). Health behavior theory and cumulative knowledge regarding health behaviors: Are we moving in the right direction? *Health Education Research*, *20*(3), 275–290. doi:10.1093/her/cyg113 PMID:15632099

Nutbeam, D. (2021). The vital role of meaningful community engagement in responding to the COVID-19 pandemic. *Public Health Research & Practice*, *31*(1), 3112101. doi:10.17061/phrp3112101 PMID:33690782

Pew Research Center. (2020). Majority of Americans now say they would get a vaccine for the coronavirus. https://www.pewresearch.org/ science/wp-content/uploads/sites/16/2020/12/. PS_2020.12.03_covid19-vaccine-intent_00-01. png.

Ptil, S., Rao, R. S., & Agarwal, A. (2013). Awareness and risk perception of hepatitis B infection among auxiliary healthcare workers. *Journal of International Society of Preventive & Community Dentistry*, *3*(2), 67. doi:10.4103/2231-0762.122434 PMID:24778982

Rogers, E. M., Vaughan, P. W., Swalehe, R. M., Rao, N., Svenkerud, P., & Sood, S. (1999). Effects of an entertainment-education radio soap opera on family planning behavior in Tanzania. *Studies in Family Planning*, *30*(3), 193–211. doi:10.1111/j.1728-4465.1999.00193.x PMID:10546311

Scales, D., Gorman, J., & Jamieson, K. H. (2021). The COVID-19 infodemic—Applying the epidemiologic model to counter misinformation. *The New England Journal of Medicine*, *385*(8), 678–681. doi:10.1056/NEJMp2103798 PMID:33979506

Seale, H., Harris-Roxas, B., Heywood, A., Abdi, I., Mahimbo, A., Chahan, A., & Woodland, L. (2023). The role of community leaders and other information intermediaries during the COVID-19 pandemic: Insights from the multicultural sector in Australia. *Humanities & Social Sciences Communications*, *9*(1), 174. doi:10.1057/s41599-022-01196-3

Seale, H., Harris-Roxas, B., Heywood, A., Abdi, I., Mahimbo, A., Chauhan, A., & Woodland, L. (2022). Speaking COVID-19: Supporting COVID-19 communication and engagement efforts with people from culturally and linguistically diverse communities. *BMC Public Health*, *22*(1), 1257. doi:10.1186/s12889-022-13680-1 PMID:35761264

Smedley, B. D., & Syme, S. L. (2000). *Promoting health: Intervention strategies from social and behavioral research*. National Academy Press.

Westoff, C. F., & Bankole, A. (1997). Mass media and reproductive behavior in Africa. https://dhsprogram.com/publications/publication-ar2-analytical-studies.cfm

WHO. (2012). Addressing the challenge of women's health in Africa. www.glowm.com

Wild, A., Kunstler, B., Goodwin, D., Onyala, S., Zhang, L., Kufi, M., Salim, W., Musse, F., Mohideen, M., Asthana, M., Al-Khafaji, M., Geronimo, M. A., Coase, D., Chew, E., Micallef, E., & Skouteris, H. (2021). Communicating COVID-19 health information to culturally and linguistically diverse communities: Insights from a participatory research collaboration. *Public Health Research & Practice*, *31*(1), 3112105. doi:10.17061/phrp3112105 PMID:33690789

World Health Organization. (2020). World Hepatitis Day 2020. https://www.who.int/campaigns/world-hepatitis-day/2020

Compilation of References

(2020). Kandel (2020). Information Disorder Syndrome and its Management. *JNMA; Journal of the Nepal Medical Association, 58*(224), 280–285. PMID:32417871

Abdul Rauf Alhassan, A.R., & Anyinzaam-Adolipore, J.N. (2021). Female Genital Mutilation in Ghana: Prevalent and Socioeconomic Predictors. *Journal of BioMed Research International.*

Abubakari, H., Assem, I. S., & Amankwah, A. S. (2021). Framing of COVID-19 safety protocols in Kusaal musical health communication: Language and literary analysis. *Language & Communication, 81*, 64–80. doi:10.1016/j.langcom.2021.09.002 PMID:36540773

Abubakhar, A., Jibrin, R., & Umar, M. A. (2022). Radio stations framing of the Covid-19 pandemic in Borno State radio stations. *Nigerian Journal of Communication, 18*(1), 138–151.

Abu-Fadili, M. (2018). Combatting Misinformation and Disinformation through Media and Information Lietracy (MIL). In C. Ireton & J. Posetti (Eds.), *Journalism, 'Fake News' and Disinformation: Handbook for Journalism Education and Training* (pp. 70–80). UNESCO.

Adane, M., Ademas, A., & Kloos, H. (2022). Knowledge, attitudes, and perceptions of COVID-19 vaccine and refusal to receive COVID-19 vaccine among healthcare workers in northeaster Ethiopia. *BMC Public Health, 22*(1), 128. doi:10.1186/s12889-021-12362-8 PMID:35042476

Adebisi, Y. A., Rabe, A., & Lucero-Prisno, D. E. III. (2021). Risk communication and community engagement strategies for COVID-19 in 13 African countries. *Health Promotion Perspectives, 11*(2), 137–147. doi:10.34172/hpp.2021.18 PMID:34195037

Adejumo, O. A., Ogundele, O. A., Madubuko, C. R., Oluwafemi, R. O., Okoye, O. C., Okonkwo, K. C., Owolade, S. S., Junaid, O. A., Lawal, O. M., Enikuomehin, A. C., Ntaji, M. I., Sokunbi, A., Timothy, A. O., Abolarin, O. S., Ali, E. O., & Ohaju-Obodo, J. O. (2021). Perceptions of the COVID-19 vaccine and willingness to receive vaccination among health workers in Nigeria. *Osong Public Health and Research Perspectives, 12*(4), 236–243. doi:10.24171/j.phrp.2021.0023 PMID:34289295

Adekunle, T. B., & Mohammed, W. F. (2022). Communication in context: How culture, structure, and agency shape health and risk communication about COVID?19 in Ghana. World Medical & Health Policy, 14(2), 437-444.

Adzer, V. C. (2012). Factors militating against the development of indigenous languages: The TIV language in perspective. *Journal Of Igbo Language & Linguistics, 5*, 76–79.

Africanews (2021). Ethiopia launches Covid vaccination in Addis Ababa. Available from: https://www.africanews.com/2021/03/14/ethiopia-launches-covid-vaccinations-in-addis-ababa

Agboli, A. (2021). Overcoming female genital mutilation and internalised social norms in the context of migration: turning points and explanatory mechanisms (Doctoral dissertation, UCL-Université Catholique de Louvain).

Agley, J., Xiao, Y., Thompson, E.E., & Golzarri-Arroyo, L. (2021). Factors associated with reported likelihood to get vaccinated for COVID-19 in a nationally representative US survey. *Public Health*. 196, 91–94. https://doi.org/.009 doi:10.1016/j.puhe.2021.05

Ahmad, R. (2020). Multilingual resources key to fighting. https://www. languageonthemove.com/multilingual-resources-key-to-fighting-covid-19/

Aïmeur, S., Amri, S., & Brassard, G. (2023). Fake News, Disinformation and Misinformation in Social Media: A Review. *Social Network Analysis and Mining*, *13*(1), 30. doi:10.1007/s13278-023-01028-5 PMID:36789378

Ajayi, J.O, Fatukasi, O & Asemah, E. S (2021). Utilisation of WhatsApp for Communicating Covid-19 Messages in Akure, Ondo State. SAU Journal of Management and Social Science, 6(2).

Ajepe, I., & Ademowo, A. J. (2016). English language dominance and the fate of indigenous languages in Nigeria. *International Journal of History and Cultural Studies*, *2*(4), 10–17.

Ajzen, I. (1991). The theory of planned behaviour. *Organizational Behavior and Human Decision Processes*, *50*(2), 179–211. doi:10.1016/0749-5978(91)90020-T

Ajzen, I. (2002). Perceived behavioural control, self-efficacy, locus of control and the Theory of Planned Behaviours. *Journal of Applied Social Psychology*, *32*(4), 665–683. doi:10.1111/j.1559-1816.2002.tb00236.x

Akpan, U. S. (2023). The role of traditional town criers using indigenous Yoruba language in COVID-19 awareness on radio for rural dwellers in Lagos. In P. Mpofu, I. A. Fadipe, & T. Tshabangu (Eds.), *African Language Media* (pp. 127–139). Routledge. doi:10.4324/9781003350194-13

Al Zou'biR. M. (2022). The Impact of Media and Information Literacy on Students' Acquisition of the Skills Needed to Detect Fake News. Journal of Media Literacy Education Pre-Prints. Retrieved from https://digitalcommons.uri.edu/jmle-preprints/28

Aleyomi, T. P. (2021). *Democratic Participant Theory. A Postgraduate Seminar of the Department of Mass Communication*. Kaduna State University.

Al-Hassan, S., Andani, A., & Abdul-Malik, A. (2011). The Role of Community Radio in Livelihood Improvement: The Case of Simli Radio. *The Journal of Field Actions*, *5*(19).

Amenaghawon, F., & Salawu, A. (2022). Mainstreaming Afro-hip-hop Music in Redressing the Spread of Infodemics on COVID-19. In Indigenous African Popular Music, Volume 2: Social Crusades and the Future (pp. 239-255). Cham: Springer International Publishing. doi:10.1007/978-3-030-98705-3_14

Anaeto, S. Onabanjo, O. & Osifeso .J. (2012*) Models and theories of communication*. United State of America. Africa Renaissance Books Incorporated, Anho, E. J & Muoboghare, N (2021). Newspaper Coverage of Coronavirus Disease (Covid-19) SAU Journal of Management and Social Science, 6(2).

Anane, A. A. (2015). *Doctor-Patient Communication in the Consulting Room: A Study of Two University Health Facilities in Ghana* (Master of Philosophy Thesis, University of Education, Winneba)

Anderson, C. (2008). *The end of theory: The data deluge makes the scientific method obsolete*. Wired.

Anderson, G. J. (2015). Children, Morality and Abusive Words: The Ghanaian Perspectives. *Humanities and Social Sciences Letters*, *3*(2), 87–93. doi:10.18488/journal.73/2015.3.2/73.2.87.93

Apuke, O.D. & Tunca, A. (2018). Social Media and Crisis Management: A review and Analysis of Existing Studies. Laű Sosyal Bilimler Dergisi (IX – II: 199 – 215).

Arora, P. (2019). *The Next Billion Users: Digital Life Beyond the West*. Harvard University Press. doi:10.4159/9780674238879

Asante, E. (1995). *Towards an African Christian Theology of the Kingdom of God: The Kingship of Onyame*. Mellen University Press.

Asekun-Olarinmoye, E. O., & Amusan, O. A. (2008). The impact of health education on attitudes towards female genital mutilation (FGM) in a rural Nigerian community. *The European Journal of Contraception & Reproductive Health Care, 13*(3), 289–297. doi:10.1080/13625180802075174 PMID:18609348

Asiedu, C. (2012). Information communication technologies for gender and development in Africa: The case for radio and technological blending. *The International Communication Gazette, 74*(3), 240–257. doi:10.1177/1748048511432606

Aston, J., & Gaudenzi, S. (2012). Interactive documentary: Setting the field. *Studies in Documentary Film, 6*(2), 125–139. doi:10.1386/sdf.6.2.125_1

Ata-Awaji, A. R., & Confidence, O. S. (2021). Exposure to broadcast media messages and knowledge of Covid-19 pandemic among residents of Port Harcourt, Nigeria. *Media Communication Currents, 5*(1), 19–37.

Atkinson, R., & Flint, J. (2016). *Accessing Hidden and Hard to Reach Populations: Snowball Research Strategies*. Available at: https://www.sru.soc.survey.ac.uk/SRU33.PDF

Austin, P. (2016). Language documentation 20 years on. In L. Filipović & M. Pütz (Eds.), *Endangered languages and languages in danger: issues of documentation, policy, and language rights* (pp. 147–170). John Benjamins Publishing Company. doi:10.1075/impact.42.07aus

Avineri, N., Laura, R., Graham, E. J., Johnson, R., Conley, R., & Jonathan, R. (2018). *Language and social justice in practice*. Routledge. doi:10.4324/9781315115702

Awolola, O.O., & Ilupeju, N.A., (2019) Female genital mutilation; culture, religion, and medicalization, where do we direct our searchlights for it eradication: Nigeria as a case study. Tzu Chi Medical Journal, 31(1), 1–4.

Ayanwale, M. A., Adewuyi, H. O., & Afolabi, O. (2023). Learning through radio and television during Covid-19: Perspectives of K12 stakeholders. *Social and Humanities, 2*(1), 61–72. doi:10.21303/2504-5571.2023.002663

Ayeomoni, O. M. (2012). A Lexico-syntactic Comparative Analysis of Ondo and Ikale Dialects of the Yoruba Language. *Theory and Practice in Language Studies, 2*(9). Advance online publication. doi:10.4304/tpls.2.9.1802-1810

Babatunde, E. D. (1998). *Women's Rights versus Women's Rites: A study of circumcision among the Ketu Yoruba of South Western Nigeria*. Africa World Press, Inc.

Balfour, R. J. (2010). 'The long walk…' in a special issue on Languages in Higher Education in South Africa. Language Learning Journal, 37(3), 249-251.

Bamgbose, A. (2011). African languages today: The Challenge of and prospects for empowerment under globalization. *Selected Proceedings of the 40th Annual Conference on African Linguistics,* 1–14.

Bandura, A. (2008). *Social Cognitive Theory of Mass Communication*. Routledge.

Baptista, J. P., & Grandim, A. (2020). Understanding Fake News Consumption: A Review. *Social Sciences (Basel, Switzerland), 9*(10), 185. doi:10.3390/socsci9100185

Baran, S. J., & Davis, D. K. (2012). *Mass Communication Theory: Foundations, Ferment, and Future.* Wadsworth Cengage Learning.

Bari, M. S., Hossain, M. J., Ahmmed, F., Sarker, M. M. R., Khandokar, L., Chaithy, A. P., Aziz, F., Mitra, S., Emran, T. B., Islam, M. S., Islam, M. R., & Mohamed, I. N. (2021). Knowledge, Perception, and Willingness towards Immunization among Bangladeshi Population during COVID-19 Vaccine Rolling Period. *Vaccines, 9*(12), 1449. doi:10.3390/vaccines9121449 PMID:34960195

Barnes, B. (1974). *Scientific knowledge and sociological theory.* Routledge & Kegan Paul.

Bates, M. J. (2010). Information behavior. Encyclopedia of library and information sciences, 3, 2381-2391.

BBC. (2021a). Coronavirus in Zimbabwe: Nick Mangwana apologises for 'medical assassins' slur. https://www.bbc.com/news/world-africa-55797903

BBC. (2021b). Tanzania President confronts anti-Covid vaccine MP. http://www.channelafrica.co.za/sabc/home/channelafrica/news/details?id=ffe1c60b-0b22-426d-b567-fe6f5e9bd118&title=Tanzania%20President%20confronts%20anti-Covid%20vaccine%20MP

Ben-Enukora, C., Oyero, O., Okorie, N., Oyesomi, K., & Adeyeye, B. (2020). Effectiveness of Yoruba language radio jingles in promoting knowledge, attitude and practices regarding Lassa fever among women in Ondo state, Nigeria. *Journal of Public Health in Africa, 11*(2). Advance online publication. doi:10.4081/jphia.2020.1323 PMID:33680412

Benkler, Y. (2006). *The Wealth of Networks.* Yale University Press.

Bennett C. (2022). Where did Victoria go so wrong with contact tracing, and have they fixed it? Melbourne: The conversation. theconversation.com/where-did-victoria-go-so-wrong-with-contact-tracing-and-have-they-fixed-it-147993

Berger, A. (1991). *Media research techniques.* Sage.

Bernard, H. R. (2002). *Research Methods in Anthropology: Qualitative and Quantitative Methods* (3rd ed.). Alta Mira Press.

Bernd-Carsten, S. (2004). Whose Discourse? A Comparison of the Foucauldian and Habermasian Concepts of Discourse in Critical IS Research. AMCIS 2004 Proceedings. 538.https://aisel.aisnet.org/amcis2004/53

Berry, R. (2014). The future of radio is the internet, not on the internet. In Radio: The Resilient Medium. (pp. 3-15). Sunderland: Centre for Research in Media and Cultural Studies.

Bhartiya, S., Kumar, N., Singh, T., Murugan, S., Rajavel, S., & Wadhwani, M. (2021). Knowledge, attitude and practice towards COVID-19 vaccination acceptance in West India. *International Journal of Community Medicine and Public Health, 8*(3), 1170. doi:10.18203/2394-6040.ijcmph20210481

Biswas, N., Mustapha, T., Khubchandani, J., & Price, J. H. (2021). The nature and extent of COVID-19 vaccination hesitancy in healthcare workers. J Community Health. https://www.ncbi.nlm.nih.gov/pubmed/33877534

Bloom, D. E., Cadarette, D., & Ferranna, M. (2021). The societal value of vaccination in the age of COVID-19. *American Journal of Public Health, 111*(6), 1049–1054. doi:10.2105/AJPH.2020.306114 PMID:33856880

Bonini, T. (2012). Doing radio in the age of Facebook. In Radio Evolution: Conference Proceedings. ECREA/University of Minho.

Bosch, T. (2003). Radio, community and identity in South Africa: A rhizomatic study of Bush radio in Cape Town (Doctoral dissertation, Ohio University). http://rave.ohiolink.edu/etdc/view?acc_ num=ohiou1079300111

Bosch, T. (2014). Social Media and Community Radio Journalism in South Africa. *Digital Journalism (Abingdon, England), 2*(1), 29–43. doi:10.1080/21670811.2013.850199

Boston University School of Public Health. (2022). Behavioral change model: Health belief model. https://sphweb.bumc.bu.edu/otlt/MPH-Modules/SB/BehavioralChangeTheories/BehavioralChangeTheories2.html

Bowles, J., Larreguy, H., & Liu, S. (2020). Countering misinformation via WhatsApp: Preliminary evidence from the COVID-19 pandemic in Zimbabwe. *PLoS One, 15*(10), e0240005. doi:10.1371/journal.pone.0240005 PMID:33052967

Bradshaw, M. B., & Stratford, E. (2010). *Qualitative research design and rigour*. Oxford University Press.

Brønholt, R. L., Langer Primdahl, N., Jensen, A. M. B., Verelst, A., Derluyn, I., & Skovdal, M. (2021). Challenges and Tactics Adopted by Migrants in Denmark When Accessing Health Risk Information about COVID-19. *International Journal of Environmental Research and Public Health, 18*(17), 8932. Advance online publication. doi:10.3390/ijerph18178932 PMID:34501520

Brown, W. (2015). Examining four processes of audience involvement with media personae: Transportation, parasocial interaction, identification, and worship. *Commun Theor.*

Brown, J., Michie, S., Walmsley, M., & West, R. (2016). An online documentary film to motivate quit attempts among smokers in the general population (4Weeks2Freedom): A randomized controlled trial. *Nicotine & Tobacco Research: Official Journal of the Society for Research on Nicotine and Tobacco, 18*(5), 1093–1100. doi:10.1093/ntr/ntv161 PMID:26220547

Brown, S., & Rosier, M. (2023). COVID-19 Vaccine Apartheid and the Failure of Global Cooperation. *British Journal of Politics and International Relations, 25*(3), 535–554. doi:10.1177/13691481231178248 PMID:38602976

Bunch, L. A. (2021). Tale of two crises: Addressing Covid-19 vaccine hesitancy as promoting racial justice. *HEC Forum, 33*(1-2), 143–154. doi:10.1007/s10730-021-09440-0 PMID:33464452

Bunyi, G. (1999). Rethinking the place of African indigenous languages in African education. *International Journal of Educational Development, 19*(4-5), 337–350. doi:10.1016/S0738-0593(99)00034-6

Burke, F. (2020). The dangers of misinformation and neglecting linguistic minorities during a pandemic. https://horizon-magazine.eu/article/dangers-misinformation-and neglecting-linguistic-minorities-during-pandemic.html

Bwire. (2021). As Tanzania Changes Tack on Covid-19, Leaders Have a Role to Play in Pushing Accurate Information. Africa Check. https://africacheck.org/fact-checks/blog/analysis-tanzania-changes-tack-covid-19-leaders-have-role-play-pushing-accurate

Cacciatore, M. A., Scheufele, D. A., & Iyengar, S. (2016). The End of Framing as We Know It… and the Future of Media Effects. *Mass Communication & Society, 19*(1), 7–23. doi:10.1080/15205436.2015.1068811

Cajetan, I. O., Jumbo, C. N., & Etumnu, W. E. (2021). Influence of Covid-19 Broadcast Media Campaigns on the Health Consciousness of Owerri Residents. SAU Journal of Management and Social Science, 6(2).

Callaghan, T., Moghtaderi, A., Lueck, J. A., Hotez, P., Strych, U., Dor, A., Fowler, E. F., & Motta, M. (2021, March). Correlates and disparities of intention to vaccinate against COVID-19. *Social Science & Medicine, 272*, 113638. doi:10.1016/j.socscimed.2020.113638 PMID:33414032

Campbell, J. (2018). Outbreak of African Swine Flu in China is One of Many. https://www.cfr.org/blog/outbreak-african-swine-flu-china-one-many

Canada: Immigration and Refugee Board of Canada,14 March 2003, South Africa: Reports on female genital mutilation (FGM) and or female circumcision; where practised (urban and/or rural areas); the tribes, religions and cultures that practise it, whether it is legal or not; the government's position and availability of state protection. Available at: https://www.refworld.org/docid/3f7d4e3e2a.html

Cappuzzo, B. (2021). The importance of multilingual information and plain English in Response to the COVID-19 pandemic. *European Scientific Journal*, *17*(30), 37–52. doi:10.19044/esj.2021.v17n30p37

Cardoso, F. M., Meloni, S., Santanchè, A., & Moreno, Y. (2019). Topical alignment in online social systems. *Frontiers in Physics (Lausanne)*, *7*, 58. doi:10.3389/fphy.2019.00058

Cassese, E. C., Farhart, C. E., & Miller, J. M. (2020). Gender Differences in COVID-19 Conspiracy Theory Beliefs. *Politics & Gender*, *16*(4), 1–10. doi:10.1017/S1743923X20000409

Catalán-Matamoros, D. (2011). The role of mass media communication in public health. *Health management-Different approaches and solutions*, 399-414.

Cauwenberg, J. V., Donder, L. D., Clarys, P., Bourdeaudhuij, I. D., Owen, N., Dury, S., Witte, N. D., Buffel, T., Verté, D., & Deforche, B. (2014). Relationships of individual, social, and physical environmental factors with older adults' television viewing time. *Journal of Aging and Physical Activity*, *22*(4), 508–517. doi:10.1123/JAPA.2013-0015 PMID:24231688

CBS. (2022). Conspiracy theorists claim bird flu is fake news: "It's just COVID for chickens". https://www.cbsnews.com/news/bird-flu-outbreak-2022-conspiracy-theories/

Cele, N. (2021). Understanding language policy as a tool for access and social inclusion in South African Higher Education: A critical policy analysis perspective. *South African Journal of Higher Education*, *35*(6), 25–46. doi:10.20853/35-6-3730

Centre for Reproductive Rights. (2006). Female Genital Mutilation, A Matter of Human Rights - An Advocate's Guide to Action. Author.

Centres for Disease Control and Prevention. (2022). *Culture and language*. https://www.cdc.gov/healthliteracy/culture.html

Chan, K. L. R. (2018). Being a 'Purist' in Trilingual Hong Kong: Code-Switching among Cantonese, English and Putonghua. *Linguistic Review*, *35*(1), 75–95. doi:10.17250/khisli.35.1.201803.003

Chattopadhyay, K., & Mohanty, S. (2022). New media and cultural disconnect: A study on the lodha tribal community of India. Asian Journal of Social Science, 50(2), 137-146.

Chen, C. M. (2020). Public health messages about COVID-19 prevention in multilingual Taiwan. *Multilingua*, *39*(5), 597–606. doi:10.1515/multi-2020-0092

Cheruiyot, D., & Conie-Ferrel, R. (2018). Fact-Checking Africa. *Digital Journalism (Abingdon, England)*, *6*(8), 964–975. doi:10.1080/21670811.2018.1493940

Chibike, J. J., & Ncube, B. J. (2023). Local radio, Covid-19 and nationalism: The role of Radio Zimbabwe in the Zimbabwean project of nationalism. In Communicating Pandemics Globally [Work in progress].

Chikanda, A., & Crush, J. (2016). The geography of refugee flows to Zimbabwe. *African Geographical Review*, *35*(1), 18–34. doi:10.1080/19376812.2014.933706

Chikowore. (2021). Zimbabwean Journalist Hopewell Chin'ono Still Fighting for Bail. Daily Maverick.https://www.dailymaverick.co.za/article/2021-01-14-zimbabwean-journalist-hopewell-chinono-still-fighting-for-bail/

Chimhundu, H. (2006). Languages and Cultures of Marginalized Groups: Challenges of Inclusion in Higher Education. Paper presented at the International Conference on the Transformation of Masvingo State University to Great Zimbabwe National University, Great Zimbabwe Hotel.

Chingono, N. (2020). Zimbabwe Health Minister Facing Coronavirus Corruption Charge Sacked. The Guardian. https://www.theguardian.com/global-development/2020/jul/09/zimbabwe-health-minister-facing-coronavirus-corruption-charge-sacked

Chio, I. (2009). Interactive Documentary: A Production Model for Nonfiction Multimedia Narratives. *Intelligent Technologies for Interactive Entertainment*, *9*, 44–55. doi:10.1007/978-3-642-02315-6_5

Chonka, P., Diepeveen, S., & Haile, Y. (2023). Algorithmic power and African indigenous languages: Search engine autocomplete and the global multilingual Internet. *Media Culture & Society*, *45*(2), 246–265. doi:10.1177/01634437221104705

Chou, A. B., & Budenz, A. (2020). Considering emotion in COVID-19 vaccine communication: Addressing vaccine hesitancy and fostering vaccine confidence. *Health Communication*, *35*(14), 1718–1722. doi:10.1080/10410236.2020.1838096 PMID:33124475

Cinelli, M., Quattrociocchi, W., Galeazzi, A., Valensise, C. M., Brugnoli, E., Schmidt, A. L., Zola, P., Zollo, F., & Scala, A. (2020). The COVID-19 social media infodemic. *Scientific Reports*, *10*(1), 1–10. doi:10.1038/s41598-020-73510-5 PMID:33024152

Citron, F. M. M., Michaelis, N., & Goldberg, A. E. (2020). Metaphorical language processing and amygdala activation in L1 and L2. *Neuropsychologia*, *140*, 107381. Advance online publication. doi:10.1016/j.neuropsychologia.2020.107381 PMID:32061649

Cloitre, M., & Shinn, T. (1985). Expository practice: social, cognitive and epistemological linkages. In T. Shinn & R. Whistler (Eds.), *Expository Science: Forms and Functions of Popularization* (pp. 31–60). Reidel. doi:10.1007/978-94-009-5239-3_2

Cohen, B. C. (1963). *The Press and Foreign Policy*. Princeton University Press.

Cohen, J. A. (Ed.). (2008). *Challenges and successes in reducing health disparities: Workshop summary*. National Academies Press.

Cohen, S., Guerra, A. W., & Miguel, J. (2022). Erratum to "social class and emotional well-being: Lessons from a daily diary study of families engaged in virtual elementary school during COVID-19.". *AERA Open*, *8*. doi:10.1177/23328584221095854

Coleman, D. (2010). Projections of the ethnic minority populations of the United Kingdom 2006-2056. *Population and Development Review*, *36*(3), 441–486. doi:10.1111/j.1728-4457.2010.00342.x PMID:20882702

Communication Authority of Kenya. (2023). Mobile Subscription Hit 66m as at March 2023. https://www.ca.go.ke/mobile-subscriptions-hit-66m-march-2023

Connor, K. M., & Davidson, J. R. T. (2003). Development of a new resilience scale: The connor-davidson resilience scale (CD-RISC). *Depression and Anxiety*, *18*(2), 76–82. doi:10.1002/da.10113 PMID:12964174

Coscieme, L., & Skodowska-Curie, M. (2020). Countries With Female Leaders Suffer Six Times Fewer COVID-19 Deaths. https://www.tcd.ie/news_events/articles/countries-with-female-leaders-suffer-six-times-fewer-covid-19-deaths/

Crandell, E. (2013). Framing in the Chinese Media: Who Framed Bo Xilai and How? American University Honors Thesis. Capstone.

Crayner, J. B. (2007). *Borbor Kunkumfi: History of the Migration of the Fantes to their Present Homes* (2nd ed.). Bureau of Ghana Languages.

Creswell, J. W. (2014). *Research design: Qualitative, quantitative and mixed methods* (4th ed.). Sage.

Creswell, J. W., & Creswell, J. D. (2023). *Research Design: Qualitative, Quantitative, and Mixed Methods Approaches* (6th ed.). Sage Publications Inc.

Crisis and Emergency Risk Communication. (2014). Atlanta: US Centers for Disease Control and Prevention. https://emergency.cdc.gov/cerc/ppt/cerc_2014edition_Copy.pdf

Croteau, D., & William, H. (2000). *Media/Society*. Pine Forge Press.

Crush, J., & Tawodzera, G. (2011). *Medical Xenophobia: Zimbabwean access to health services in South Africa*. Idasa.

Cuadrado, D. C. (2022). Corruption During Covid-19 Trends, Drivers, And Lessons Learned For Reducing Corruption In Health Emergencies. Chr. *Michelsen Institute*, *U4*(CMI), 16.

Cunliffe-Jones, P. (2021). The State of Media Literacy In Sub-Saharan Africa 2020 and a Theory of Misinformation Literacy. In Misinformation Policy In Sub-Saharan Africa: From Laws and Regulations to Media Literacy. London: University of Westminster Press. doi:10.16997/book53.a

Dahal, S., & Aram, I. A. (2013). Empowering Indigenous Community through Community Radio: A Case Study from Nepal. *The Qualitative Report*, *18*(41), 1–26. doi:10.46743/2160-3715/2013.1456

Damasceno, C. S. (2021). Multiliteracies for Combating Information Disorder and Fostering Civic Dialogue. *Social Media + Society*, *7*(1), 1–10. doi:10.1177/2056305120984444

Daniele, F. (2021). The centrality of language in health communication. *European Scientific Journal*, *17*(30), 24–36. doi:10.19044/esj.2021.v17n30p24

Daniyan, B., Ekwedigwe, K., Sunday-Adeoye, I., Yakubu, E., Uguru, S., & Dantani, D. (2018). Review of the Practice of Female Genital Mutilation in Nigeria. *Journal of Epidemiology*, *8*(4), 356.

Dare, F. O., Oboro, V. O., Fadiora, S. O., Orji, E. O., Sule-Odu, A. O., & Olabode, T. O. (2004). Female genital mutilation: An analysis of 522 cases in South-Western Nigeria. *Journal of Obstetrics & Gynaecology*, *24*(3), 281–283. doi:10.1080/01443610410001660850 PMID:15203627

Dasgupta, S. (2019). Impact of exposure to mass media on female empowerment: Evidence from India. *International Journal of Development Issues*, *18*(2), 243–258. doi:10.1108/IJDI-10-2018-0156

Davies, S. E., & Wenham, C. (2020). Why the COVID-19 response needs International Relations. *International Affairs*, *96*(5), 1227–1251. doi:10.1093/ia/iiaa135 PMID:34191916

Davis, C. R., Baker, C. N., Osborn, J., & Overstreet, S. (2022). Understanding teacher self-efficacy to address students' social-emotional needs in the COVID-19 pandemic. *Urban Education*, *004208592210998*. Advance online publication. doi:10.1177/00420859221099834

Daymon, C., & Holloway, I. (2011). Choosing Between Different Types of Research. *Qualitative Research Methods in Public Relations and Marketing Communication*, *2*, 99–113.

De Golbéry, L., & Chappuis, A. (2000). Underprivileged minorities in India: Dalits and tribals. A cartographic Approach. *Essays on Population and Space in India.* French Institute of Pondicherry.

de Lange, N., Olivier, T., & Wood, T. (2008). Participatory video documentary: Just for whom? *Education as Change*, *12*(2), 109–122. doi:10.1080/16823200809487210

de Las Heras-Pedrosa, C., Jambrino-Maldonado, C., Rando-Cueto, D., & Iglesias-Sánchez, P. P. (2022). COVID-19 study on scientific articles in health communication: A science mapping analysis in web of science. *International Journal of Environmental Research and Public Health*, *19*(3), 1705. doi:10.3390/ijerph19031705 PMID:35162726

de Las Heras-Pedrosa, C., Rando-Cueto, D., Jambrino-Maldonado, C., & Paniagua-Rojano, F. J. (2020). Exploring the social media on the communication professionals in public health. Spanish official medical colleges case study. *International Journal of Environmental Research and Public Health*, *17*(13), 4859. doi:10.3390/ijerph17134859 PMID:32640598

de-Lima-Santos, M.-F., & Ceron, W. (2022). Artificial Intelligence in News Media: Current Perceptions and Future Outlook. *Journalism and Media*, *3*(1), 13–26. doi:10.3390/journalmedia3010002

Department of Higher Education and Training. (2017). *Language Policy for Higher Education*. Department of Higher Education and Training.

Department of Public Service and Administration. (2021). Postponement of Cash allowances. Available at: www.gov.za/covid-19/resources/fake-news-coronavirus-covid-19

Depoux, A., Martin, S., Karafillakis, E., Preet, R., Wilder-Smith, A., & Larson, H. (2020). The pandemic of social media panic travels faster than the COVID-19 outbreak. *Journal of Travel Medicine*, *27*(3), taaa031. doi:10.1093/jtm/taaa031 PMID:32125413

Derakhshan, A, (2020). Information Disorder: Toward an Interdisciplinary Framework for Research and Policymaking. Council of Europe.

Desa, U. (2018). Promoting Inclusion through Social Protection: Report on the World Social Situation 2018. New York: United Nations.

Di Carlo, P. (2020). Message- vs. community-centered models in risk communication [internet]. Sydney: Language on the Move. https://www.languageonthemove.com/message-vs-community-centered-models-in-risk-communication/

Di Carlo, P., McDonnell, B., Vahapoglu, J., Good, J., Seyfeddinipur, M., & Kordas, K. (2021). Building climate-sensitive nutrition programmes. *Bulletin of the World Health Organization*, *100*(1), 78–80. doi:10.2471/BLT.21.285617 PMID:35017760

Dilbeck, K. E. (2008). *Rhetorical Sensitivity and Communication Competence: A Test for Convergent Validity* (Doctoral Dissertation, Bangkok University).

Dinleyici, E. C., Borrow, R., Safadi, M. A. P., van Damme, P., & Munoz, F. M. (2020). Vaccines and routine immunization strategies during the COVID-19 pandemic. *Human Vaccines & Immunotherapeutics*, *17*(2), 400–407. doi:10.1080/21645515.2020.1804776 PMID:32845739

Dludla, N. (2020). South Africa's chief justice unrepentant for linking vaccines to Satanism. https://www.reuters.com/article/health-coronavirus-safrica-vaccine-idUSL8N2IR2VW

Dobson, M. W., & Ha, D. (2007). Exploring interactive stories in an HIV/AIDS learning game: HEALTHSIMNET. *Simulation & Gaming*, *39*(1), 39–63. doi:10.1177/1046878107308093

Docrat, Z., & Kaschula, H. (2015). Meaningful engagement: Towards a language rights paradigm for effective language policy implementation. *Southern African Linguistics and Applied Language Studies*, *5*(1), 1–9.

Docrat, Z., & Kaschula, R. H. (2020). Transformative power of language policies in higher education: A legal English approach or a linguistic African language approach. In R. H. Kaschula & E. Wolff (Eds.), *The Transformative Power of Language: From Postcolonial to Knowledge Societies in Africa* (pp. 85–108). Cambridge University Press. doi:10.1017/9781108671088.006

Dohaney, J., de Róiste, M., Salmon, R. A., & Sutherland, K. (2020). Benefits, barriers, and incentives for improved resilience to disruption in university teaching. *International Journal of Disaster Risk Reduction*, *50*, 101691. doi:10.1016/j.ijdrr.2020.101691 PMID:32509512

Dolczewski, M. (2022). Semi-structured interview for self-esteem regulation research. *Acta Psychologica*, *228*, 103642. doi:10.1016/j.actpsy.2022.103642 PMID:35716626

Do-Santos, F. O., & Brasil, A. (2020). Broadcasting the Covid-19 pandemic in Central Africa: A content analysis of United Nations Peacekeeping Radio. *Radiofonas*, *11*(2), 89–128.

Dwivedi, P. (2016). An Introduction To Katkari Tribes Of Maharashtra. Retrieved from https://indiafellow.org/blog/all-posts/an-introduction-to-katkari-tribes-of-maharashtra/

Dzinamarira, T., Nachipo, B., Phiri, B., & Musuka, G. (2021). COVID-19 vaccine roll-out in South Africa and Zimbabwe: urgent need to address community preparedness, fears and hesitancy. Vaccines, 9(3), 250.

Eberhard, D. M., Simons, G. F., & Fennig, C. D. (2020) (eds). Ethnologue: Languages of the World. 23rd ed. Dallas: SIL International.

Edge, D. (1988). The social shaping of technology. Edinburgh PICT Working Paper No. 1, Edinburgh University.

Ehreth, J. (2003). The value of vaccination: A global perspective. *Vaccine*, *21*(27), 4105–4117. doi:10.1016/S0264-410X(03)00377-3 PMID:14505886

Eke, N., & Nkanginieme, E. O. (1999). Female Genital Mutilation: A Global Bug That Should Not Cross the Millennium. *World Journal of Surgery*, *23*(10), 1082–1083. doi:10.1007/s002689900627 PMID:10512951

Ekezie, W., Maxwell, A., Byron, M., Czyznikowska, B., Osman, I., Moylan, K., ... Pareek, M. (2022). Health communication and Inequalities in primary care access during the COVID-19 pandemic among ethnic minorities in the United Kingdom: lived experiences and recommendations. International Journal of Environmental Research and Public Health, 19(22), 15166.

El-Defrawi, M. H., Lotfy, G., Dandash, K. F., Amany, H., Refaat, A. H., & Eyada, M. (2001). Female Genital Mutilation and its Psychosexual Impact. *Journal of Sex & Marital Therapy*, *27*(5), 465–473. doi:10.1080/713846810 PMID:11554208

Emeka-Nwobia, N. U. (2015). The place of indigenous Nigerian languages in National development. *Research on Humanities and Social Sciences*, *5*(12), 112–116.

Endangered Languages Project. (2020). COVID-19 information in indigenous, endangered, and under-resourced languages. https://endangeredlanguagesproject.github.io/COVID-19

Entmann, R.M. (2007). Framing Bias: Media in the Distribution of Power. Academic Press.

Entmann, R. M. (2003). Cascading Activation: Contesting the White House's Frame After 9/11. *Political Communication*, *20*(4), 415–432. doi:10.1080/10584600390244176

Entman, R. M. (1993). Framing: Towards Clarification of A Fractured Paradigm. *Journal of Communication*, *43*(4), 51–58. doi:10.1111/j.1460-2466.1993.tb01304.x

Epundu, U. U., Emelumadu, O. F., Nwabueze, A., Nebue, C. C., & Ilika, A. (2018). The Epidemiology of Female Genital Mutilation in Nigeria-A Twelve Year Review. Afrimedic Journal, 6(1), 1-10.

Eshiett, M., & Parry, E. (2003). Migrants and health: A cultural dilemma. *Clinical Medicine*, *3*(3), 229–231. doi:10.7861/clinmedicine.3-3-229 PMID:12848255

EWN. (2021). Madagascan Leader in Covid Vaccine U-Turn. https://ewn.co.za/2021/03/26/madagascan-leader-in-covid-vaccine-u-turn

Ezeh, A., Oyebode, O., Satterthwaite, D., Chen, Y.-F., Ndugwa, R., Sartori, J., Mberu, B., Melendez-Torres, G. J., Haregu, T., Watson, S. I., Caiaffa, W., Capon, A., & Lilford, R. J. (2017). The history, geography, and sociology of slums and the health problems of people who live in slums. *Lancet*, *389*(10068), 547–558. doi:10.1016/S0140-6736(16)31650-6 PMID:27760703

Eze, O. J., Ajah, B. O., Nwonovo, O. S., & Atama, C. S. (2022). Health sector corruption and COVID-19 outbreak: Evidence from Anambra and Enugu States, Nigeria. *Journal of Contemporary African Studies*, *40*(1), 34–46. doi:10.1080/02589001.2021.1921129

Fadipe, I. A., & Salawu, A. (2021). Influence of African Indigenous language media in COVID-19 digital health messaging. *Catalan Journal of Communication & Cultural Studies*, *13*(2), 267–284. doi:10.1386/cjcs_00053_1

Fadipe, I. A., & Salawu, A. (2022). 'Coronavirus, you are a Stranger,'Examining Yoruba Indigenous Music in the Quest to Tackle COVID-19 Pandemic. *Journal of African Films and Diaspora Studies*, *5*(1), 75–99. doi:10.31920/2516-2713/2022/5n1a4

Fatahi, N. (2010). *Cross-cultural encounters through interpreter: experiences of patients, interpreters and healthcare professionals*. Geson Hylte Tryck.

Federal Ministry of Health. (2007). Elimination of Female Genital Circumcision in Nigeria. Author.

Ferrante, L., & Fearnside, P. M. (2020). Protect Indigenous peoples from COVID-19. Science, 368(6488), 251-251.

Filio Marineli, F., Tsoucalas, G., Karamanou, M., & Androutsos, G. (2013). Mary Mallon (1869-1938) and the History of Typhoid Fever. Hellenic Society of Gastroenterology. *Annals of Gastroenterology*, *26*(2), 132–134. PMID:24714738

Fishbein, M., & Ajzen, I. (1975). *Belief, attitude, intention, and behaviour: An introduction to theory and research.* Addison-Wesley.

Fishman, J. (1972). *The sociology of language: An interdisciplinary social science approach to language in society.* Newbury House.

Fleisch, B. (2008). *Primary Education in Crisis: Why South African School Children Underachieve in Reading and Mathematics*. Juta and Co.

Forum on Information & Democracy. (2021). A New Deal for Journalism. https://informationdemocracy.org/working-groups/sustainability-of-journalism/

Foss, K. A. (2020). #TyphoidMary – Now a Hashtag – Was a Maligned Immigrant Who Got a Bum Rap. https://theconversation.com/typhoidmary-now-a-hashtag-was-a-maligned-immigrant-who-got-a-bum-rap-136571

Fox, N. (2009). *Using Interviews in Research Projects*. National Institute for Health Science.

France, S. (2020). Drogba Slam Medical Professors Over 'Racist' Remarks Coronavirus Vaccine Tests Should be Conducted in Africa. https://www.goal.com/en/news/etoo-drogba-medical-professors-racist-coronavirus-vaccine-tests-conducted-africa/1wuqs7zifvehm19gl6fq36yqgo

Fraudulent Coronavirus Disease. (2019). (COVID-19) Products. Available at: 11: 41 pm on 25/08/2023 https://www.fda.gov/consumers/health-fraud-scams/fraudulent-coronavirus-disease-2019-covid-19-products

Freimuth, V. S., & Mettger, W. (1990). Is there a hard-to-reach audience? *Public Health Reports*, *105*(3), 232–238. PMID:2113680

Frieden, T. R., Buissonnière, M., & McClelland, A. (2021). The world must prepare now for the next pandemic. *BMJ Global Health*, *6*(3), e005184. doi:10.1136/bmjgh-2021-005184 PMID:33727280

Fung, I. C. H., & Cairncross, S. (2006). Effectiveness of handwashing in preventing SARS: A review. *Tropical Medicine & International Health*, *11*(11), 1749–1758. doi:10.1111/j.1365-3156.2006.01734.x PMID:17054756

Furlong, A. (2023). WHO COVID Origins Investigation is 'Stymied'. https://www.politico.eu/article/who-abandon-covid-origin-investigation-china-data/

Fynn, J. K. (1987). The Political System of the Fante of Ghana during the Pre-Colonial Period. *Universitas*, *9*(1), 108–120.

Gaganakis, M. (2006). Language and ethnic group relations in de-segrated South African Schools. . doi:10.1080/0159630940150103

Gagnon, V. B., Larsen, R., Graves, L., & Westlund, O. (2023). Knowledge Work in Platform Fact-Checking Partnerships. *International Journal of Communication*, *17*, 1169–1189.

Gallotti, R., Valle, F., Castaldo, N., Sacco, P., & De Domenico, M. (2020). Assessing the risks of "infodemics" in response to COVID-19 epidemics. *Nature Human Behaviour*, *4*(12), 1285–1293. doi:10.1038/s41562-020-00994-6 PMID:33122812

Gamson, W. A., & Modigliani, A. (1989). Media Discourse and Public Opinion on Nuclear Power: A Constructionist Approach. *American Journal of Sociology*, *95*(1), 1–37. doi:10.1086/229213

García-Álvarez, D., Soler, M. J., & Achard-Braga, L. (2021). Psychological well-being in teachers during and post-covid-19: Positive Psychology Interventions. *Frontiers in Psychology*, *12*, 769363. Advance online publication. doi:10.3389/fpsyg.2021.769363 PMID:34975659

Garcia, O. (2009). *Bilingual Education in the 21st Century: A Global Perspective*. Wiley-Blackwell.

Gazzola, M., & François, G. (2013). Is ELF more effective and fair than translation? An evaluation of the EU's multilingual regime. *International Journal of Applied Linguistics*, *23*(1), 93–107. doi:10.1111/ijal.12014

Gert, B., & Gert, J. (2020). The Definition of Morality. *The Stanford Encyclopedia of Philosophy*. https://plato.stanford.edu/archives/fall2020/entries

Ghani, A., & Khan, S. (2020). *Disorder in the Newsroom: The Media's Perceptions and Response to the Infodemic*. Media Matter for Democracy.

Giles, H., & Ogay, T. (2009). Communication accommodation theory. Explaining Communication: Contemporary theories and examples. Lawrence Erlbaum Associates.

Glanz, K., & Oldenburg, B. (2001). Utilizing theories and constructs across models of behavior change. In R. Patterson (Ed.), *Changing patient behavior: Improving outcomes in health and disease management*. Jossey-Bass.

Glesne, C. (2016). *Becoming Qualitative Researchers: An Introduction* (5th ed.). Pearson.

Global Compact Media, U. N. 2020. COVID-19: What makes a good leader during a crisis. https://unglobalcompact.org/take-action/20th-anniversary-campaign/covid-19-what-makes-a-good-leader-during-a-crisis

Global Preparedness Monitoring Board. (2020). Building trust within and across communities for health emergency preparedness. Geneva and Washington, DC. https://apps.who.int/gpmb/assets/thematic_papers_2020/tp_2020_3.pdf

Gochman, D. S. (1997). Health behavior research: Definitions and diversity. In D. S. Gochman (Ed.) Handbook of health behavior research, Vol. I. Personal and social determinants. Plenum Press.

Goffman, E. (1956). *The Presentation of Self in Everyday Life*. Doubleday.

Gonah, L., Corwin, A., January, J., Shamu, S., Jokomo, Z. N., & Putten, M. (2016). Barriers to Healthcare Access and Coping Mechanisms among Sub-Saharan African Migrants living in Bangkok, Thailand: A Qualitative Study. *Medical Journal of Zambia*, *43*(4), 238–246. doi:10.55320/mjz.43.4.315

Goodrich, S. (2021). *Transparency International (TI). Track and Trace.: Identifying Corruption Risks in UK Public Procurement for the COVID-19 Pandemic*. Transparency International.

Gordon-Brilla, S., & Rogers, D., *Higginbottom, J. Ensha, L., & Sutherland, R. (n.d.). The Colour of Covid-19. The Racial Inequality of Marginalised Communities*. Routledge.

Gore, F., Bloem, P. J. N., Patton, G. C., Ferguson, J., & Joseph, V. (2014). *Global burden of disease in young people aged 10–24 years: a systematic analysis*. Routledge.

Gore, M., Kawade, A., Smith, P., Pinnock, H., & Juvekar, S. (2022). Working as frontline health facilitators, service providers, program supporters, and social health activists in Indian hilly terrain areas: A qualitative study of accredited social health activists' experiences before and during the COVID-19 pandemic. *Journal of Global Health*, *12*, 12. doi:10.7189/jogh.12.05052 PMID:36579668

Goswami, M. P. (2017). Mobile Phone, Entertainment and Tribal Life. Media Mimansa.

Govere, E. (2017). *Exploring the perception of refugees and asylum seekers regarding access to mental health service in Zimbabwe: A case study of Tongogara Refugee Camp*. Unpublished Master's Thesis. University of Witwatersrand.

Granziera, H., Collie, R., & Martin, A. (2020). Understanding teacher wellbeing through job demands-resources theory. *Cultivating Teacher Resilience*, 229–244. doi:10.1007/978-981-15-5963-1_14

Grey, A. (2017). How do language rights affect minority languages in China? An ethnographic investigation of the Zhuang minority language under conditions of rapid social change (PhD). Macquarie University. http://www.languageonthemove.com/ wpcontent/uploads/2017/05/Grey_How_do_language_rights_affect_minority_languages.pdf

Grey, A. (2020). How to improve Australia's public health messaging about. https://www.languageonthemove.com/how-to-improve-australias-public health-messaging-about-covid-19/

Gualtieri, A. E. (2021). New York Mayor Bill de Blasio tempts New Yorkers with free fries: "Mmm, vaccinations. Available at: https://www.cbsnews.com/news/covid-vaccine-new-york-shake-shack-fries/

Guangming, P. (2020). Mais de 3.000 Equipes Médicas em Hubei Foram Infectadas no Estágio Inicial da Epidemia, Atualmente não há Relatos de Infecção Entre as Equipes de Assistência Médica. https://politics.gmw.cn/2020-03/06/content_33626862.htm

Gyekye, K. (1996). *African Cultural Values: An Introduction*. Sankofa Publishing Corp.

Habermas, H. (1998). *The Inclusion of the Other: Studies in Political Theory*. MIT Press.

Haimovich, G., & Márquez Mora, H. (2020). Why it's important to use Indigenous languages in health communication. https://www.languageonthemove.com/ why-its-important-to-use-indigenous-languages-in-health-communication/

Hajj Hussein, I., Chams, N., Chams, S., El Sayegh, S., Badran, R., Raad, M., Gerges-Geagea, A., Leone, A., & Jurjus, A. (2015). Vaccines Through Centuries: Major Cornerstones of Global Health. *Frontiers in Public Health*, *3*, 269. doi:10.3389/fpubh.2015.00269 PMID:26636066

Hall, G., & Gandolfo, A. (2016). Poverty and exclusion among Indigenous Peoples: The global evidence. World Bank Blogs. Retrieved from https://blogs.worldbank.org/voices/poverty-and-exclusion-among-indigenous-peoples-global-evidence

Hallin, D. C., & Mancini, P. (2004). *Comparing media systems: Three models of media and politics*. Cambridge University Press. doi:10.1017/CBO9780511790867

Hannock, B., Ockleford, E., & Windridge, K. (2013). *An Introduction to Qualitative Research*. Available at: https://www.rds-yh.nihr.ac.uk/wpcontent/uploads/2013/05/05/introduction-to-qualitative-reserch.pdf

Hart, R. P., & Burks, D. M. (1972). Rhetorical Sensitivity and Social Interaction. *Speech Monographs*, *39*(2), 75–91. doi:10.1080/03637757209375742

Haug, N., Geyrhofer, L., Londei, A., Dervic, E., Desvars-Larrive, A., & Loreto, V. (2020). Ranking the effectiveness of worldwide COVID-19 government interventions. Academic Press.

Hawthorn, A. (2021). Apocalypse Then. Germ Warfare: Weaponizing an Illness Is Older Than You Might Think. https://www.cbc.ca/news/canada/newfoundland-labrador/apocalypse-then-germ-warfare-1.6052178

Healthy People . (2010). US Dept of Health and Human Services. https://professionals.wrha.mb.ca/old/extranet/publichealth/priorities-communication.php

Hecht, M. L., & Choi, H. (2012). The communication theory of identity as a framework for health message design. Health communication message design. *Theory into Practice*, 137–152.

Henley, J. (2020. Female-led Countries Handled Coronavirus Better, Study Suggests. The Guardian. https://www.theguardian.com/world/2020/aug/18/female-led-countries-handled-coronavirus-better-study-jacinda-ardern-angela-merkel

Hennigh, L. (1970). Functions and Limitions of Alaskan Eskimo Wife Trading. *Open Journal Systems*, *23*(1), 24–34. doi:10.14430/arctic3151

Hermans, M. P. J., Kooistra, J., Cannegieter, S. C., Rosendaal, F. R., Mook-Kanamori, D. O., & Nemeth, B. (2017). Healthcare and disease burden among refugees in long-stay refugee camps at Lesbos, Greece. *European Journal of Epidemiology*, *32*(9), 851–854. doi:10.1007/s10654-017-0269-4 PMID:28597126

Himma-Kadakas, M., & Ojamets, I. (2022). Debunking False Information: Investigating Journalists' Fact-Checking Skills. *Digital Journalism (Abingdon, England)*, *10*(5), 866–887. doi:10.1080/21670811.2022.2043173

Hornberger, N. H. (2002). Multilingual language policies and the continua of biliteracy: An ecological approach. *Language Policy*, *1*(1), 27–51. doi:10.1023/A:1014548611951

Horowitz, M. A., & Lowe, G. F. (2020). Public service media in the era of information disorder: Collaboration as a solution for achieving universalism. In P. Savage, M. Medina, & G. F. Lowe (Eds.), *Universalism in public service media* (pp. 175–190). Nordicom, University of Gothenburg.

Hotez, P. J. (2023). *The Deadly Rise of Anti-science: A Scientist's Warning*. JHU Press. doi:10.56021/9781421447223

Howard, J. (2016). The Truth About 'Patient Zero' and HIV's Origins. CNN. https://edition.cnn.com/2016/10/27/health/hiv-gaetan-dugas-patient-zero/index.html

Hudnall Stamm, B. (2004). Considering a theory of cultural trauma and loss. *Journal of Loss and Trauma*, *9*(1), 89–11. doi:10.1080/15325020490255412

Hugulius, K., Adams, M., & Romo-Murphey, E. (2019). The Power of Radio to Promote Health and Resilience in Natural Disasters: A Review. *International Journal of Environmental Research and Public Health*, *16*(14), 2526. doi:10.3390/ijerph16142526 PMID:31311142

Human Rights Watch. (2020). China: Covid-19 Discrimination Against Africans. https://www.hrw.org/news/2020/05/05/china-covid-19-discrimination-against-africans

Hunter-Adams, J., & Rother, H. A. (2017). A Qualitative study of language barriers between South African health care providers and cross-border migrants. *BMC Health Services Research*, *17*(97), 97. Advance online publication. doi:10.1186/s12913-017-2042-5 PMID:28143514

Huppert, F. A. (2009). Psychological well-being: Evidence regarding its causes and consequences. *Applied Psychology. Health and Well-Being*, *1*(2), 137–164. doi:10.1111/j.1758-0854.2009.01008.x

Hu, S., Wang, S., Luo, W., Zhang, M., Huang, X., Yan, Y., Liu, R., Ly, K., Kacker, V., She, B., & Li, Z. (2021). Wang, W. Luo, M. Zhang, X. Huang, Y. Yan (2021).Revealing public opinion towards COVID-19 vaccines with Twitter data in the United States: Spatiotemporal perspectiveJ Med. *Internet Research*, *23*(9), e30854. doi:10.2196/30854 PMID:34346888

Hussey, N. (2012). The Language Barrier: The overlooked challenge to equitable health care. *SAHR*, 13, 189 – 195. https://journals.co.za/doi/pdf/10.10520/EJC133688

Hwang, G.-J., Wang, S.-Y., & Lai, C.-L. (2021). Effects of a Social Regulation-based online learning framework on students' learning achievements and behaviors in mathematics. *Computers &amp. Computers & Education*, *160*, 104031. doi:10.1016/j.compedu.2020.104031

Hymes, D. (1970). Linguistic Method of Ethnography. In P. Garvin (Ed.), *Method and Theory in Linguistics*. Mouton. www.academia.edu/16312703/

Idowu, A. A. (2008). Effects of female genital-mutilation on human rights of women and female children: The Nigerian situation. *Research Journal of International Studies*, *8*, 13–26.

Ilesanmi, O. S., Akosile, P. O., Afolabi, A. A., & Ukwenya, V. O. (2023). Handling distrust on risk communication in Nigeria: A strategy to strengthening the COVID-19 outbreak response. *Disaster Medicine and Public Health Preparedness*, *17*, e27. PMID:34308825

Infoscipedia. (2023). *What is remote learning*. IGI Global. https://www.igi-global.com/dictionary/character-development/97112

Institute of Medicine. (2003). *The Future of the Public's Health in the 21st Century*. National Academy Press.

International Covenant on Civil and Political Rights, adopted 16th December, 1966 (entry into force, 23 March 1976).

Islam Md, S., Siddique, A. B., Akter, R., Tasnim, R., Sujan Md, S. H., & Ward, P. R. (2021). Knowledge, attitudes and perceptions towards COVID-19 vaccinations: A cross-sectional community survey in Bangladesh. *BMC Public Health*, *21*(1), 1851. doi:10.1186/s12889-021-11880-9 PMID:34645399

Islam, M. S., Kamal, A.-H. M., Kabir, A., Southern, D. L., Khan, S. H., Hasan, S. M. M., Sarkar, T., Sharmin, S., Das, S., Roy, T., Harun, M. G. D., Chughtai, A. A., Homaira, N., & Seale, H. (2021, May 12). COVID-19 vaccine rumors and conspiracy theories: The need for cognitive inoculation against misinformation to improve vaccine adherence. *PLoS One*, *16*(5), e0251605. doi:10.1371/journal.pone.0251605 PMID:33979412

Islary, J. (2014). Health and health seeking behaviour among tribal communities in India: A socio-cultural perspective. Journal of Tribal Intellectual Collective India, 1-16.

Ivan Krastev & Mark Leonard. (2021). Every major crisis of the past decade has divided Europe. COVID is no different. Euronews. https://www.euronews.com/2021/09/08/every-major-crisis-of-the-past-decade-has-divided-europe-covid-is-no-different-view

Iyamu, I., Apantaku, G., Yesufu, Z., Oladele, E. A., Eboreime, E., Afirima, B., ... Mpofu, M. (2022). Is social media, as a main source of information on COVID-19, associated with perceived effectiveness of face mask use? Findings from six sub-Saharan African countries. Global Health Promotion, 29(3), 86-96.

Iyengar, S. (1992). How Television News Affects Voters: From Setting Agendas to Defining Standards, 6 Notre Dame J.L. *Ethics & Public Policy,* 33.

Iyengar, S. (1991). *Is anyone responsible? How television frames political issues*. University of Chicago Press. doi:10.7208/chicago/9780226388533.001.0001

Iyengar, S., & Kinder, D. R. (1987). *News that Matters: Television and American opinion.* University of Chicago Press.

Iyinolakan, O. (2023). Exploring the Potential of Artificial Intelligence for Supporting Indigenous Language Journalism Pedagogy in Nigeria. Symposium on African Journalism Education in the Post-COVID-19 digital era, 1-8. 10.31730/osf.io/jak43

Jacob, C., Hausemer, P., Zagoni-Bogsch, A., & Diers-Lawson, A. (2023). Policy Department for Economic, Scientific and Quality of Life Policies Directorate-General for Internal Policies. https://www.medicalbrief.co.za/as-tanzania-changes-tack-on-covid-19-leaders-have-a-role-to-play-in-pushing-accurate-information/

Ji, D., & Liu, L. (2022). Fighting Covid-19 by National Mobilization: A Communicative Analysis of the Roles of the Chinese Government. In Manufacturing Government Communication on Covid-19. A Comparative Perspective. Paris: Springer. doi:10.1007/978-3-031-09230-5_3

Johnson & Mandara. (2004). An Exploration of Attitudes Toward Female Genital Cutting in Nigeria. *Journal of Population Research and Policy Review,* 26(1).

Jones, S., Ehiri, J., & Anyanwu, E. (2004). Female Genital Mutilation in Developing Countries: An Agenda for Public Health Response. *European Journal of Obstetrics, Gynecology, and Reproductive Biology, 116*(2), 144–151. doi:10.1016/j.ejogrb.2004.06.013 PMID:15358454

Jones, S., Torres, V., & Arminio, J. (2009). *Negotiating the complexities of qualitative research in higher education: Fundamental Elements and Issues.* Routledge.

Kamwangamalu, N. M. (2003). Globalization of English, language maintenance and shift in South Africa. *International Journal of the Sociology of Language, 2003*(164), 65–81. doi:10.1515/ijsl.2003.056

Kandala, N.B., Nwakeze, N., Spatial, Ngianga, S., & Kandala, I.I. (2009). Distribution of Female Genital Mutilation in Nigeria. *Journal of the American Society of Tropical Medicine and Hygiene, 81*(5), 784–792.

Karlsson, L. C., Soveri, A., Lewandowsky, S., Karlsson, L., Karlsson, H., Nolvi, S., Karukivi, M., Lindfelt, M., & Antfolk, J. (2021). Fearing the disease or the vaccine: The case of COVID-19. *Personality and Individual Differences, 2021*, 172. doi:10.1016/j.paid.2020.110590 PMID:33518869

Kar, S. B., Alcalay, R., & Alex, S. (2000). *Health communication: A multicultural perspective.* Sage publications.

Kasl, S. V., & Cobb, S. (1966). Health behavior, illness behavior, and sick-role behavior: Health and illness behavior. *Archives of Environmental Health, 12*(2), 246–266. doi:10.1080/00039896.1966.10664365 PMID:5322534

Kawade, A., Gore, M., Lele, P., Chavan, U., Pinnock, H., & Smith, P. (2021). Interplaying role of healthcare activist and homemaker: a mixed-methods exploration of the workload of community health workers (Accredited Social Health Activists) in India. Human Resources for Health, 19, 1-12.

Kelly, A & Johnson, T. (2020). Research and Data Section. UN Women.

Kimhi, S., Marciano, H., Eshel, Y., & Adini, B. (2020). Recovery from the COVID-19 pandemic: Distress and resilience. *International Journal of Disaster Risk Reduction, 50*, 101843. doi:10.1016/j.ijdrr.2020.101843 PMID:32953439

Kissi, S., & van Eck, E. (2017). Reading Hebrews through Akan Ethnicity and Social Identity. *Hervormde Teologiese Studies, 73*(3), a4490. doi:10.4102/hts.v73i3.4490

Kitui, B. (2012) *Female Genital Mutilation in South Africa.* AfricLaw: Advancing the rule and role of law in Africa. https://africlaw.com/2012/06/07/female-genital-mutilation- in-south-africa/

Klouman, E., Manongi, R., & Klepp, K. I. (2005). Self-reported and observed female genital cutting in rural Tanzania: Associated demographic factors, HIV and sexually transmitted infections. *Tropical Medicine & International Health, 10*(1), 105–115. doi:10.1111/j.1365-3156.2004.01350.x PMID:15655020

Kluge, H. H. P., Jakab, Z., & Bartovic, J. (2020). Comment refugee and migrant health in the COVID-19 response. *Lancet, 2019*, 2019–2020.

Kokaliari, E., Catanzarite, G., & Berzoff, J. (2013). It is called a mother tongue for a reason: A qualitative therapists' perspective on bilingual psychotherapy – Treatment implications. *Smith College Studies in Social Work, 83*(1), 97–118. doi:10.1080/00377317.2013.747396

Kolawole, O (2015) Social distancing and the coronavirus outbreak in Nigeria: what's the bigger picture? Techpoint Africa Newsletter.

Kolawole, A. O. D., & Anke, V. K. (2010). A review of determinants of female genital mutilation in Nigeria. *Journal of Medicine and Medical Sciences, 1*(11), 510–515.

Koon, A. D., Hawkins, B., & Mayhew, S. H. (2016). Framing and the health policy process: A scoping review. *Health Policy and Planning, 31*(6), 801–816. doi:10.1093/heapol/czv128 PMID:26873903

Koshoedo, S. A., Paul-Ebhohimhen, V. A., Jepson, R. G., & Watson, M. C. (2015). Understanding the complex interplay of barriers to physical activity amongst black and minority ethnic groups in the United Kingdom: A qualitative synthesis using meta-ethnography. *BMC Public Health, 15*(643), 643. doi:10.1186/s12889-015-1893-0 PMID:26164652

Kott, A., & Limaye, R. J. (2016). Delivering risk information in a dynamic information environment: framing authoritative voice in centres of disease control (CDC) and Prime time broadcast news 211

Krishnatray, P & Shrivastava, S. (2021). Asia Pacific Media Educator. Coronavirus Pandemic: How National Leaders Framed Their Speeches to Fellow Citizen. University of Wollongong. doi. doi:10.1177/1326365X211048589journals.sagepub.com/home/ame

Kuckartz, U. (2019). Qualitative text analysis: A systematic approach. *Compendium for early career researchers in mathematics education*, 181-197.

Kudzayi. (2020). Zimbabwe: Covid-19 Drugs Scandal Lays Bare the Rot in The System. https://www.theafricareport.com/30676/zimbabwe-covid-19-drugs-scandal-lays-bare-the-rot-in-the-system/

Kugarakuripi, J., & Ndoma, S. (2022). Lack of trust in government, reliance on social media may drive vaccine hesitancy in Zimbabwe. Findings from the most recent Afrobarometer survey in Zimbabwe

Kumar, M. M., Pathak, V. K., & Ruikar, M. (2020). Tribal population in India: A public health challenge and road to future. Journal of family medicine and primary care, 9(2), 508.

Lane, D.S., & Rubinstein, R.A. (1996). Judging the Other: Responding to Traditional Female Genital Surgeries. doi:10.2307/3527930

Larsson, L., Chikwari, C. D., Simms, V., Tembo, M., Mahomva, A., Mugurungi, O., ... Kranzer, K. (2023). Addressing sociodemographic disparities in COVID-19 vaccine uptake among youth in Zimbabwe. *BMJ Global Health*, *8*(7), e012268. doi:10.1136/bmjgh-2023-012268 PMID:37407229

Lashko, G. (2006). Meeting the needs of black and minority ethnic communities. *Housing Care Support.*, *9*(1), 2–4. doi:10.1108/14608790200600001

Leask, J., Hooker, C., & King, C. (2010). Media coverage of health issues and how to work effectively with journalists: A qualitative study. *BMC Public Health*, *10*(535), 1–7. doi:10.1186/1471-2458-10-535 PMID:20822552

Lee, C. T., Kanji, R., Wang, A. H., Mamuji, A., Rozdilsky, J., & Chu, T. (2021). Cultural Contexts During a Pandemic: A Qualitative Description of Cultural Factors that Shape Protective Behaviours In The Chinese Canadian Community. *BMC Public Health*, *21*(1), 1897. doi:10.1186/s12889-021-11928-w PMID:34666726

Leopold Munhende. (2021). Ministers Clash Over Covid Jabs. https://www.newzimbabwe.com/ministers-clash-over-covid-jabs/

Liang, R.Y.H., Chen, D.T. (2012). Online learning: Trends, potential and challenges. Academic Press.

Li, J. (2020). Transnational migrant students between inclusive discourses and exclusionary practices. *Multilingua*, *39*(2), 192–212. doi:10.1515/multi-2019-0125

Li, J., Ai, B., & Zhang, J. (2019). Negotiating language ideologies in learning Putonghua: Myanmar ethnic minority students' perspectives on multilingual practices in a borderland school. *Journal of Multilingual and Multicultural Development*, 1–14. doi:10.1080/01434632.2019.1678628

Li, J., Xie, P., Ai, B., & Li, L. (2020, September 25). Multilingual communication experiences of international students during the Covid-19 pandemic. *Multilingua*, *39*(5), 529–539. doi:10.1515/multi-2020-0116

Lindsey, L. L., & Beach, S. (2002). *Sociology* (2nd ed.). Prentice Hall.

Lin, L., Savoia, E., Agboola, F., & Viswanath, K. (2014). What have we learned about communication inequalities during the H1N1 pandemic: A systematic review of the literature. *BMC Public Health*, *14*(484), 1–13. doi:10.1186/1471-2458-14-484 PMID:24884634

Li, S., Wang, Y., Xue, J., Zhao, N., & Zhu, T. (2020). The Impact of COVID-19 Epidemic Declaration on Psychological Consequences: A Study on Active Weibo Users. *International Journal of Environmental Research and Public Health*, *17*(6), 2032. doi:10.3390/ijerph17062032 PMID:32204411

Lising, L. (2020). COVID-19 health information campaigns in the Philippines. https://www.languageonthemove.com/covid-19-health-information-campaigns-in-the philippines/

Lister, M., Jon, D., Giddings, S., Grant, I., & Kieran, K. (2003). *New Media: A Critical Introduction*. Routledge.

Littlejohn, S. W., Foss, K. A., & Oetzel, J. G. (2017). *Theories of Human Communication* (11th ed.). Waveland Press Incorp.

Liu, J., & McLeod, D. M. (2019). Counter-Framing Effects of User Comments. *International Journal of Communication*, 13.

Lubenow, T. A. (2012). The public sphere 50 years later: Public Sphere and Mass Media in Jurgen Habermas. *Revista Transformacao*, *35*(3), 229–274. doi:10.7443/15110

Lucas, J. M., Targema, T. S., Jibril, A., Sambo, E. O., & Istifanus, B. A. (2020). Combating COVID-19 infodemic in Nigerian rural communities: The imperatives of Traditional Communication Systems. *ASEAN Journal of Community Engagement*, *4*(2), 360–385. doi:10.7454/ajce.v4i2.1102

Lucas, S. (2000). The River: A journey back to the source of HIV and AIDS. *BMJ (Clinical Research Ed.)*, *320*(7247), 1481A. PMID:10827067

Lyu, J. C., Le Han, E., & Luli, G. K. (2021). COVID-19 vaccine-related discussion on Twitter: Topic modeling and sentiment analysis. *Journal of Medical Internet Research*, *23*(6), e24435. doi:10.2196/24435 PMID:34115608

Maarek, P. (2022). Similar and Dissimilar Patterns of Government Communication on Covid-19. In Manufacturing Government Communication on Covid-19. A Comparative Perspective. Springer. doi:10.1007/978-3-031-09230-5_1

Machaya, P. (2021). Zimbabwe Plays Vaccine Politics, Rejects Western Vaccines. https://www.zimlive.com/zimbabwe-plays-vaccine-politics-rejects-western-vaccines/

Mackay, H., & Gillespie, G. (1992). Extending the social shaping of technology approach: Ideology and appropriation. *Social Studies of Science*, *22*(4), 685–716. doi:10.1177/030631292022004006

MacKenzie, D. (1981). Interests, positivism and history. *Social Studies of Science*, *11*(4), 498–505. doi:10.1177/030631278101100405

Mackworth-Young, C. R., Chingono, R., Mavodza, C., McHugh, G., Tembo, M., Chikwari, C. D., ... Ferrand, R. A. (2021). Community perspectives on the COVID-19 response, Zimbabwe. Bulletin of the World Health Organization, 99(2), 85.

Macleod, A., & McCabe, M. P. (2020). Defining Sexuality in Later Life: A Systematic Review. *Australasian Journal on Ageing*, *39*(S1), 6–15. doi:10.1111/ajag.12741 PMID:32567178

Madiba, M. (2014). Promoting concept literacy through multilingual glossaries: A translanguaging approach. In Multilingual Teaching and Learning in Higher Education in South Africa. Multilingual Matters. doi:10.21832/9781783091669-007

Magson, N. R., Freeman, J. Y., Rapee, R. M., Richardson, C. E., Oar, E. L., & Fardouly, J. (2020). Risk and protective factors for prospective changes in adolescent mental health during the COVID-19 pandemic. *Journal of Youth and Adolescence*, *50*(1), 44–57. doi:10.1007/s10964-020-01332-9 PMID:33108542

Mahmud, S., Mohsin, Md., & Dewan, Md. N., & Muyeed, A. (2021). *The Global Prevalence of Depression, Anxiety, Stress and Insomnia among General Population during COVID-19 Pandemic: A Systematic Review and Meta-Analysis*. doi:10.21203/rs.3.rs-1136589/v1

Makalela, L. (2015). Moving out of the linguistic boxes: The effects of translanguaging strategies for multilingual classrooms. *Language and Education*, *29*(3), 200–217. doi:10.1080/09500782.2014.994524

Makinana, A. (2020). Stella Ndabeni-Abrahams Pays R1,000 & Gets A Criminal Record for Lockdown Lunch. https://www.timeslive.co.za/politics/2020-04-22-stella-ndabeni-abrahams-pays-r1000-fine-after-covid-19-lunch-in-lockdown/

Makoni, M. (2021). Tanzania Refuses COVID-19 Vaccines. *Lancet*, *397*(10274), 566. doi:10.1016/S0140-6736(21)00362-7 PMID:33581810

Malinowski, B. (1947). *Freedom and Civilisation*. George Allen.

Mandara, M. (2012). Family planning in Nigeria and Prospects for the Future. *International Journal of Gynaecology and Obstetrics: the Official Organ of the International Federation of Gynaecology and Obstetrics*, *117*(1), 1–4. doi:10.1016/j.ijgo.2012.01.002 PMID:22342053

Manno, F. A. M. III, Lively, M. B., Manno, S. H. C., Cheng, S. H., & Lau, C. (2018). Health risk communication message comprehension is influenced by image inclusion. *Journal of Visual Communication in Medicine*, *41*(4), 157–165. doi:10.1080/17453054.2018.1480321 PMID:29987960

Mano, W. (2012). Why radio is Africa's medium of choice in the global age. In D. Ligaga, D. Moyo, & L. Gunner (Eds.), *Radio in Africa: cultures, publics and communities* (pp. 102–117). Johannesburg Wits University Press.

Marani, M., Katul, G. G., Pan, W. K., & Parolari, A. J. (2021). Intensity and frequency of extreme novel epidemics. *Proceedings of the National Academy of Sciences of the United States of America*, *118*(35), e2105482118. doi:10.1073/pnas.2105482118 PMID:34426498

Mare, A., Mabweazara, H. M., & Moyo, D. (2019). "Fake News"and Cyber-Propaganda in Sub-Saharan Africa: Recentering the Research Agenda. African Journalism Studies, 40(4), 1–12. doi:10.1080/23743670.2020.1788295

Marino, I. M., Adogba, O., & Tilli, N. (2020). Mental health interventions: Reflections on a radio program as alternative for stigma reduction and social integration. *Frontiers in Communication*, *5*, 550912. doi:10.3389/fcomm.2020.550912

Markowitz, D. M., Levine, T. R., Serota, K. B., & Moore, A. D. (2023). Cross-checking journalistic fact- checkers: The role of sampling and scaling in interpreting false and misleading statements. *PLoS One*, *18*(7), e0289004. doi:10.1371/journal.pone.0289004 PMID:37490489

Markus, H. R., & Kitayama, S. (2010). Cultures and selves: A cycle of mutual constitution. *Perspectives on Psychological Science*, *5*(4), 420–430. doi:10.1177/1745691610375557 PMID:26162188

Martin Rojo, L. (2010). *Constructing Inequality in Multilingual Classrooms*. Walder De Gruyter. doi:10.1515/9783110226645

Martin, B. (2014). Semiotics and the Media. In R. S. Fortner & P. M. Fackler (Eds.), *The Handbook of Media and Mass Communication Theory* (pp. 56–73). Wiley Blackwell. doi:10.1002/9781118591178.ch4

Mashiri, P. (2002). Shona–English Code-Mixing in the Speech of Students at the University of Zimbabwe. *Southern African Linguistics and Applied Language Studies*, *20*(4), 245–262. doi:10.2989/16073610209486314

Mason, C., Lazenby, S., Stuhldreher, R., Kimball, M., & Bartlein, R. (2022). Lessons learned from implementing digital health tools to address COVID-19 in LMICs. Frontiers in Public Health, 10, 859941.

Mathe & Motsaathebe. (2023d). Play on Twitter During a Health Crisis in Non-Democratic Context. Gratification or Dissent? Social Media and Society.

Mathe, L. (2023). Women's political participation in Zimbabwe: Play and content creation on Twitter. *Information Communication and Society*, *26*(13), 2598–2613. Advance online publication. doi:10.1080/1369118X.2023.2250442

Mathe, L., & Motsaathebe, G. (2023a). African multilingual public sphere: A critical analysis of minority indigenous language(s) representation on Breeze FM talk radio in Zimbabwe. *African Identities*, 1–17. Advance online publication. doi:10.1080/14725843.2023.2251700

Mathe, L., & Motsaathebe, G. (2023b). The political economy of indigenous local media for minority languages in Zimbabwe: A case of Lyeja FM community radio. *Journal of Asian and African Studies*. Advance online publication. doi:10.1177/00219096231160233

Mathe, L., & Motsaathebe, G. (2023c). Dissemination of Community Radio Content in Facebook Posts: Limitations and Opportunities for Indigenous Languages. *Forthcoming in Communicatio.*

Mavuso, S. (2020). Ramaphosa Backs Dlamini-Zuma in Cigarette Ban War. https://www.iol.co.za/news/politics/ramaphosa-backs-dlamini-zuma-in-cigarette-ban-war-47507125

Mazzoleni, G. (2015). The International Encyclopedia of Political Communication. London: Wiley Blackwell.

Mbiti, J. S. (1975). *The Prayers of African Religion.* SPCK.

McAbee, L., Tapera, O., & Kanyangarara, M. (2021). Factors associated with COVID-19 vaccine intentions in eastern Zimbabwe: A cross-sectional study. *Vaccines, 9*(10), 1109. doi:10.3390/vaccines9101109 PMID:34696215

McCombs, M., & Ghanem, S. I. (2001). The Convergence Of Agenda Setting and Framing. In S. D. Reese, O. H. Gandy, & A. E. Grant (Eds.), Framing public life. Academic Press.

McCoy, S. (2020). Africa's Elite Build VIP Hospitals for Themselves, Leaving Workers to Die. https://www.wsws.org/en/articles/2020/04/08/elit-a08.html

McGuire, K. (2021, March). COVID-19, Contagion, and Vaccine Optimism. *The Journal of Medical Humanities, 42*(1), 51–62. doi:10.1007/s10912-021-09677-3 PMID:33587203

McQuail, D. (1987). *Mass communication theory: An introduction.* Sage Publications, Inc.

Mendes, L., Dos Santos, H. B., & Ichikawa, E. Y. (2017). Health and safety at work: Analysis from the Brazilian documentary film Flesh and Bone. *Safety and Health at Work, 8*(4), 347–355. doi:10.1016/j.shaw.2017.01.003 PMID:29276633

Merriam, S. B., & Tsdell, E. J. (2016). Qualitative Research: A Guide to Design and Implementation (4th ed.). Jossy Bass.

Merriam, S. (2002). *Qualitative research in practice: Examples for discussion and analysis.* Jossey-Bass.

Mhute, I., Mangeya, H., & Jakaza, E. (2021). Endangering the endangered: Impact of fake covid-19 social media communications in Zimbabwe. *Pharos Journal of Theology, 102*(2), 1–11. doi:10.46222/pharosjot.102.211

Mignolo, W. D. (2007). Delinking. *Cultural Studies, 21*(2–3), 449–514. doi:10.1080/09502380601162647

Mirbabaie, M., Bunker, D., Stieglitz, S., Marx, J., & Ehnis, C. (2020). Social media in times of crisis: Learning from Hurricane Harvey for the coronavirus disease 2019 pandemic response. *Journal of Information Technology, 35*(3), 195–213. doi:10.1177/0268396220929258

Mkhize, D., & Balfour, R. (2017). Language rights in education in South Africa. *South African Journal of Higher Education, 31*(6), 133–150. doi:10.20853/31-6-1633

Mkhize, T. (2020). The role of African languages in decolonizing South African universities. In R. H. Kaschula & E. Wolff (Eds.), *The Transformative Power of Language: From Postcolonial to Knowledge Societies in Africa* (pp. 33–42). Cambridge University Press. doi:10.1017/9781108671088.003

Mohamud, M., Kaba, M., & Tamire, M. (2016). Assessment of Barriers of Behavioural Change to Stop FGM Practice among Women of Kebribeyah District, Somali Regional State, Eastern Ethiopia. *Global Journals Inc,* 16(6).

Mohanty, S. N. (Ed.). (2020). *Emotion and information processing: a practical approach.* Springer International Publishing AG. doi:10.1007/978-3-030-48849-9

Montgomery, J., Stathopoulou, T., & Eikemo, T. A. (2019). Asylum-seeking parents' reports of health deterioration in their children since fleeing their home country. *Journal of Refugee Studies, 32*(Special_Issue_1), 52–62. doi:10.1093/jrs/fez018

Moore, A., & MacKenzie, M. K. (2020, October 26). Policy making during crises: How diversity and disagreement can help manage the politics of expert advice. *BMJ (Clinical Research Ed.)*, *371*, m4039. doi:10.1136/bmj.m4039 PMID:33106231

Moscadelli, A., Albora, G., Biamonte, M. A., Giorgetti, D., Innocenzio, M., Paoli, S., Lorini, C., Bonanni, P., & Bonaccorsi, G. (2020). Fake news and Covid-19 in Italy: Results of a quantitative observational study. *International Journal of Environmental Research and Public Health*, *17*(16), 5850. doi:10.3390/ijerph17165850 PMID:32806772

Motsaathebe, G. (2010). Language, Afrikology and the Tremor of the Political Moment: English as the Main Language of Discourse in Africa. *Indilinga*, *9*(1), 96–109.

Mpofu, P., & Salawu, A. (2020). African language use in the digital public sphere: Functionality of the localised Google webpage in Zimbabwe. *South African Journal of African Languages*, *40*(1), 76–84. doi:10.1080/02572117.2020.1733833

Mufandauya, R. (2015). *Effectiveness of the refugee encampment policy in Zimbabwe; a study of Tongogara Refugee Camp (2013-2014).*

Muliyah, P., Aminatun, D., & Septiyana, L. (2022). Teaching in pandemic: Teachers' experiences during coronavirus outbreak. *Journal of Research on Language Education*, *3*(1), 1. doi:10.33365/jorle.v3i1.1894

Murewanhema, G., Burukai, T. V., Chireka, B., & Kunonga, E. (2021). Implementing national COVID-19 vaccination programmes in sub-Saharan Africa-early lessons from Zimbabwe: A descriptive cross-sectional study. *The Pan African Medical Journal*, *40*(1). Advance online publication. doi:10.11604/pamj.2021.40.180.30824 PMID:35018213

Murhula, P. B. B., & Singh, S. B. (2022). The Impact of COVID-19 Vaccine Nationalism on Global Health and Human Rights to Health Standards. *The Oriental Anthropologist*, *22*(1), 93–101. doi:10.1177/0972558X221096263

Murrrey., R. (2015). Merit vs Equality? The argument that gender quotas violate meritocracy is based on fallacies. Academic Press.

Mutanga, M. B., Ureke, O., & Chani, T. (2021). Social media and the COVID-19: South African and Zimbabwean netizens? response to a pandemic. Indonesian Journal of Information Systems, 4(1), 1-14.

Mutingwende. (2023). Religious sects shun health services as cholera spreads in Zvimba. Spiked Media. https://spiked-media.co.zw/religious-sects-shun-health-services-as-cholera-spreads-in-zvimba/

Mwaniki, M. (2012). Language and social justice in South Africa's higher education: Insights from a South African university. *Language and Education*, *26*(3), 213–232. doi:10.1080/09500782.2011.629095

Mwansoko, H. J. M. (2006). Kitangulizi cha Tafsiri: Nadharia na Mbinu. Dar es Salaam: TUKI.

Nabea, W. (2007). Language Policy in Kenya: Negotiation with Hegemony. *The Journal of Pan African Studies*, *1*(3), 121–138.

Naffi, N., Davidson, A., & Jawhar, H. (2023). (5). ways to help stop the "infodemic," the increasing misinformation about coronavirus. *Retrieved*, (August), 21.

Nagler, R. H., Vogel, R. I., Gollust, S. E., Rothman, A. J., Fowler, E. F., & Yzer, M. C. (2020). Public Perceptions of Conflicting Information Surrounding COVID-19: Results from a Nationally Representative Survey of U.S. Adults. *PLoS One*, *15*(10), e0240776. doi:10.1371/journal.pone.0240776 PMID:33085719

Najafi, S., Tofigh, S., & Sobczyk. (2023). Covid 19: Virology. In Corona Virus Disease 2019 (Covid-19). A Clinical Guide. Wiley Blackwell.

Namyalo, S., & Nakayiza, J. (2015). Dilemmas in implementing language rights in multilingual Uganda. *Current Issues in Language Planning*, *16*(4), 409–424. doi:10.1080/14664208.2014.987425

Nash, S., & Arora, A. (2021). Interventions to improve health literacy among Aboriginal and Torres Strait Islander Peoples: a systematic review. BMC Public Health, 21(1), 1-15.

National Bureau of Statistics, United Nations Children's Fund, and United Nations Population Fund (UNFPA). (2017). Nigeria Multiple Indicator Cluster Survey 2011. Abuja, Nigeria: NBS. Available at https://www.unicef.org/nigeria/media/1376/file

National Commission For Scheduled Tribes. (n.d.). https://ncst.nic.in/sites/default/files/documents/NCST.pdf

National Population Commission and ORC Macro. (2014). *Nigeria Demographic and Health Survey 2003.* National Population Commission and ORC Macro.

Naz, N., Gulab, F., & Aslam, M. (2022). Development of qualitative semi-structured interview guide for case study research. *Competitive Social Science Research Journal, 3*(2), 42–52.

Ncube, B. J. (2019). *Radio Mthwakazi and the Construction of Ndebele Ethnic Identity.* Doctoral Thesis. Johannesburg: University of Johannesburg.

Nesen, J. N., & Bakar, A. Y. A. (2021). Coping strategies for parents with special need children during COVID-19 lockdown in Malaysia. *Journal of Management Information and Decision Science, 24*(SI1), 1–9.

News, Z. B. C. (2021). Covid-19 Weekly Update [Video playlist]. YouTube. https://www.youtube.com/playlist?list=PL-R_K60Fu927gvzDlcNRtVoLKoKbG_J6N

NewZWire. (2020). 'Open for all': Outrage as Sakunda Steps in to Revive Two Idle Hospitals For Coronavirus. https://newzwire.live/open-for-all-outrage-as-sakunda-steps-in-to-revive-two-idle-hospitals-for-coronavirus

Ngondo, P. S., & Klyueva, A. (2022). Toward an ubuntu-centered approach to health communication theory and practice. Review of Communication, 22(1), 25-41.

Nichols, B. (2001). *Introduction to documentary.* Indiana University Press.

Njuguna, C. (2006). Globalisation, media and culture: The role of the broadcast media in promoting a national identity in Kenya, MA thesis, University of Nairobi.

Nkoala, S. (2022). Educators' experiences of using multilingual pedagogies during emergency remote teaching: A case study of South African universities. *International Journal of Multilingualism.* Advance online publication. doi:10.1080/14790718.2022.2074012

Nkosi, Z. P. (2014). Postgraduate students' experiences and attributes towards isiZulu as a medium of instruction at the University of KwaZulu-Natal. *Current Issues in Language Planning, 15*(3), 245–264. doi:10.1080/14664208.2014.915456

Nnamdi, S. U. (2019). FGM in Nigeria: Combative Legislation and the Issue's Impact on the Economic Growth of Women. https://impakter.com/female-genital-mutilation-in- nigeria-combative-legislation-and-the-issues-impact-on-the-economic-growth-of- women/

Nnorom, C. C. (2000). *Female Genital Mutilation Practice in Nigeria: Patterns.* Preference and Remedies.

Noar, S. M., & Zimmerman, R. S. (2005). Health behavior theory and cumulative knowledge regarding health behaviors: Are we moving in the right direction? *Health Education Research, 20*(3), 275–290. doi:10.1093/her/cyg113 PMID:15632099

Norton, R. (1983). *Communicator Style: Theory, Applications, and Measures.* Sage publications.

Nutbeam, D. (2021). The vital role of meaningful community engagement in responding to the COVID-19 pandemic. *Public Health Research & Practice, 31*(1), 3112101. doi:10.17061/phrp3112101 PMID:33690782

O'Brien, S., Federici, F., Cadwell, P., Marlowe, J., & Gerber, B. (2018). Language translation during disaster: A comparative analysis of five national approaches. *International Journal of Disaster Risk Reduction, 31*, 627–636. doi:10.1016/j.ijdrr.2018.07.006

O'Brien, S., & Federico, M. F. (2019). Crisis translation: Considering language needs in multilingual disaster settings. Disaster Prevention and Management. *Disaster Prevention and Management, 29*(2), 129–143. Advance online publication. doi:10.1108/DPM-11-2018-0373

O'Flynn, S. (2012). Documentary's metamorphic form: Webdoc, interactive, transmedia, participatory and beyond. *Studies in Documentary Film, 6*(2), 141–157. doi:10.1386/sdf.6.2.141_1

Obagwu, P. U., & Idris, K. M. (2019). Social responsibility theory of the press: A critique of it application and constraints. *International Journal of Innovative Research and Development, 8*(12), 26–35. doi:10.24940/ijird/2019/v8/i12/DEC19010

Obiorah, K. E. (2021). The role of Nigerian indigenous languages in COVID-19 discourse. *Journal of Language and Health, 2*(2), 43–52. doi:10.37287/jlh.v2i2.514

Obukadeta, F. M. (2019). *Language Policy and Planning in the Broadcast Media of a Multilingual Context: A Case Study of Kogi State, Nigeria* (Doctoral dissertation, University of Sheffield).

Office for the Coordination of Humanitarian Affairs – OCHA. (2021). South Africa Reckons with Its Status as a Top Immigration Destination, Apartheid History, and Economic Challenges. https://reliefweb.int/report/south-africa/south-africa-reckons-its-status-top-immigration-destination-apartheid-history

Ofosuhene, M. (1993). *Women Traders as Heads of Households in Larteh Akwapim* (Thesis, University of Ghana).

Ogbujah, C. (2017). Ideals and Values: Pivots to Meaningful Intercultural Dialogue. *Dialogue and Universalism, 1*(1), 67–81. doi:10.5840/du20172717

Ogechi, N. (2002). The Reality and Challenges of Publishing in Kiswahili in Kenya. In Utafiti wa Kiswahili,. Eldoret: Moi University Press.

Ogechi, N. (2005). On Lexicalization in Sheng. *Nordic Journal of African Studies, 3*(14), 334–335.

Ogola, O. (2003). The National Language Policy Implementation and Experience: The Case of Kiswahili in the Parliament of Kenya. Dissertation Zur Erlangung des Doktorgrades der Philosophie, Universitat Wien.

Ogone, J. O. (2020). Mobile Phones in Africa: The Politics of Cultural And Material Integration into Local Economies. *International Journal of Cultural Studies, 23*(4), 531–546. doi:10.1177/1367877920903739

Okeke, T. C., Anyaehie, U. S. B., & Ezenyeaku, C. C. K. (2012). An overview of female genital mutilation in Nigeria. *Annals of Medical and Health Sciences Research, 2*(1), 70–73. doi:10.4103/2141-9248.96942 PMID:23209995

Okunaa, C. S., & Omenugha, K. A. (2012). Introduction to Mass Communication (3rd Edition). Enungu: New Generation Books.

Olaoye, A. A. (2013). The role of indigenous languages in national development: A case study of Nigerian linguistic situation. *International Journal of Applied Linguistics and English Literature, 2*(3), 29–34. doi:10.7575/aiac.ijalel.v.2n.3p.29

Onwukwe, A. C, Onyebuchi, A. C, Chikwe, U. O & Ihekwoaba, U. P (2021). Owerri Residents Perception of the Transmission of Information via Social Media during covid-19. SAU Journal of Management and Social Science, 6(2).

Onyebuchi, A. C, Onyebuchi, A. C Chikwe, U. O & Ihekwoaba, U. P (2021). Influence of Radio Messages on Adoption of Covid-19 Preventive Measures among Residents of Owerri Municipality using Hot FM. SAU Journal of Management and Social Science, 6(2).

Onyenankeya, K. (2022). Indigenous language newspapers and the digital media conundrum in Africa. *Information Development*, *38*(1), 83–96. doi:10.1177/0266666920983403

Orji, E. O., & Babalola, A. (2006). Correlates of Female Genital Mutilation and Its Impact on Safe Motherhood. *Journal of the Turkish German Gynecological Association*, *7*(4), 319–324.

Osterholm, M. T. (2020). Preparing for the next pandemic. In *The Covid-19 Reader* (pp. 11–20). Routledge. doi:10.4324/9781003141402-2

Paravala, V. (2003). Building solidarities- A case of community Radio in Zharkhand. *Economic and Political Weekly*, *37*(22), 2188–2197.

Parr, H. (2007). Collaborative film-making as process, method and text in mental health research. *Cultural Geographies*, *14*(1), 114–138. doi:10.1177/1474474007072822

Pascucci, M. A., Chu, N., & Leasure, A. R. (2012). Health promotion for the oldest of old people. *Nursing Older People*, *24*(3), 22–28. doi:10.7748/nop2012.04.24.3.22.c9017 PMID:22567772

Patrick. (2023). "We can't do this alone": Nigerian fact-checkers teamed up to debunk politicians' false claims at this year's election. https://reutersinstitute.politics.ox.ac.uk/news/we-cant-do-alone-nigerian-fact-checkers-teamed-debunk-politicians-false-claims-years-election

Patton, M. Q. (2002). *Qualitative Research and Evaluation Methods*. Sage.

Pavlik, J. (2001). *Journalism and New Media*. Columbia University Press. doi:10.7312/pavl11482

Peter van Garderen. (2007). Archival Materials: A practical Definition. Van Garderen, P. (2007). Archival materials: a practical definition. *Blog. Archivemati. Ca.* https://vangarderen.net/posts/archival-materials-a-practical-definition.html

Pew Research Center. (2020). Majority of Americans now say they would get a vaccine for the coronavirus. https://www.pewresearch.org/ science/wp-content/uploads/sites/16/2020/12/. PS_2020.12.03_covid19-vaccine-intent_00-01. png.

Pieri, E. (2019). Media Framing and the Threat of Global Pandemics: The Ebola Crisis in UK Media and Policy *Response. Sociological Research Online*, *24*(1), 73–92. doi:10.1177/1360780418811966 PMID:34285639

Piller, I. (2016). *Linguistic diversity and social justice*. Oxford University Press. doi:10.1093/acprof:oso/9780199937240.001.0001

Piller, I. (2016b). Monolingual way of seeing multilingualism. *Journal of Multicultural Discourses*, *11*(1), 25–33. doi:10.1080/17447143.2015.1102921

Piller, I. (2019). On the conditions of authority in academic publics. *Journal of Sociolinguistics*, *23*(5), 521–528. doi:10.1111/josl.12393

Piller, I., & Cho, J. (2013). Neoliberalism as language policy. *Language in Society*, *42*(1), 23–44. doi:10.1017/S0047404512000887

Piller, I., Zhang, J., & Li, J. (2020). Linguistic diversity in a time of crisis: Language challenges of the COVID-19 pandemic. *Multilingua*, *39*(5), 503–515. doi:10.1515/multi-2020-0136

Pindula. (2020). Zambia's Opposition Leader Says Sacking Health Minister Came ' a Little Too Late'. https://www.pindula.co.zw/2021/01/11/zambias-opposition-leader-says-sacking-health-minister-came-a-little-too-late/

Pinsky, P. F., Ford, M., Gamito, E., Higgins, D., Jenkins, V., Lamerato, L., Tenorio, S., Marcus, P. M., & Gohagan, J. K. (2008). Enrollment of racial and ethnic minorities in the prostate, lung, colorectal and ovarian cancer screening trial. *Journal of the National Medical Association, 100*(3), 291–298. doi:10.1016/S0027-9684(15)31241-4 PMID:18390022

Piscopo, J. M. (2021). Working Paper Effective, Decisive, and Inclusive: Women's Leadership In Covid-19 Response And Recovery. Leadership And Governance Section UN Women.

Pluddemann, P. (2015). Unlocking the grid: Language-in-education policy realization in post-apartheid South Africa. *Language and Education, 29*(3), 186–199. doi:10.1080/09500782.2014.994523

Porat, T., Nyrup, R., Calvo, R. A., Paudyal, P., & Ford, E. (2020). Public health and risk communication during COVID-19—Enhancing psychological needs to promote sustainable behavior change. *Frontiers in Public Health, 8*, 637. doi:10.3389/fpubh.2020.573397 PMID:33194973

Posetti, J. (2018). News Industry Transformation: Digital Technology, Social Platforms and the Spread of Misinformation and Disinformation. In C. Ireton & J. Posetti (Eds.), *Journalism, 'Fake News' and Disinformation: Handbook for Journalism Education and Training* (pp. 55–69). UNESCO.

Preece, S. (2019). Elite bilingual identities in higher education in the anglophone world: The stratification of linguistic diversity and reproduction of socio-economic inequalities in the multilingual student population. *Journal of Multilingual and Multicultural Development, 40*(5), 404–420. doi:10.1080/01434632.2018.1543692

Prezi, G. O. (2022). Language Attitudes of the Igbo: A Threat to the Igbo Language. *Styles of Communication, 14*(1).

Ptil, S., Rao, R. S., & Agarwal, A. (2013). Awareness and risk perception of hepatitis B infection among auxiliary healthcare workers. *Journal of International Society of Preventive & Community Dentistry, 3*(2), 67. doi:10.4103/2231-0762.122434 PMID:24778982

Puntoni, S., De Langhe, B., & Van Osselaer, S. M. (2009). Bilingualism and the emotional intensity of advertising language. *The Journal of Consumer Research, 35*(6), 1012–1025. doi:10.1086/595022

Pym, A. (2012). *On Translator Ethics. Principles for Mediation Between Cultures* (Revised Edition). John Benjamins Publishing Company. doi:10.1075/btl.104

Quinn, N., Shulman, A., Knifton, L., & Byrne, P. (2011). The impact of a national mental health arts and film festival on stigma and recovery. *Acta Psychiatrica Scandinavica, 123*(1), 71–81. doi:10.1111/j.1600-0447.2010.01573.x PMID:20491719

Quinn, P. (2018). Crisis communication in public health emergencies: The limits of 'legal control' and the risks for harmful outcomes in a digital age. *Life Sciences, Society and Policy, 14*(4), 1–40. doi:10.1186/s40504-018-0067-0 PMID:29404722

Raghunathan, S., Darshan Singh, A., & Sharma, B. (2022). Study of resilience in learning environments during the COVID-19 pandemic. *Frontiers in Education, 6*, 677625. Advance online publication. doi:10.3389/feduc.2021.677625

Rahman, M. M, Chisty, M. A, Alam A, Sakib, M. A, Quader, M. A, Shobuj, I. A, Abdul Halim, M., & Rahman, F (2022). Knowledge, attitude, and hesitancy towards COVID-19 vaccine among university students of Bangladesh PLUS ONE Collection Psychology. doi:10.1371/journal.pone.0270684

Rahman, A., & Toubia, N. (Eds.). (2000). *Female genital mutilation: a guide to laws and policies worldwide*. Zed books.

Raju, E., & Ayeb-Karlsson, S. (2020). Covid-19: How do you isolate in a refugee camp. *International Journal of Public Health, 65*(5), 515–517. doi:10.1007/s00038-020-01381-8 PMID:32385541

Ramalingareddy, K. (2016). Improving health services for tribal populations. International Journal of Research in Social Sciences, 6(11), 345-357.

Ramirez de la Piscina, T., Zabalondo, B., Aiestaran, A., & Agirre, A. (2016). The Future of Journalism—Who to Believe? *Journalism Practice*, *10*(1), 71–92. doi:10.1080/17512786.2015.1006932

Rasmussen, B., Hutchinson, A., Lowe, G., Wynter, K., Redley, B., Holton, S., Manias, E., Phillips, N., McDonall, J., McTier, L., & Kerr, D. (2022). The impact of covid-19 on psychosocial well-being and learning for australian nursing and midwifery undergraduate students: A cross-sectional survey. *Nurse Education in Practice*, *58*, 103275. doi:10.1016/j.nepr.2021.103275 PMID:34922092

Rauchfleisch, A., Vogler, D., & Eisenegger, M. (2021). Public Sphere in crisis mode: How the COVID-19 pandemic influenced public discourse and user behaviour in the Swiss twitter-sphere. *Javnost (Ljubljana)*, *28*(2), 129–148. doi:10.1080/13183222.2021.1923622 PMID:34393592

Ravi, K. (2012). Media and Social Responsibility: A critical Perspective with Special Reference to Television. *Academic Research International*, *2*(1), 306–325.

Reese, S.D. (2007). The Framing Project: A Bridging Model for Media Research Revisited. Academic Press.

Rhodes University. (2019). *Language Policy*. Accessed on 22nd September 2023 from World Wide Web < https://www.ru.ac.za/media/rhodesuniversity/content/institutionalplanning/documents/Language_Policy_2019.pdf>

Riebling, J.R., & von der Wense, I. (2019). Framing The Mass Media: Exploring 'Fake News' As a Frame Embedded In Political Discourse. *Journal of Alternative and Community*, 4.

Rikard, R. V., Thompson, M. S., McKinney, J., & Beauchamp, A. (2016). Examining health literacy disparities in the United States: a third look at the National Assessment of Adult Literacy (NAAL). BMC public health, 16, 1-11.

Rimal, R. N., & Lapinski, M. K. (2009). Why health communication is important in public health. Bulletin of the World Health Organization, 87, 247-247a. doi:10.2471/BLT.08.056713

Ritschel, C. (2020). Hulk Hogan Sparks Backlash For Suggesting Coronavirus Is Punishment From God: 'Maybe We Don't Need A Vaccine'. https://www.independent.co.uk/news/world/americas/hulk-hogan-coronavirus-vaccine-god-punishment-plagues-instagram-wwe-wrestling-a9452851.html

Rodrigues, C. M. C., & Plotkin, S. A. (2020). Impact of Vaccines; Health, Economic and Social Perspectives. *Frontiers in Microbiology*, *11*, 1526. doi:10.3389/fmicb.2020.01526 PMID:32760367

Rogers, E. M., Vaughan, P. W., Swalehe, R. M., Rao, N., Svenkerud, P., & Sood, S. (1999). Effects of an entertainment-education radio soap opera on family planning behavior in Tanzania. *Studies in Family Planning*, *30*(3), 193–211. doi:10.1111/j.1728-4465.1999.00193.x PMID:10546311

Rohloff, P., & Henderson, B. (2015). Development, language revitalization, and culture: the case of Mayan languages of Guatemala, and their relevance for African languages. In J. Essegbey, B. Henderson, & F. Mc Laughlin (Eds.), *Language documentation and endangerment in Africa* (pp. 177–194). John Benjamins Publishing Company. doi:10.1075/clu.17.07roh

Rosenfield, L. W., Hayes, L. S., & Frentz, T. S. (1976). *The Communicative Experience*. Allyn and Baycon.

Rosli, A. M., & Bakar, A. Y. (2021). The Mental Health State and psychological well-being of school teachers during COVID-19 pandemic in Malaysia. *Bisma The Journal of Counseling*, *5*(3), 182–195. doi:10.23887/bisma.v5i3.42015

Rota, P. A., Oberste, M. S., Monroe, S. S., Nix, W. A., Campagnoli, R., Icenogle, J. P., Peñaranda, S., Bankamp, B., Maher, K., Chen, M., Tong, S., Tamin, A., Lowe, L., Frace, M., DeRisi, J. L., Chen, Q., Wang, D., Erdman, D. D., Peret, T. C. T., ... Bellini, W. J. (2003). Characterization of a Novel Coronavirus Associated with Severe Acute Respiratory Syndrome. *Science, 300*(5624), 1394–1399. doi:10.1126/science.1085952 PMID:12730500

Rothe, C., Schunk, M., Sothmann, P., Bretzel, G., Froeschl, G., Wallrauch, C., Zimmer, T., Thiel, V., Janke, C., Guggemos, W., Seilmaier, M., Drosten, C., Vollmar, P., Zwirglmaier, K., Zange, S., Wölfel, R., & Hoelscher, M. (2020). Transmission of 2019-nCoV infection from an asymptomatic contact in Germany. *The New England Journal of Medicine, 382*(10), 970–971. doi:10.1056/NEJMc2001468 PMID:32003551

Rubel, P. G. (1978). *Your own pigs you may not eat: A comparative study of New Guinea societies.* Australian National University Press.

Rubin, E. J., Baden, L. R., Morrissey, S., & Campion, E. W. (2020). Medical journals and the 2019-nCoV outbreak. *The New England Journal of Medicine, 382*(9), 866. doi:10.1056/NEJMe2001329 PMID:31986242

Rudwick, S., Sijadu, Z., & Turner, I. (2021). Politics of language in COVID-19: Multilingual perspectives from South Africa. *Politikon: South African Journal of Political Studies, 48*(2), 242–259. doi:10.1080/02589346.2021.1917206

Rusike, T. (2023). My Mission is to Save Lives. https://www.sundaynews.co.zw/my-mission-is-to-save-lives/

Sabato, T. M. (2018). Utilization of media-driven technology for health promotion and risk reduction among American Indian and Alaska Native young adults: An exploratory study. Journal of Health Disparities Research and Practice, 12(1), 4.

Salawu, A. (2022). Toward a Model of Indigenous Language for Development Communication. *Indigenous Language for Development Communication in the Global South*, 13.

Salawu, A. (2006). Indigenous Language Media: A Veritable Tool for African Language Learning. *Journal of Multicultural Discourses, 1*(1), 86–95. doi:10.1080/10382040608668533

Salawu, A. (2015). A political economy of sub-Saharan African language press: The case of Nigeria and South Africa. *Review of African Political Economy, 42*(144), 299–313. doi:10.1080/03056244.2014.988695

Salawu, A., Tsutsa, F., & Mpofu, P. (2022). Adoption of Digital Media by African Language Print Newspapers: The Case of Isolezwe. *Journal of Social Sciences and Humanities, 19*(5), 24–35.

Samad, A., Al Jerjawi, K., & Dadich, A. (2023). A. Crisis Leadership: Political Leadership during the COVID-19 Pandemic. *Sustainability (Basel), 15*(1), 266. doi:10.3390/su15010266

Scales, D., Gorman, J., & Jamieson, K. H. (2021). The COVID-19 infodemic—Applying the epidemiologic model to counter misinformation. *The New England Journal of Medicine, 385*(8), 678–681. doi:10.1056/NEJMp2103798 PMID:33979506

Schäfer, M. S. (2015). Digital public sphere. The international encyclopedia of political communication, 15, 1-7.

Scheufele, D. (2004). Framing-effects Approach: A Theoretical and Methodological Critique. doi:10.1515/comm.2004.29.4.401

Scheufele, D. A., & Iyengar, S. (2012). The State of Framing Research: A Call for New Directions. In The Oxford Handbook of Political Communication Theories. Oxford University Press.

Scheufele, D. (1999). Framing as a Theory of Media Effects. *Journal of Communication, 49*(1), 103–122. doi:10.1111/j.1460-2466.1999.tb02784.x

Schmidt, T., Cloete, A., Davids, A., Makola, L., Zondi, N., & Jantjies, M. (2020). Myths, Misconceptions, Othering and Stigmatizing Responses to Covid-19 in South Africa: A Rapid Qualitative Assessment. *PLoS One*, *15*(12), e0244420. doi:10.1371/journal.pone.0244420 PMID:33351852

Schoch-Spana, M., Brunson, E. K., Long, R., Ruth, A., Ravi, S. J., Trotochaud, M., Borio, L., Brewer, J., Buccina, J., Connell, N., Hall, L. L., Kass, N., Kirkland, A., Koonin, L., Larson, H., Lu, B. F., Omer, S. B., Orenstein, W. A., Poland, G. A., ... White, A. (2021). The public's role in COVID-19 vaccination: Human-centered recommendations to enhance pandemic vaccine awareness, access, and acceptance in the United States. *Vaccine*, *39*(40), 6004–6012. doi:10.1016/j.vaccine.2020.10.059 PMID:33160755

Schwerdtle, P., Bowen, K., & McMichael, C. (2017). The health impacts of climate-related migration. *BMC Medicine*, *16*(1), 1–7. doi:10.1186/s12916-017-0981-7 PMID:29301536

Seale, H., Harris-Roxas, B., Heywood, A., Abdi, I., Mahimbo, A., Chahan, A., & Woodland, L. (2023). The role of community leaders and other information intermediaries during the COVID-19 pandemic: Insights from the multicultural sector in Australia. *Humanities & Social Sciences Communications*, *9*(1), 174. doi:10.1057/s41599-022-01196-3

Seale, H., Harris-Roxas, B., Heywood, A., Abdi, I., Mahimbo, A., Chauhan, A., & Woodland, L. (2022). Speaking COVID-19: Supporting COVID-19 communication and engagement efforts with people from culturally and linguistically diverse communities. *BMC Public Health*, *22*(1), 1257. doi:10.1186/s12889-022-13680-1 PMID:35761264

Seeger, M. W. (2006, August). Best Practices in Crisis Communication: An Expert Panel Process. *Journal of Applied Communication Research*, *34*(3), 232–244. doi:10.1080/00909880600769944

Segre, G., Campi, R., Scarpellini, F., Clavenna, A., Zanetti, M., Cartabia, M., & Bonati, M. (2021). Interviewing children: The impact of the covid-19 quarantine on children's perceived psychological distress and changes in routine. *BMC Pediatrics*, *21*(1), 231. Advance online publication. doi:10.1186/s12887-021-02704-1 PMID:33985448

Shamsi, H. A. (2020). Implications of Language Barriers for Healthcare: A Systematic Review. *Oman Medical Journal*, *35*(2), e122. Advance online publication. doi:10.5001/omj.2020.40 PMID:32411417

Shank, G. (2002). *Qualitative Research. A Personal Skills Approach*. Merrill Prentice Hall.

Shawcross, A. (2016). *Facts We Can Believe in: How to Make Fact-Checking Better*. Beyond Propaganda Series. Legatum Institute.

Shaw, J., & Robertson, C. (1997). *Participatory video: A practical approach to using video creatively in group development work*. Routledge.

Shaw, S. M., & Lee, J. (2018). *Gendered Voices, Feminist Visions: Classic and Contemporary Readings* (8th ed.). Oxford University Press.

Shell-Duncan, B., Moreau, A., Wander, K., & Smith, S. (2018). The role of older women in contesting norms associated with female genital mutilation/cutting in Senegambia: A factorial focus group analysis. *PLoS One*, *13*(7), e0199217. doi:10.1371/journal.pone.0199217 PMID:30044770

Shigemura, J., Ursano, R. J., Morganstein, J. C., Kurosawa, M., & Benedek, D. M. (2020). Public responses to the novel 2019 coronavirus (2019-ncov) in Japan: Mental health consequences and target populations. *Psychiatry and Clinical Neurosciences*, *74*(4), 281–282. doi:10.1111/pcn.12988 PMID:32034840

Shilts, R. (2007). *And the Band Played On* (20th ed.). St Martin Press.

Showtack, R., Santos, M. G., Feuerherm, E., Jacobson, H., & Martinez, G. (2019*). Language as a social determinant of health: An applied linguistics perspective on health equity*. https://www.aaal.org/news/language-as-a-social-determinant-of-health-an-applied-linguistics-perspective-on-health-equity##

Siebert, F., Peterson, T., & Schramm, W. (1956). Four theories of the papers. The authoritarian, libertarian, social responsibility and soviet community concepts of what the press should do. Urban: University of Illinois.

Singer, M. K., Dressler, W., & George, S. (2016). Culture: The missing link in health research. *Social Science & Medicine*, *170*, 237–246. doi:10.1016/j.socscimed.2016.07.015 PMID:27542574

Singh, P., & Kumari, R. (2019). Usage pattern of mobile phone among tribals of Jharkhand. Mass Communicator: International Journal of Communication Studies, 13(1), 27-31.

Sinha, A. (n.d.). Communication Anthropology: A realization. World Anthropology Congress. Retrieved from https://wac.kiss.ac.in/blog/communication-anthropology-a-realization/

Skutnabb-Kangas, T. (2006). Language policy and linguistic human rights. In T. Ricento (Ed.), *An Introduction to Language Policy: Theory and Method* (pp. 78–94). Blackwell.

Smedley, B. D., & Syme, S. L. (2000). *Promoting health: Intervention strategies from social and behavioral research.* National Academy Press.

Smith, M. L., Menn, M., Lisako, J., & McKeyer, J. (2011). Effectiveness of Radio as a Health Information Source. *Journal of Radio & Audio Media*, *18*(2), 196–211. doi:10.1080/19376529.2011.615776

Sneath, D. (2016). Tribe. Cambridge Encyclopedia of Anthropology. doi:10.29164/16tribe

Sokhela, D. G., Makhanya, N. J., Sibiya, N. M., & Nokes, K. M. (2013). Experiences of Fast Queue health care users in primary health care facilities in eThekwini district, South Africa. *Curationis*, *36*(1). Advance online publication. doi:10.4102/curationis.v36i1.60 PMID:23902165

Solvoll, M., & Høiby, M. (2023). Framing the Covid-19 Pandemic. *Mediekultur*, *73*(73), 6–27. doi:10.7146/mk.v38i73.131934

Stathopoulou, T., Avrami, L., Kostaki, A., Cavounidis, J., & Eikemo, T. A. (2019). Safety, health and trauma among newly arrived refugees in Greece. *Journal of Refugee Studies*, *32*(Special_Issue_1), 22–35. doi:10.1093/jrs/fez034

Steinbuka, I. (2022). Pros and Cons of the EU Response and Communication during Covid-19 Crisis. In Manufacturing Government Communication on Covid-19. A Comparative Perspective. Paris: Springer. doi:10.1007/978-3-031-09230-5_2

Stieglitz, S., Mirbabaie, M., Schwenner, L., Marx, J., Lehr, J., & Brűnker, F. (2017). Sensemaking and Communication roles in Social Media Crisis Communication. Academic Press.

Stout, C., & McGlynn, A. (2020). Necessity as the Mother of Invention: Attempts to Overcome the Digital Divide During the Covid-19 Pandemic. In S. Navarro & S. Hernandez (Eds.), *The Colour of Covid-19. The Racial Inequality of Marginalised Communities* (pp. 29–45). Routledge.

Talabi, F. O., Oyedeji, K. A., Adelabu, O., & Bernice, O. (2022). Public perception of radio campaign messages in managing COVID-19 pandemic in selected states. *Human Vaccines & Immunotherapeutics*, *18*(5), 1–6. doi:10.1080/21645515.2022.2085958 PMID:35714340

Tambo, E., Djuikoue, I. C., Tazemda, G. K., Fotsing, M. F., & Zhou, X. N. (2021). Early-stage risk communication and community engagement (RCCE) strategies and measures against the coronavirus disease 2019 (COVID-19) pandemic crisis. *Global Health Journal (Amsterdam, Netherlands)*, *5*(1), 44–50. doi:10.1016/j.glohj.2021.02.009 PMID:33850632

Tandwa, L. (2020). Cigarette Sales Ban: DA Labels Nkosazana Dlamini-Zuma A 'Liar', Says Ramaphosa Should 'Fire' Her. https://www.news24.com/news24/southafrica/news/cigarette-sales-ban-da-labels-nkosazana-dlamini-zuma-a-liar-says-ramaphosa-should-fire-her-20200529

Taruvinga, M. (2020). Mahomva's Reassignment Raises Stink. newzimbabwe.com.

Teicher A. (2023). Super-spreaders: A Historical Review. *Lancet Infect Dis.* . doi:10.1016/S1473-3099(23)00183-4

Terry, G., Hayfield, N., Clarke, V., & Braun, V. (2017). Thematic analysis. The SAGE handbook of qualitative research in psychology, 2, 17-37.

The Chanzo Reporter. (2021). Is This the End of Gwajima's Campaign Against COVID-19 Vaccines? The Chanzo. https://thechanzo.com/2021/08/17/is-this-the-end-of-gwajimas-campaign-against-covid-19-vaccines/

The Nigeria Fact-Checkers' Coalition showed how collaborative journalism can work in West Africa. (n.d.). https://www.niemanlab.org/2023/10/the-nigeria-fact-checkers-coalition-showed-how-collaborative-journalism-can-work-in-west-africa/

The Standard. (2020). Makandiwa, Bill Gates, vaccines and microchips. https://www.newsday.co.zw/thestandard/2020/04/12/makandiwa-bill-gates-vaccines-microchips

The Zimbabwe Mail. (2021). Outrage as Makandiwa blames vaccines for poverty in Africa https://www.thezimbabwemail.com/religion/outrage-as-makandiwa-blames-vaccines-for-poverty-in-africa/

Thompson, R. G., Nutor, J. J., & Johnson, J. K. (2021). Communicating awareness about COVID-19 through songs: An example from Ghana. *Frontiers in Public Health*, *8*, 607830. doi:10.3389/fpubh.2020.607830 PMID:33537281

Tijani-Adenle, G. (2021). *Information Disorder and Future of Journalism in Nigeria*. Centre for Journalism Innovation and Development.

Titilayo, A., Palamuleni, M. E., & Anuodo, O. O. (2015). Female Genital Mutilation/Cutting in Nigeria: Any Abandonment yet? *Ife Social Sciences Review*, *24*(2), 109–122.

Tkach, B., & Williams, A. A. (2018). Mobile (in) security? Exploring the realities of mobile phone use in conflict areas. *Information Communication and Society*, *21*(11), 1639–1654. doi:10.1080/1369118X.2017.1348531

Tobin, E. A., Okonofua, M., & Azeke, A. (2021). Acceptance of a COVID-19 Vaccine in Nigeria: A Population-Based Cross-Sectional Study. *Annals of Medical and Health Sciences Research*, *11*(5).

Tongco, M. D. C. (2007). Purposive Sampling as a Tool for Informant Selection. *Ethnobotany Research and Applications*, *5*, 147–158. doi:10.17348/era.5.0.147-158

Toubia & Sharief. (2003). Female Genital Mutilation (FGM). Have we Made Progress? International Journal of Gynecology and Obstetrics, September; 82(3), 251-261.

Transparency International. (2021). Transparency International UK 2020-21. Impact report. file:///C:/Users/roya.witness/Downloads/Transparency%20International%20UK%20Annual%20Imapct%20Report%20and%20Accounts%20ye%20 31%20March%202021.pdf

Tshabangu, T., & Salawu, A. (2021). Indigenous-language Media Research in Africa: Gains, Losses, Towards a New Research Agenda, African. *Journalism Studies*. Advance online publication. doi:10.1080/23743670.2021.1998787

Türkili, C. (2022). Role of media framing on the formation of opinion. Master of Science Media and Cultural Studies Thesis. Çankaya Ankara: Middle East Technical University.

Turner, N., & Wildsmith-Cromarty, R. (2014). Challenges to the implementation of bilingual/multilingual language policies at tertiary institutions in South Africa (1995-2012). *Language Matters (Pretoria)*, *45*(3), 295–312. doi:10.1080/10228195.2014.961525

Tyng, C. M., Amin, H. U., Saad, M. N. M., & Malik, A. S. (2017). The influences of emotion on learning and memory. *Frontiers in Psychology*, *24*(8), 1454. doi:10.3389/fpsyg.2017.01454 PMID:28883804

Ude-Akpeh, C. E., & Onyima, T. (2020). Influence of Indigenous Language and authority figures in broadcast of COVID-19 Pandemic messages among rural dwellers in south East Nigeria. *Nnamdi Azikiwe University Journal of Communication and Media Studies, 1*(2).

Uekusa, S. (2019). Disaster linguicism: Linguistic minorities in disasters. *Language in Society*, *48*(3), 353–375. doi:10.1017/S0047404519000150

Ufuophu-Biri, E. (2017). Relationship between exposure to media campaigns on family planning and adoption of family planning methods among women in delta state. *Journal of Social Management Science*, *12*, 153–162.

Ugande, G. B. (2008). An evaluation of radio Benue's role in HIV/AIDS awareness creation in Vandiekya Local Government Area of Benue State. *The Nigerian Journal of Communication*, *6*, 122–140.

UNESCO. (2001). *UNESCO Universal Declaration on Cultural Diversity*. UNESCO.

Unicef, OECD, & UNESCO. (2020, January 1). *Education: From school closure to Recovery*. UNESCO.org. https://www.unesco.org/en/covid-19/education-response

UNICEF. (2005). *Female Genital Mutilation/Female Genital Cutting: A Statistical Report*. UNICEF.

UNICEF. (2013). Female Genital Mutilation/Cutting: A Statistical Overview and Exploration of the Dynamics of Change. UNICEF.

UNICEF. (2017) Approach to the Elimination of Female General Mutilation: A Decade of Action to Achieve Gender Equality. https://www.unicef.org/media/88751/file/FGM- Factsheet-2020.pdf

UNICEF. (2019). Statistical Profile on Female Genital Mutilation. https://www.unicef.org/

Union, A. (2003). *Protocol to the African Charter on Human and People's Rights on the Rights of Women in Africa*. African Union.

UNNews. (2020). None of us is safe until we all are, says UN chief at EU push to end COVID-19 pandemic. https://news.un.org/en/story/2020/05/1063132

Uwom, O. O., Ajaegbu, C., Oloyede, D. B., & Sowemimo-Coker, S. (2014). Prospects of Internet technology in news production: A study of Voice of Nigeria and Nigeria television authority. *Global Journal of Arts Humanities and Social Sciences*, *2*(1), 56–66.

Van Damme, W., Dahake, R., Delamou, A., Ingelbeen, B., Wouters, E., Vanham, G., van de Pas, R., Dossou, J.-P., Ir, P., Abimbola, S., Van der Borght, S., Narayanan, D., Bloom, G., Van Engelgem, I., Ag Ahmed, M. A., Kiendrébéogo, J. A., Verdonck, K., De Brouwere, V., Bello, K., ... Assefa, Y. (2020). The COVID-19 pandemic: Diverse contexts; different epidemics—how and why? *BMJ Global Health*, *5*(7), e003098. doi:10.1136/bmjgh-2020-003098 PMID:32718950

van Liempt, I., & Mieke, K. (2020). Coronavirus: Misinformation is leading to 'fake news' anxieties in Dutch refugee communities. The Conversation. https:// theconversation.com/coronavirus-misinformation-is-leading-to-fake-news-anxieties-indutch-refugee-communities-141830

Veareyi, J. (2017). Towards a migration-aware health system in South Africa: a strategic opportunity to address health inequity. SAHR. https://www.hst.org.za/publications/South%20African%20Health%20Reviews/9_Towards%20a%20migration%20aware%20health%20system%20in%20South%20Africa_a%20strategic%20opportunity%20to%20address%20health%20inequity.pdf

Villani, L., Pastorino, R., Molinari, E., Anelli, F., Ricciardi, W., Graffigna, G., & Boccia, S. (2021). Impact of the COVID-19 pandemic on psychological well-being of students in an Italian university: A web-based cross-sectional survey. *Globalization and Health, 17*(1), 1–14. doi:10.1186/s12992-021-00680-w PMID:33823897

Villanueva, S. (2015). Collaborative practices in the contemporary documentary: A proposed analysis and revision of the participatory mode in documentary theory. *L'Atalante. Revista de estudios cinematográficos,* 20.

Vita, V. (2020). Bridging new and traditional media in the fight against Covid-19. Sydney: Language on the Move. https://www.languageonthemove.com/bridging-new-and-traditional-media-in-the-fight-against-covid-19/

Voice of America. (2020). Panic Grips Faithful After Cameroon COVID Pastor Dies. https://www.voanews.com/a/covid-19-pandemic_panic-grips-faithful-after-cameroon-covid-pastor-dies/6189445.html

Vonen, H., Olsen, M. L., Eriksen, S. S., & Eikemo, T. A. (2021). Refugee Camps and Covid-19: Can we prevent a humanitarian crisis. *Scandinavian Journal of Public Health, 49*(1), 27–28. doi:10.1177/1403494820934952 PMID:32522120

Waigwa, S., Doos, L., Bradbury-Jones, C., & Taylor, J. (2018). Effectiveness of health education as an intervention designed to prevent female genital mutilation/cutting (FGM/C): A systematic review. *Reproductive Health, 15*(1), 1–14. doi:10.1186/s12978-018-0503-x PMID:29650025

Waisbord, S., & Mellado, C. (2014). De-westernizing communication studies: A reassessment. *Communication Theory, 24*(4), 361–372. doi:10.1111/comt.12044

Wakefield, M. A., Loken, B., & Hornik, R. C. (2010). Use of mass media campaigns to change health behaviour. *Lancet, 376*(9748), 1261–1271. doi:10.1016/S0140-6736(10)60809-4 PMID:20933263

Wald, P. (2008). Contagious Cultures, Carriers, and the Outbreak Narrative WHO. Supporting Madagascar's COVID-19 vaccine uptake at 78. https://www.afro.who.int/countries/madagascar/news/supporting-madagascars-covid-19-vaccine-uptake-78

Walker, A., & Parmar, P. (1996). *Warrior marks: Female genital mutilation and the sexual blinding of women*. Harvest Books.

Wardle, C. (2019). Understanding Information Disorder. First Draft. https://creativecommons.org/licenses/by-nc-nd/4.0/

Wardle, C., & Derakhshan, H. (2017). *Information Disorder: Towards an Interdisciplinary Framework for Research and Policymaking*. Council of Europe.

Wasserman, H. (2005). Renaissance and Resistance: Using ICTs for social change in South Africa. *African Studies, 64*(2), 177–199. doi:10.1080/00020180500355686

Wasserman, H., & Madrid-Morales, D. (2022). *An Assessment of Media Literacy and Fact-Checking Training Needs of South African Schools and Universities. African Check.*

Waters, D., James, R., & Darby, J. (2011). Health promoting community radio in rural Bali: An impact evaluation. *Rural and Remote Health, 11*(2), 1555–2011. doi:10.22605/RRH1555 PMID:21375357

Watts, R., & Pattnaik, J. (2022). Perspectives of parents and teachers on the impact of the COVID-19 pandemic on children's socio-emotional well-being. *Early Childhood Education Journal*. Advance online publication. doi:10.1007/s10643-022-01405-3 PMID:36285153

Westoff, C. F., & Bankole, A. (1997). Mass media and reproductive behavior in Africa. https://dhsprogram.com/publications/publication-ar2-analytical-studies.cfm

Whitehorn, J., Ayorinde, O., & Samantha, M. (2002). Female Genital Mutilation: Cultural and Psychological Implications. *Sexual and Relationship Therapy*, *17*(2), 161–170. doi:10.1080/14681990220121275

WHO Commission on Social Determinants of Health. (2008). Closing the gap in a generation. Health equity through action on the social determinants of health. Geneva: WHO. https://www.who.int/social_determinants/en/

WHO. (2012). Addressing the challenge of women's health in Africa. www.glowm.com

WHO. (2015). World report on aging and health. Geneva: World Health Organization.

WHO. (2020). WHO issues its first emergency use validation for a COVID-19 vaccine and emphasizes need for equitable global access. Available from: https://www.who.int/news/item

Wieman, J. M. (1975). *An Exploration of Communicative Competence in Initial Interaction: An Experimental Study*. Purdue University.

Wild, A., Kunstler, B., Goodwin, D., Onyala, S., Zhang, L., Kufi, M., Salim, W., Musse, F., Mohideen, M., Asthana, M., Al-Khafaji, M., Geronimo, M. A., Coase, D., Chew, E., Micallef, E., & Skouteris, H. (2021). Communicating COVID-19 health information to culturally and linguistically diverse communities: Insights from a participatory research collaboration. *Public Health Research & Practice*, *31*(1), 3112105. doi:10.17061/phrp3112105 PMID:33690789

Willems, W., & Mano, W. (2016). Decolonizing and provincializing audience and internet studies: Contextual approaches from African vantage points. In W. Willems & W. Mano (Eds.), *Everyday Media Culture in Africa* (pp. 15–40). Routledge. doi:10.4324/9781315472775

Willingham, E. (n.d.). COVID Vaccines Show No Signs of Harming Fertility or Sexual Function. Scientific American. https://www.scientificamerican.com/article/covid-vaccines-show-no-signs-of-harming-fertility-or-sexual-function/

Wingfield, M. (2021). Faith leaders are key to reaching herd immunity in U.S., researchers say. Baptist News Global. https://baptistnews.com/article/faith-leaders-are-key-to-reaching-herd-immunity-in-u-s-researchers-say/#.YxVUWuzMKNY

Winograd, D. M., Fresquez, C. L., Egli, M., Peterson, E. K., Lombardi, A. R., Megale, A., Tineo, Y. A. C., Verile, M. G., Phillips, A. L., Breland, J. Y., Santos, S., & McAndrew, L. M. (2021). Rapid review of virus risk communication interventions: Directions for COVID-19. *Patient Education and Counseling*, *104*(8), 1834–1859. doi:10.1016/j.pec.2021.01.024 PMID:33583651

Wiredu, K. (1992). *Person and Community: Ghanaian Philosophical Studies* (Vol. 1). CRVP.

Wodak, R. & Meyer. (2009). Methods for Critical Discourse Analysis (2nd ed.). London: Sage.

Women, U. N. (2020) COVID-19 and Women's Leadership: From an Effective Response to Building Back Better. Policy Brief (18). https://www.unwomen.org/en/digital-library/publications/2020/06/policy-brief-covid-19-and-womens-leadership

Wood, M. L., Stoltz, D. S., Van Ness, J., & Taylor, M. A. (2018). Schemas and frames. *Sociological Theory*, *36*(3), 244–261. doi:10.1177/0735275118794981

World Bank Group. (2023, March 30). *Remote learning during COVID-19: Lessons from Today, principles for Tomorrow*. World Bank. https://www.worldbank.org/en/topic/edutech/brief/how-countries-are-using-edtech-to-support-remote-learning-during-the-covid-19-pandemic

World Bank. (2023). Indigenous Peoples. Retrieved from https://www.worldbank.org/en/topic/indigenouspeoples

World Health Organisation. (1998a). Gender and Health: Technical Paper. WHO.

World Health Organisation. (2023). Malaria. https://www.who.int/news-room/fact-sheets/detail/malaria

World Health Organization. (1998b). Female Genital Mutilation: An Overview. WHO.

World Health Organization. (2008). *Sixty-First World Health Assembly: Resolutions and Decisions*. World Health Organization.

World Health Organization. (2017). Communicating risk in public health emergencies. A WHO guideline for emergency risk communication (ERC) policy and practice. Retrieved from https://apps.who.int/iris/bitstream/handle/10665/259807/9789241550208-eng.pdf?sequence=2

World Health Organization. (2020). World Hepatitis Day 2020. https://www.who.int/campaigns/world-hepatitis-day/2020

World Health Organization. (2021). Weekly epidemiological update on COVID-19—14 September 2021. https://www.who.int/publications/m/item/weekly-epidemiological-update-on-covid-19---14-september-2021

World Health Organization. (n.d.). WHO Coronavirus (COVID-19) Dashboard. Available online: https://covid19.who.int/

Worobey, M., Watts, T.D., McKay, R.A., Suchard, M.A., Granade, T., Teuwen, D.E., Koblin, B.A., Heneine, W., Lemey, P., & Jaffe, H.W. (2016). 1970s and 'Patient 0' HIV-1 genomes illuminate early HIV/AIDS history in North America. *Nature*. 539(7627), 98–101. doi:10.1038/nature19827

Wouters, O. J., Shadlen, K. C., Salcher-Konrad, M., Pollard, A. J., Larson, H. J., Teerawattananon, Y., & Jit, M. (2021). Challenges in ensuring global access to COVID-19 vaccines: Production, affordability, allocation, and deployment. *Lancet*, *397*(10278), 1023–1034. doi:10.1016/S0140-6736(21)00306-8 PMID:33587887

Xiang, Y., Li, W., Zhang, Q., Jin, Y., Rao, W.-W., Zeng, L.-N., Lok, G. K. I., Chow, I. H. I., Cheung, T., & Hall, B. J. (2020). Timely research papers about COVID-19 in China. *Lancet*, *395*(10225), 684–685. doi:10.1016/S0140-6736(20)30375-5 PMID:32078803

Yaya, S., & Ghose, B. (2018). Female genital mutilation in Nigeria: A persisting challenge for women's rights. *Social Sciences (Basel, Switzerland)*, *7*(12), 244. doi:10.3390/socsci7120244

Ye, F. T.-F., Gao, X., Sin, K.-F., & Yang, L. (2023). Remote learning and mental health during the societal lockdown: A study of primary school students and parents in times of covid-19. *BMC Public Health*, *23*(1), 1106. Advance online publication. doi:10.1186/s12889-023-16040-9 PMID:37286984

Yin, R. K. (2014). *Case study research: Design and methods*. Sage Publication.

Yin, R. K. (2018). *Case Study Research and Applications: Designs and Methods* (6th ed.). Sage Publications Incorp.

Yu, L. (2020). Fighting the coronavirus in local languages. https://www. languageonthemove.com/fighting-the-coronavirus-in-local-languages/

Yule, G. (1996). *Pragmatics*. Oxford University Press.

Zarocostas, J. (2020). How to fight an infodemic. *Lancet*, *395*(10225), 676. doi:10.1016/S0140-6736(20)30461-X PMID:32113495

Zhou, Q., Tian, T., Ni, J., Zhao, X., Li, H., Yang, Y., Zhang, Y., & Pan, J. (2021, November 25). COVID-19 Vaccination Acceptance in China after It Becomes Available: A Cross-Sectional Study. *Vaccines*, *9*(12), 1398. doi:10.3390/vaccines9121398 PMID:34960144

Zimmerman, B. J. (2005). Attaining self-regulation: A sociocognitive perspective. In M. Boekaerts, P. R. Pintrich, & M. Zeidner (Eds.), *Handbook of self-regulation* (pp. 13–39). Elsevier Inc.

Zou, R., Zeb, S., Nisar, F., Yasmin, F., Poulova, P., & Haider, S. A.ZOU. (2022). The impact of emotional intelligence on career decision-making difficulties and generalized self-efficacy among university students in China. *Psychology Research and Behavior Management*, *15*, 865–874. doi:10.2147/PRBM.S358742 PMID:35422664

About the Contributors

Kealeboga Aiseng holds a PhD in African Languages and Linguistics from the University of the Witwatersrand. He is a senior lecturer in journalism and media studies at Rhodes University, Makhanda. Aiseng's research interests are sociolinguistics, language policy, African popular culture, new media, and film studies. Aiseng is the author of "The Sociolinguistics of South African Television: Language Ideologies in Selected Case Studies" and a co-editor of "Political Economy of Contemporary African Culture: The Political Interplay."

Israel Fadipe is lecturer at Ajayi Crowther University, Faculty of Communication and Media Studies, Oyo, Nigeria. He specialises in communication, cultural and gender studies, and has published articles, chapters and books in both local and international journals and publishers such as Palgrave Macmillan, Springer International, Taylor and Francis Ltd, Malthouse Press Limited, Lexington Books, IGI Global, Ibadan Journal of Humanistic Studies, Journal of Communication and Media Research, International Journal of Communication, Muziki-Journal of Music Research in Africa, Africology: Journal of Pan-African Study, Journal of Culture and Environment, Journal of Communication and Language Arts, EJOTMAS and The Journal of Society and Media, Catalan Journal of Communication and Cultural Studies, Gender and Behaviour, Communicare, Journal of African Films and Diaspora Studies, Performance Arts and Communication Studies in these areas. He graduated from the Department of Communication and Language Arts, University of Ibadan, with BA, MA and PhD in Communication and Language Arts.

* * *

Babatunde Adeyeye is a faculty member in the Department of Mass Communication at Covenant University. He is also a Postdoctoral Research Fellow in the Indigenous Language Media in Africa research entity at North-West University, Mafikeng Campus, South Africa. He obtained his B.Sc, M.Sc and PhD Degrees from Kogi State University, Anyigba, Benue State University, Makurdi and Covenant University, Ota, respectively. He is a member of the International Association for Media and Communication Research (IAMCR), the African Council for Communication Education (ACCE), and the Nigerian Institute of Public Relations (NIPR). His research interest includes Indigenous Language use in Development Communication, Journalism, and Public Relations.

Kwesi Aggrey is senior lecturer, and heads the Department of Development Communication in the School of Communication and Media Studies, University of Education, Winneba, Ghana. His research interest spans development and cultural issues, media anthropology, political economy of the media, and health and development communication. He has over twenty years experience in both academic and administrative domains of higher educational teaching and learning. He is currently a member of the Communication Educators Association of Ghana (CEAG), International Association for Media and Communication Research (IAMCR), International Communication Association (ICA), and African Studies Association of Africa (ASAA).

Priscilla Aboagyewaa Boateng is a doctoral student at the Department of Strategic Communication in the School of Communication and Media Studies, University of Education, Winneba, Ghana. Her areas of research primarily focuses on health communication, social media, campaign, public health of marginalised communities, and strategic communication. She is a member of the International Association for Media and Communication Research (IAMCR).

Jennings Joy Chibike is Media and Communication Lecturer at Lupane State University and a DPhil student at Midlands State University in Zimbabwe. He holds a Master of Science Degree in Journalism and Media Studies from the National University of Science and Technology. His research interests are in indigenous language media, identity politics, memory studies, audio studies, human rights and democracy and political communication.

Ogechi Okanya Cookey holds a PhD in Communication Studies and has great interest in corporate communication, environmental/climate communication and research. She teaches in the Department of Mass Communication, Edwin Clark University, Nigeria. She is an environmental and climate justice advocate, undertaking research activities in the area of climate change. She champions for research-based policy making, as well as community-centred, applied and action research as reliable ways of unravelling and tackling the polycrisis confronting human society.Her interest is also in the Niger Delta and other regions in Africa that are suffering environmental degradation, conflict and security threats.

Manisha Nitin Gore, Academician, researcher, and results-driven public health professional with a distinguished career in implementing public health interventions. Proficient in HIV/AIDS, Maternal and Child Health, Non-Communicable Diseases, Community Nutrition, and Mental Health. Strong program/project management skills, budget oversight, and international NGO experience. Expertise in social determinants of HIV/AIDS, mental health in adolescents, reproductive health, and rural food security. Skills include Epidemiology, Anthropology, Proposal Writing, Quantitative and Qualitative Research, software proficiency, Capacity Building, Project Management, Health Policy, and Training & Development.

Kedmon Hungwe is a Professor of Psychology and Education at Michigan Technological University. He was recently awarded a Carnegie Fellowship at Rhodes University in South Africa, where the initial work on this chapter began. He has published in several media journals, including Media & Society, Journal of Popular Film and Television, and the Historical Journal of Film, Radio and Television.

Zikhona Mamase is a Language Practioner, a dedicated professional pursuing Masters in Education. Completed Joint Honours degree in African Languages and Journalism and Media Studies, with Language Planning and Intellectualisation, Human Language Technology, Sociolinguistics, and Digital Media as course components. Accomplished in various areas, including Drama, Directing, Acting, Photo and

Videography, with a focus on graphic design, and Creative Arts education. Possess a strong educational foundation with a Bachelor of Arts degree and a Postgraduate Certificate in Education, with 2 teaching methods: Creative Arts for Grades 7 to 9 and isiXhosa Home Language from Grades 7 to 12. Skilled in teaching and mentorship, curriculum development, and fostering creativity and language proficiency among students. Currently advancing knowledge in Initial Teacher Education for Foundation Phase at Masters Level, with focus in Exploring the Development of IsiXhosa Home Language Knowledge in Student Teachers. Analysing how these types of knowledge are integrated into the teacher education program can shed light on strengths and weaknesses in preparing teachers for the Foundation Phase.

Stephen S. E. Masote is currently involved in teaching and learning, research, community engagement and academic citizenship. Dr Masote has contributed to translations from English to Setswana in a book entitled Stitching a whirlwind, An Anthology of Southern African poems and translations: Africa Pulse 2018. Oxford. Supervising Honours and PhD students. Research outputs 1.An aspect of moral education in "Molefi Kgafela": A traditional poem from collection of praise poems of Tswana Chiefs by I. Schapera. South African Journal of African Languages vol.35.Issue 2.2015 2. Implementation of Value education in the foundation phase. Journal of Education Studies. Vol 16 Issue 2. 2017. Papers read: • Dr Masote has presented a paper at the 9th Malaysia International Conference on Languages and Cultures: Engaging Threads and Trends: 16 – 18 August 2016. • Read a paper: Use of Facebook as a potential platform to promote African Languages: Puo ya Setswana in perspective at Bloemfontein in 2015. • Read a paper during the Africa speaks event at Unisa in 2017.

Limukani Mathe is a Lecturer and Research Fellow attached to the Entity of Indigenous Language Media in Africa (ILMA) at the University of North-West in South Africa. Previously, he was a Lecturer and Research Fellow in the Department of Communication and Media at the University of Johannesburg. His research interests are at the intersection of democracy and digital technologies with particular focus on web-based communities (commentary forums, social media) news sites, indigenous language media and journalism practices in the Global South.

Gilbert Motsaathebe is an NRF rated Research Professor attached to the Entity of Indigenous Langauge Media in Africa (ILMA) at the University of North-West in South Africa.

Felix Mukono is studying for a Masters degree in Sociology at Midlands State University. This work reflects his emerging interests in individual, community, and societal well-being, as well as the ways in which social work can play a role in public health research and interventions.

Samuel Muzhingi is an independent researcher who holds a Master of Arts in Communication (Development Communication) from Daystar University in Nairobi, Kenya. He is also a holder of a Bachelor of Science (Honors) Degree in Journalism and Media Studies from the National University of Science and Technology in Bulawayo, Zimbabwe. His research interests are in media representation, climate change communication, mediated communication and development communication.

Iniobong Courage Nda is a lecturer in the Faculty of Communication and Media Studies, University of Uyo, Uyo, Akwa Ibom State, Nigeria, where she has taught communication and media studies since 2012. As a scholar who has garnered practical expertise from both the print (The Sensor Newspaper) and broadcast media (The Nigerian Television Authority, NTA) respectively, Dr. Nda has been able to integrate her field experience with the classroom demands for effective and efficient teaching of mass communication and has published her researches in several national and international journals including contributing chapters to books.

Abigail Odozi Ogwezzy-Ndisika is the first female professor in the Department of Mass Communication, University of Lagos. At different times, she had served as the Head of this Department. She is an expert in Development Communication, Public Relations and Advertising, with research interest in the gender dimension to development and strategic communication. She has worked on multi-sector projects and with a number of international organizations across Nigeria.

Adenike Omotayo Okeya-Olayinka PhD is a lecturer in the Department of Broadcasting Information and Media Science, Faculty of Communication and Media Studies at the Ajayi Crowther University, Oyo, Nigeria. She had her first degree from the Joseph Ayo Babalola University (JABU) in Ikeji Arakeji, Osun State in 2012 emerging as the Best Graduating Student and was given the Lateef Jakande Award for the Best Graduating Student in the Department of Mass Communication. Thereafter, she was awarded the Master of Science (MSc) Degree in Mass Communication by the Babcock University, Ilishan-Remo, Ogun State in 2015. In 2018, she was awarded the Doctor of Philosophy (PhD) in Mass Communication with specialization in Broadcasting and Development Communication from the Babcock University where she got the Senior Vice President's Award for being the Best Overall Graduating Student with the highest CGPA at the Doctor of Philosophy Level. Dr. Okeya-Olayinka has to her credits, scholarly publications in academic journals and associated scholarly outlets and has also attended learned conferences. She has a strong passion for research, teaching and community service. Her major areas of research include Broadcast Journalism, Film and Cinematography, Health Communication, Development Communication Studies and Media and Society. She is an active member of African Council for Communication Education (ACCE), Association of Communication Scholars and Professionals of Nigeria (ACSPN), Advertising Practitioners Council of Nigeria (APCON), International Literacy Association (ILA), Association of Media and Communication Researchers of Nigeria (AMCRON), International Association of Religion Journalists (IARJ's) and Gender and African Studies Group (BUGAS).

Josephine Otiende is a distinguished figure in the field of Development Communication, renowned for her tireless efforts in leveraging communication strategies to drive positive social change. Josephine has spearheaded numerous strategic communication initiatives in Africa. Through this venture, she has provided strategic communication advisory services to a range of non-profits, NGOs, and governmental organizations globally. Josephine remains committed to fostering the next generation of development communicators. She imparts her expertise in strategic communication and communication strategy through mentorship and professional training sessions, inspiring the next generation of development communicators.

Violet Maphefo Sefolaro Pule is currently teaching Setswana undergrade and beginning postgraduate in 2023. Dr Pule has 12 years' teaching experience supervision in higher education. Published paper: Pule, V. and Theledi, K. (2023) "The Impact of the Presence of Prosodic Features (Tone Markings) on Comprehending Setswana Words in Reading", African Journal of Inter/Multidisciplinary Studies, 5(1), pp. 1–12. doi: 10.51415/ajims. v5i1.1076. Presented papers and on pending publication: • Studying

African Languages for who and for what? The awareness of language profession and its employability with reference to South African indigenous languages • The use of dictionaries in promoting reading in African languages with special reference to Setswana • Gamification as a supporting tool in the learning of Setswana Grammar for Distance learning students.

Ashley Rakatsinzwa earned her Master's degree in Applied Linguistics from the University of Zimbabwe. Her research interests have continually evolved, mirroring the complexity and multifaceted nature of language use. Her primary areas of focus are pragmatics, emphasizing how context influences language interpretation, and language teaching and curriculum development. She has designed methods, materials, and curricula for language instruction.

Witness Roya is a postdoctoral fellow with the Department of Communication at Mangosuthu University of Technology. He holds a PhD in Communication from the University of Fort Hare and has lectured English, Media and Communication in Zimbabwe and South Africa. Witness has interests in areas such as Governance, Political Communication, Indigenous Knowledge Systems, Afrocentricity, Apartheid Studies, Visual Anthropology, Ethics and ChatGPT among others. His 2024 publications include "The Influence of African Oral Art Forms in Raising Climate Change Awareness in Oliver Mtukudzi's 'Pindirai'" In. Student's Journal of Health Research Africa Vol. 5 No. 3 (2024): March 2024 Issue, "Newsday and the Herald's Inclusion of Disabled People in the Use of Digital Media in Zimbabwe" (Chapter 5). In. Digitisation, AI and Algorithms in African Journalism and Media Contexts: Practice,Policy and Critical Literacies Edited by Dralega, C.A (both co-authored with Prof S. Ngcobo) and "Realist. or chauvinist? A critique of Tawona Shadaya Knight's Tweets concerning objectification of women" (Chapter 15) In. Political Economy of African Popular Culture edited by Aiseng, K and Fadipe, I.A. Witness has a few papers which are in press and are set to be published later this year (2024). One of these, a book chapter "Neocolonial Framing of Developing and Developed Countries Attitudes Towards Covid-19 in The Guardian and Al-Jazeera Newspapers" will appear in Decolonizing Africa in a Digitized Age edited by Akpan, U and Onwumechili, C.

Bismark Odum Sackey is Lecturer and doctoral candidate at the Department of Development Communication, School of Communication and Media Studies, University of Education, Winneba, Ghana. His research interest include stakeholder engagement, festival for development, gender, and intersectionality.

Abiodun Salawu is a Professor of Journalism, Communication, and Media Studies and Director of the research entity, Indigenous Language Media in Africa (ILMA) at the North-West University, South Africa. He has taught and researched journalism, media, and communication for close to three decades in Nigeria and South Africa. Prior to his academic career, he practised journalism in a number of print media organisations in Nigeria. He has to his credit, well over a gross of scholarly publications in academic journals and books. He has also edited/co-edited eleven books and authored one. He is a regular presenter of papers at local and international conferences. He is a co-vice chair of the journalism section of the International Association for Media and Communication Research (IAMCR) and a member of editorial/advisory boards of a number of journals. He was involved in the founding of the International Association for Minority Language Media Research. He is rated by the NRF as an established researcher at the level of C1 (with international recognition) and he is a member of Codesria's College of Senior Academic Mentors.

Maureen Samuel is a public health physician with over 8 years experience in research and community development. She is a resident doctor with the Lagos State University Teaching Hospital. Her research interests are in adolescent health, health policy, and maternal and child health.

Didunloluwa Tella, PhD, is a scholar and early-career academic in the field of Media and Communication. She is a lecturer in the Department of Mass Communication, KolaDaisi University, Ibadan, Nigeria. Her research interests focus on development communication in Africa; interactive (new) media and democracy; and environmental communication. Didunloluwa Tella has participated and presented at several academic conferences. She is currently working on upcoming peer-reviewed journal articles and conference proceedings.

Kgomotso K. Theledi is currently teaching undergraduate students African Languages and Linguistics (Sotho language group) and supervising postgraduate students who are doing research in Language and Linguistics, sociolinguistic and South African Language Policy at the University of Witwatersrand in the Department of African Languages. Dr Theledi was head of the Department of Setswana at North - West University from 2017 to 2019. Dr Theledi was also Head of the Department of African Languages at the University of Witwatersrand in 2020 to 2022. Dr Theledi has produced 9 Honours degree students, 5 MAs degree students and 1 PhD. Ongoing supervision: 6 MAs and 4 PhDs in 2023. Reviewed articles for SAJAL in 2019 and 2020, Tydskrif vir Litterkunde Journal in 2022. Dr Theledi is currently, an editor of Frontiers in Communication Journal. Dr Theledi has presented papers locally and internationally: * Bicultural identities expressionism in hip-hop: The case of Motswako sub-genre at UNISA colloquium in 2022. *Language and Culture at Botswana University in 2018. * Practical issues of Translation: Structure of language in Diphosophoso at Bolu Abant Izzet Baysal University in 2022. * Language planning and Policy at BAALA conference (Vanderbiljpark) in 2023. Dr Theledi published the following articles: *Theledi, K. M. A 'The Effect of proverbs and portrayal of women in society'. Published by International Journal of Education, Culture and Society in 2021- available at: . Doi.). *Theledi, KMA. 'Syntactic differences between adjectives and relative words in Setswana and isiZulu'. South African Journal of African Languages in 2022. *Pule, MV and Theledi, KMA. 'The Impact of the Presence of Prosodic features (Tone Marking)': African Journal of Inter/Multidisciplinary Studies in 2023.

Ganiyat Tijani-Adenle (Ph.D.) is a postdoctoral research fellow in the Indigenous Language Media in Africa (ILMA) research entity at North-West University, South Africa. She obtained a Ph.D. in Media, Gender and Communication from De Montfort University, Leicester, United Kingdom. She practiced as a journalist at Voice of Nigeria (VON) before joining the academia. ORCID ID: 0000-0002-2348-6926.

Index

G

H

I

J

K

L

M

N

Ensure Quality Research is Introduced to the Academic Community

Become a Reviewer for IGI Global Authored Book Projects

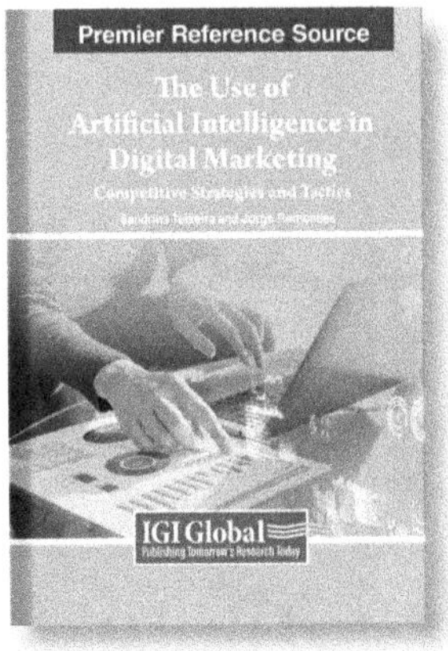

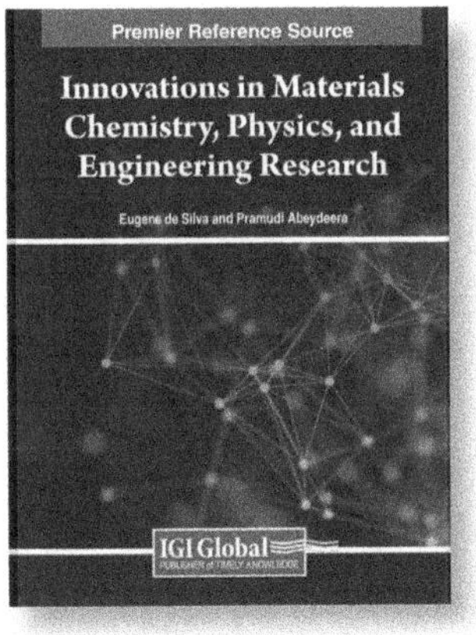

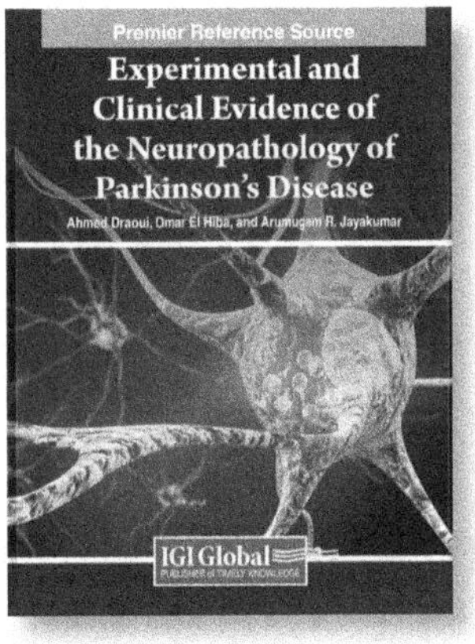

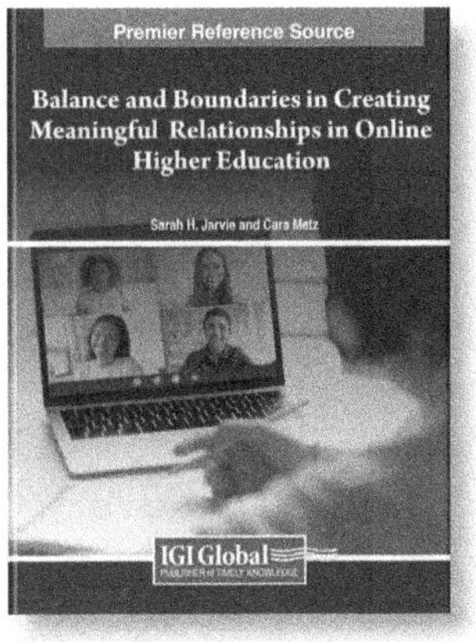

The overall success of an authored book project is dependent on quality and timely manuscript evaluations.

Applications and Inquiries may be sent to:

development@igi-global.com

Applicants must have a doctorate (or equivalent degree) as well as publishing, research, and reviewing experience. Authored Book Evaluators are appointed for one-year terms and are expected to complete at least three evaluations per term. Upon successful completion of this term, evaluators can be considered for an additional term.

If you have a colleague that may be interested in this opportunity, we encourage you to share this information with them.

www.ingramcontent.com/pod-product-compliance
Lightning Source LLC
LaVergne TN
LVHW062139300926
849161LV00010B/2577